AF478070

Interstitial Pneumonia of Unknown Etiology

Organizing Committee

Chairman

Michiyoshi Harasawa, M.D.   General Director, Tokyo Teishin Hospital, Professor Emeritus, University of Tokyo

Members

Yoshinosuke Fukuchi, M.D.   Associate Professor, Department of Geriatrics, Faculty of Medicine, University of Tokyo

Yutaka Hosoda, M.D.   Clinical Study Adviser, Radiation Effects Research Foundation, Hiroshima

Takateru Izumi, M.D.   Professor, Department of Medicine and Clinical Immunology, Chest Disease Research Institute, Kyoto University

Ikuro Kimura, M.D.   Professor, Department of Medicine, Okayama University Medical School

Masahisa Kyougoku, M.D.   Professor, Department of Pathology, Tohoku University School of Medicine

Riichiro Mikami   Director, Sagamihara National Hospital

Terumasa Miyamoto, M.D.   Professor, Department of Medicine and Physical Therapy, Faculty of Medicine, University of Tokyo

Takao Takizawa, M.D.   Professor, Department of Medicine, Respiratory Division, Tokyo Women's Medical College

Masahiko Yamamoto, M.D.   Professor, Department of Medicine, Nagoya City University Medical School

Tetsuro Yokoyama, M.D.   Professor, Department of Medicine, School of Medicine, Keio University

Hajime Morinari, M.D.   Director, Department of Respiratory Diseases, Tokyo Teishin Hospital

JAPAN INTRACTABLE DISEASES RESEARCH FOUNDATION PUBLICATION NO. 27

INTERSTITIAL PNEUMONIA OF UNKNOWN ETIOLOGY

Edited by
Michiyoshi Harasawa/Yoshinosuke Fukuchi/Hajime Morinari

UNIVERSITY OF TOKYO PRESS

JAPAN INTRACTABLE DISEASES RESEARCH FOUNDATION PUBLICATION NO. 27

Proceedings of the International Symposium "Interstitial Pneumonia of Unknown Etiology," October 24th–26th, 1988, Tokyo. The symposium was sponsored by the Japan Intractable Diseases Research Foundation.

Published by
UNIVERSITY OF TOKYO PRESS
ISBN 4-13-068151-6
ISBN 0-86008-452-3

Printed in Japan

Contents

V. Treatment

VI. Clinical Assessment

Foreword

The development of modern medicine has contributed to clarifying the etiology and treatment of various diseases as well as to improving public health and welfare. However, there are many diseases of unknown etiology, which still leave large numbers of patients in a chronic incurable state. In order to promote research on the etiology and treatment of such intractable diseases, non-governmental funding, as well as governmental support, is very important. The Japan Medical Research Foundation was established in October 1973 in order to meet this need with aid from non-governmental financial sources. One of the Foundation's main activities is to hold annual symposia and seminars on various diseases.

The International Symposium on Interstitial Pneumonia of Unknown Etiology was held as one of the Foundation's activities, and this book is an outcome of the Symposium, at which many investigators gathered and exchanged their scientific knowledge and experiences.

The Foundation is very pleased to have sponsored this Symposium, and would like to express its gratitude to Dr. Michiyoshi Harasawa, Director, Tokyo Teishin Hospital and Chairman of the Organizing Committee, and to the Committee members and all those involved for their contributions to the Symposium.

The name of the Foundation was changed in 1984 to the Japan Intractable Diseases Research Foundation; we shall continue our efforts to promote research, with more emphasis on intractable diseases.

I am hopeful that the publication of these proceedings will make the Foundation's work available to a wide scientific readership.

October 1989

Masayoshi Yamamoto
President
Japan Intractable Diseases Research Foundation

Preface

It is a great pleasure to be able to open the three-day international symposium on interstitial pneumonia of unknown etiology with the participation of seven distinguished guests from overseas. I believe it appropriate to explain to the audience the background of the planning and organization of this symposium before starting it.

Since 1972, the Ministry of Health and Welfare of Japan has been promoting projects which aim at finding cures medically and socially for those affected by intractable diseases, in other words, syndromes of unknown etiology and unsolved therapeutic modalities with more than a little probability of disabling sequelae. The target disease number was initially eight, but later was expanded to the present number of forty-three. The Japan Intractable Diseases Research Foundation was established in 1974 to further support these investigative studies. The foundation has held since then a number of symposia on different themes under its auspices.

In 1974, "pulmonary fibrosis of unknown etiology" was named one of these intractable diseases by the Ministry of Health and Welfare, which decided to organize a "research committee on pulmonary fibrosis". Professor Makoto Murao of Hokkaido University was appointed to be the chairman and immediately assembled a committee consisting of twenty members. It conducted a six-year cooperative study of the epidemiology, etiology, pathophysiology, and treatment of this disease. In 1980, Professor Hiomi Honma of Juntendo University succeeded to the chairmanship, and a "research committee on interstitial lung disease" was renewed to continue the study of this disease.

In 1983, two previously existing research committees were merged into a new "research committee on interstitial lung disease", and I was named to be its chairman. I intended to expand the subjects of study to include interstitial lung disease in general so as to propose a more meaningful classification of this illness. This approach, I believe, may shed some light on some of the characteristics of "interstitial pneumonia of unknown etiology", and the committee has engaged in cooperative studies for the past five years.

It was fortunate that interstitial pneumonia was selected last year to be a theme for an international symposium sponsored by the Japan Intractable Diseases Research Foundation, and this symposium on "interstitial pneumonia of unknown etiology" is the result. It was hoped that the symposium would reach as large an audience as possible, and we planned it as a tandem symposium of the first congress of the Asian Pacific Society of Respirology, which was scheduled to be held in October this year. This decision made it possible to form an organizing committee which included core members of the research committee, the treasurer and the chairman of the scientific program of the APSR. The program of this meeting was the product of the efforts of this organizing committee.

Let me summarize the concept of "interstitial pneumonia of unknown etiology" as it is understood in this country, based on the results of our study and a review of the literature.

The etiology of the disease is unknown and pathologic changes are mainly observed in alveolar septae, characterized by diffuse alveolitis (interstitial pneumonia) in the early stage, stiffening and shrinking of the lung as it progresses, and extensive honeycomb formation at the end. Common clinical symptoms include cough and progressive dyspnea on exertion. Chest roentgenograms of patients with IIP show diffusely distributed fine nodules, large as well as small ring shadows associated with a notable degree of volume loss. Pulmonary function tests indicate restrictive ventilatory disturbance, impaired diffusing capacity, and hypoxemia. The majority of patients with the disease succumb to respiratory failure or cor pulmonale in the terminal stage.

This disease is given a diagnosis of idiopathic pulmonary fibrosis in North America, cryptogenic fibrosing alveolitis in Britain, and idiopathic interstitial pneumonia (IIP) in Japan. Our reason for the application of the term IIP since 1981 is the observation that it is inflammation in the interstitium, rather than the fibrosing process, that is critical to influence the clinical picture and prognosis of this illness.

An epidemiological study indicated that the prevalence of the disease in this country is three per one hundred thousand, with peak onset in the fifties and sixties. There is no characteristic pattern regarding gender or regional distribution in Japan.

In 1984, a nationwide survey was conducted of cases with interstitial lung diseases under the care of the members of the research committee. The total number of cases amounted to eleven hundred and six. We then tried to categorize these cases according to etiological considerations, and classified them into three major categories: known etiology, unknown etiology, and associated with systemic diseases. IIP was most common, followed by cases of connective tissue disease, sarcoidosis, hypersensitivity pneumonia, and pneumoconiosis in order of decreasing frequency.

The recent introduction of broncho-alveolar lavage for the study of interstitial lung disease has made it possible for methods developed in cell biology to be applied to further elucidate the etiology as well as the pathophysiology of interstitial pneumonia of unknown etiology. In view of these research developments, this symposium is suitable and timely to provide a forum for discussion among various investigators.

It is my sincere hope that this symposium will be meaningful and instrumental to facilitate understanding among research scientists on every aspect of this intractable disease. Finally, I wish wholeheartedly that the patients suffering from this illness will benefit by the advances in research produced as a result of this symposium.

Michiyoshi Harasawa
Chairman, Organizing Committee of International Symposium
on Interstitial Pneumonia of Unknown Etiology

I
CLINICAL PICTURE

The Clinical Concept and Revised Criteria for the Classification of Idiopathic Interstitial Pneumonia

Masashi Tamura

The Third Department of Internal Medicine, Iwate Medical College, Iwate, Japan

The preliminary criteria (1974) for the classification of idiopathic interstitial pneumonia (IIP) were revised and updated to improve disease classification. The revised criteria consited of five items, that is, clinical symptoms and signs, chest X-ray findings, pulmonary function disorders, blood chemistry and immunological disorders and pathological findings. The revised criteria were 92.7% sensitive and 77.4% specific when tested with IIP and control patient data.

Idiopathic interstitial pneumonia (IIP) is one of the interstitial lung diseases of unknown etiology. Hamman and Rich[1,2] reported five patients with dyspnea, diffuse infiltration on chest roentgenogram, cor pulmonale and death occurring within six months. However, it is now evident that this subacute fatal form of the disease is uncommon. IIP is, more commonly, a chronic disease with slowly progressive interstitial pneumonia.[3,4] A Research Committee of Interstitial Lung Disease (RCILD) was organized in 1974, supported by the Japanese Ministry of Health and Welfare. At first, survey of IIP according to clinical diagnostic criteria for screening IIP was conducted for the past three years (1974-1976) on a nationwide scale. A total of 176 clinically and pathologically definite case were collected.[5] All X-ray films and pathological specimens collected were reviewed and classified by the RCILD according to Nobechi's radiological diagnostic criteria and Yamanaka's pathological criteria.[5]   Then, the RCILD have proposed the clinical concept of IIP for cross reference to other clinical data. "IIP is one of the interstitial lung disease of unknown etiology. Patients with IIP have a insidous onset of a nonproductive cough and exertional dyspnea and their chest roentgenogram reveals a bilateral diffuse reticulonodular shadow. Histological findings show the diffuse interstitial pneumonia (UIP) with fibrosing process. The rationale for the use of corticosteroid is to stabilize or prevent disease progression, but the majority of patients are dead from the progression to respiratory failure with cor pulmonale."

Because the preliminary criteria did not incorporate various tests currently widely used in diagnosis of IIP, the subcommittee for IIP criteria was charged with updating and revision of the 1974 criteria. In this paper, the revised criteria for the classification of IIP are presented.

Method

The subcommittee first met in 1979 with task of defining the individual varialbles. Eighty four criteria variables, including symptoms, physical signs, chest roentgenographic findings, serologic tests, pulmonary function tests and histopathological findings were subjected to this study. The subcommittee obtained reports on 103 patients with IIP and same control patients from eighteen institutes. IIP group and control groups with interstitial lung disease, composing of connective tissure disease or collagen vascular disease (CTD) and hypersensitivity pneumonitis (HP) and drug-induced pneumonitis (DP) were studied. The sensitivity and specificity of individual criteria were analyzed for clinically and satisfically significant difference, using chi square contingency table analysis.

Results

The sensitivity of elements for diagnostic criteria of IIP are shown in Table 1. The sensitivity was determined on the IIP population and is expressed as the number of patients who were positive or abnormal for the element over the number patients in whom the test was determined. Cough, dyspnea and fine crackle were a high degree of sensitivity, and also reticulonodular shadows, dominant dis-

tribution at lower lung fields and lower lobe volume loss
of chest X-ray findings were prominent sensitivity. In
this table, the low sensitivity elements were excluded.
In pulmonary function tests and serological tests, pulmonary diffusion disorder, increased maximum esophageal
pressure and alveolar arterial oxygen pressure difference
were a high degree of sensitivity, and erythrocyte sedi-
mentary rate and CRP were similar to these elements.

Table 1. Sensitivity of elements in patients with IIP

Elements	Sensitivity (%)
Symptoms and signs:	
Cough	84.8
Dyspnea	91.7
Cyanosis	44.8
Clubbed fingers	61.6
Fine crackle	96.7
Chest X-ray:	
Fine nodular	60.0
Nodular	29.4
Mottling	42.4
Reticulonodular	67.7
Coarse reticular	61.3
Dominant lower lung	60.7
Dominant outer lung	45.7
Lower love volume loss	71.4
Emphysematous bullae	34.1
Pulmonary function:	
% VC	76.0
% DLco	84.9
Peso max	85.7
PaO_2	79.5
$A-aDO_2$	83.3
Blood chemistry and immunologic:	
ESR	88.9
CRP	76.9
$\gamma-G1$	65.1
IgG	50.5
LDH	53.8
Rheumatoid factor	45.6

The specificity of elements for differential diagnosis to control patients are shown in Table 2. The specificity was determined on the control patients and is expressed as percent of the number of patients who were negative or normal for the elements. Cyanosis and clubbed fingers were a high degree of specificity, and also, nodular and coarse

Table 2. Specificity of elements in control patients

Elements	Specificity (%)	
	CTD	HP·DP
Symptoms and signs:		
Cough	40.4	25.5
Dyspnea	23.8	38.8
Cyanosis	89.8	87.8
Clubbed fingers	81.5	87.2
Fine crackle	29.3	40.8
Chest X-ray:		
Fine nodular	22.8	25.0
Nodular	98.2	100.0
Mottling	75.0	75.0
Reticulonodular	75.9	79.2
Coarse reticular	82.8	95.8
Dominant lower lung	49.1	91.7
Dominantouter lung	55.6	91.7
Lower lobe volume loss	25.5	54.2
Emphysematous bullae	94.8	100.0
Pulmonary function:		
% VC	29.1	47.7
% DLco	30.6	34.6
Peso max	62.5	64.3
PaO_2	59.3	10.7
$A-aDO_2$	50.0	78.6
Blood chemistry and immunologic:		
ESR	10.2	33.3
CRP	40.4	76.1
$\gamma-G1$	32.8	47.4
IgG	41.7	65.9
LDH	59.6	68.2
Rheumatoid factor	51.8	61.9

reticular shadows and secondary emphysematous bullae at
apex were prominent specificity. In pulmonary function
tests and serological tests, the increased maximum esophageal pressure and A-aDo$_2$ were a relative high degree of
specificity, and the increased lactic dehydrogenase was a
high specificity. The subcommittee performaed these analyses and presented the revised criteria for classification
of IIP. (Table 3) This criteria consists of five items,
that is, clinical symptoms and signs, chest X-ray findings,
pulmonary function disorders, blood chemistry and immunological disorder and pathological findings.

The sensitivity and specificity of the revised IIP
criteria were tested against the current patients data
base. It is noted that the sensitivity to the IIP pa-

Table 3. The revised criteria for classification of IIP

I Clinical symptoms and signs
  a) Dry cough
  b) Dyspnea
  c) Clubbed fingers
  d) Fine crackle (Velcro râle)

II Chest X-ray findings
  a) Distribution: diffuse, predominant outer and
    lower lung zone
  b) Roentgenographic patterns: nodular, reticulonodular
    and coarse reticular shadows (honeycombing)
  c) Lung shrinkage: elevation of diaphragmatic dome
    and lower lobe volume loss

III Pulmonary function disorders
  a) Restrictive changes: % VC↓, % TCL↓
  b) Decreased diffusing capacity: DLco↓,
    % DLco/VA↓
  c) Hypoxemia: PaO$_2$↓, A-aDO$_2$↑

IV Blood chemistry and immunological disorder
  a) Increased ESR
  b) Increased LDH value
  c) Positive RA test

V Pathological findings (autopsy or lung biopsy)
  Compatible with pathological criteria of IIP
    (definite or probable)

---

tients was 92.7% and specificity against the patients of
CTD was 77.4%, HP and DP 56.5%, when item II and any three
or more items are present. (Tables 4,5)

Table 4. Sensitivity of revised IIP criteria

	item II + any 2 items	item II + any 3 or more items
IIP (*n*=51)	100%	92.7%

Table 5. Sensitivity of revised IIP criteria

	item II + any 2 items	item II + any 3 or more items
CTD (*n*=53)	37.7%	77.4%
HP·DP (*n*=23)	13.0%	56.5%

The clinical criteria for diagnosis of IIP are shown in
Table 6. Definite criteria requires postitive item II
and V or positive item any 3 or more items, and probable
criteria item II and any 2 items. However, because of
low specificity against the control groups, some diffuse
pulmonary diseases must be excluded. IIP cannot be diagnosed until diffuse pulmonary disease of known etiology
(pneumoconiosis, tuberculosis, chronic bronchitis, diffuse
panbronchiolitis, pneumonia, lung cancer, hypersensitivity
pneumonitis, radiation pneumonitis, drug-induced pneumonitis)
and sarcoidosis, connective tissue diseases have been excluded.

Table 6. Clinical criteria for diagnosis of IIP*

	Item
Definite	item II + item V item II + any 3 or more items
Probable	item II + any 2 items

(1980, Tamura M *et al.*)[7)]

Discussion

Since RCILD have been organized in Japan in 1974, numbers of IIP patients are increasing. Although the Committee have been studying on elucidation of the pathogenesis, clinical and therapeutic approach to IIP, the inciting factors in the development of IIP are still unknown. Among the interstitial lung diseases, IIP is a "Diagnosis of exclusion"[6]; namely, there is few clinicopathological findings that is specific for this entity. However, the revised criteria set composed of clinical history, symptoms, physiocal signs, laboratory findings and pathohistological findings has good discriminating power against connective tissue diseases, drug-induced pneumonitis and hypersensitivity pneumonitis. Its potential as a turely diagnostic criteria set in IIP should await the results of more extensive tests against a wider variety of diseases.

References

1. Hamman, L. and Rich, A.R. Trans Am Clin Climatol Assoc 51, 154-163, 1935.
2. Hamman, L. and Rich, A.R. Bull Johns Hopkins Hosp 74, 177-212, 1944.
3. Crystal, R.G., Fulmer, J.D., Roberts, W.C., Moss, M.L., Line, B.R., and Reynolds, H.Y. Ann Intern Med 85, 769-788, 1976.
4. Turner-Warwick, M., Burrows, B., and Johnson, A. Thorax 35, 171-180, 1980.
5. Murao, M. Proceedings of XIIIth World Congress on Diseases of the Chest, pp 234-246, 1976.
6. Gadek, J.E. and Allen, J.D. Pulmonary Perspectives 5, 1-4, 1988.
7. Tamura, M. In: Report of the project team research on idiopathic interstitial pneumonia in Japan. (Honma, H. ed.), Tokyo, pp 4-6, 1980. (in Japanese)

Clinical Pictures of Idiopathic Interstitial Pneumonia (IIP) Based on a Nationwide Study in Japan

Yoshinosuke Fukuchi*, Kiyoshi Ishida*, Takeshi Matsuse*, and Michiyoshi Harasawa**

* *Department of Geriatrics, Faculty of Medicine, University of Tokyo, Tokyo, Japan*
** *Tokyo Teishin Hospital, Tokyo, Japan*

Clinical pictures of 351 cases of idiopathic interstitial pneumonia (IIP) and 78 cases of interstitial pneumonia associated with connective tissue disease (IPCTD) were studied. Cough, fine crackles and clubbed fingers were more common in IIP. Fever, arthralgia and skin eruptions were more frequent in IPCTD. The chest roentgenogram showed more diffuse shadows with peripheral predominance in IIP. The prevalence of bronchogenic carcinoma was 10.7% in IIP and 2.6% in IPCTD. The prognosis remained worse for IIP than for IPCTD even after controlling the difference in age, pulmonary function and accompanying lung cancers of the two diseases.

In most of earlier investigations which examined the clinical pictures of interstitial pneumonia, direct comparison between idiopathic interstitial pneumonia(IIP) and interstitial pneumonia associated with connective tissue disease(IPCTD) were difficult to achieve. This was partly because only limited number of cases were available for analysis to define the characteristics of these two maladies. The special taskforce group for the study of interstitial lung disease conducted a nationwide survey in 1984 with a grant from the ministry of health and welfare of Japan. This provided us the opportunity to examine the clinical pictures of these two illness in more details. This report describes a part of its result with special emphasis on symptomatology and prognosis of the diseases.

Subjects and Method

Surveysheets specially designed for this purpose included over 350 items of data in clinical as well as pathological findings. They were distribued to the hospitals throughout Japan and 60 hospitals complied with the request of filling out of the sheet by the staff who are in close association with the members of the research group for the study of interstitial lung disease. The decision as to whether or not to enroll a case was made by the staff based on the criteria proposed by this research group. Those who were thought to have IIP all met the criteria elaborated in the previous report on the concept of IIP.

Those cases who were categorized as IPCTD basically satisfied the criteria set by American Rheumatoid Association for the diagnosis of connective tissue disease in addition to the presence of overt interstitial lung disease. Only those cases with confirming histologic diagnosis were included for the final statistical analysis. All data were fed into a computer, processed and calculated using SAS program to test a statistical significance.

Results

Detailed data sheets were available in 1106 cases of interstitial lung disease. IIP was the most common clinical diagnosis(52.4%) followed by IPCTD(12.6%). Histologic confirmation of IIP was possible in 351 cases by transbronchial lung biopsy(TBLB, 55.8%), autopsy(35.3%) and open lung biopsy(8.8%). In 78 cases of IPCTD, morphological diagnosis was made by TBLB(84.6%), autopsy(12.8%) and open lung biopsy(2.6%). The breakdown of histology proven IPCTD disclosed rheumatoid arthritis (43.6%), progressive systemic scleroderma(17.9%), polymyositis (11.5%), SLE (6.4%), dermatomyositis (5.1%) and others. Male was predominant in IIP patients(M/F=243/108) but female was in excess of man in IPCTD(M/F=29/49). Mean age at the first visit was 60.2 ± 11.8 years for IIP and

52.4±10.9 for IPCTD. The summary of symptoms and signs on the first visit is shown in Fig.1.

Fig.1 Symptoms and Signs (First Vist)

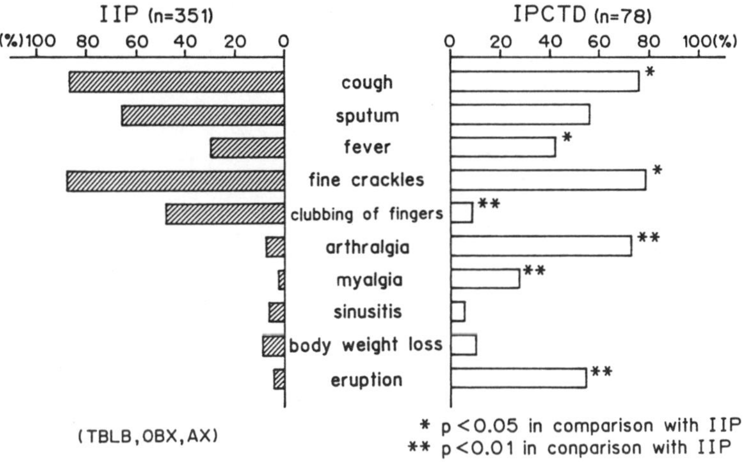

Cough (87%), sputum (66%), fine crackles (88%) and clubbing of fingers(48.2%) were more frequent in IIP than in IPCTD. On the other hand, fever(42.1%), arthralgia (73%), myalgia(27.4%) and eruption(49.3%) were more common in IPCTD than in IIP. There was no significant difference between these two illnesses regarding blood cell count, hepatic and renal function. The erythrocyte sedimentaion rate(ESR) in IPCTD (63±42mm/h) was significantly higher than in IIP. The RA factor was positive in 29.2% of IIP and 74.7% of IPCTD. Gallium scan was also positive in 62.5% of IIP and 54.5% of IPCTD. Arterial blood gas analysis at the time of first visit revealed significantly lower PaO2 (72.8±15.1Torr) for IIP than IPCTD (81.9±11.7Torr) with comparable PaCO2 and PH.

Pulmonary function study disclosed reduction in %VC (IIP/IPCTD; 69.0±20.6% / 69.2±19.3%), %DLCO (IIP/IPCTD; 51.0±21.1%/55.1±15.4%) and static compliance (IIP// IPCTD; 0.11±0.08 L/cmH2O// 0.12±0.09). Flow limitation was not present with normal FEV1% and flow volume curve. Some difference of characteristic findings in chest roentgenographic finding were observed(Fig.2).

Diffuse distribution of fine nodular or reticulonodular shadow were common both in IIP and IPCTD. But diffuse

nature in the former (90.1%) is significantly more
notable than in the latter (75.0%) with greater preference (67.7%) for peripheral distribution as compared to
IPCTD (34.8%). Volume loss of lower lung field accompanying elevated diaphragm was characteristic in 55-57% of
IIP and 43-47% of IPCTD.

Fig.2 Chest Roentgenographic Findings (First Visit)

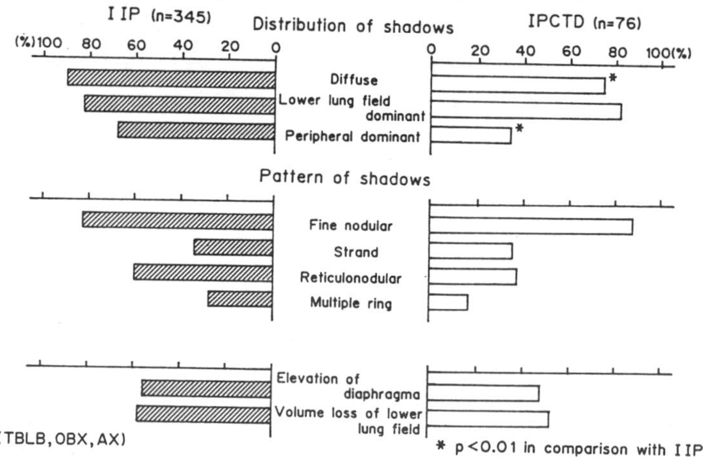

The prevalence of carcinoma was markedly higher in IIP
when compared to IPCTD as indicated in table 1.

Table 1   Prevalence of Carcinoma in IIP and IPCTD

	IIP (n=336) No. cases(%)	IPCTD (n=77) No. cases(%)
Bronchogenic carcinoma	36 (10.7%) *	2 (2.6%)
Other carcinoma	8 (2.4%)	0 (0%)

* p<0.05 in comparison with IPCTD   (TBLB,OBX,AX)

When the histologic findings of lung cancer associated
with IIP were further analyzed, epidermoid (squamous
cell) carcinoma was most common (36.1%) followed by

undifferentiated carcinoma (small cell; 22.2%, large cell; 8.3%), adenocarcinoma (22.2%) and alveolar cell carcinoma(5.6%) (Fig.3).

Table 2 represents a comparison of parameters which may influence the survival of IIP and IPCTD. As previously described, IIP patients had higher age, greater number of male population and lower PaO2.

The cumulative survival curve was obtained by Kaplan-Meir method for IIP and IPCTD (Fig.4).

Fig.3 Histologic Findings of Lung Cancer (36cases of IIP)

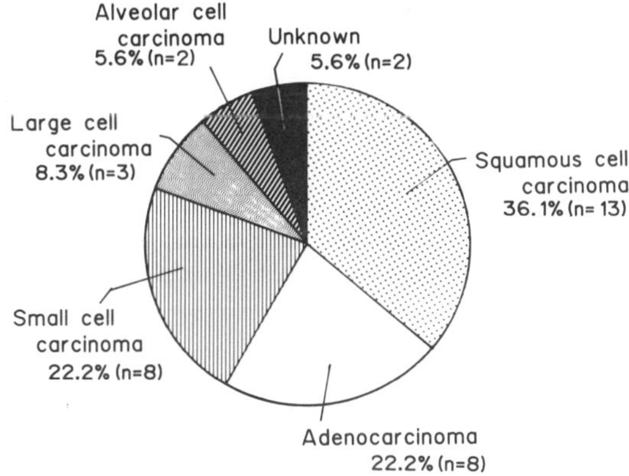

Table 2. Subjects (in all cases)

		IIP (n=351)	IPCTD (n=78)	
AGE	(y.o.)	60.2±11.8	52.4±10.9	p<0.001
Male	(%)	69.2	37.2	p<0.001
%VC	(%)	69.0±20.6	69.2±19.3	NS
%TLC	(%)	73.3±19.8	78.7±18.5	NS
FEV1%	(%)	81.9± 9.8	81.4±13.2	NS
%DLco	(%)	51.0±21.1	55.1±15.4	NS
PaO2	(Torr)	72.4±15.6	81.0±12.5	p<0.001
PaCO2	(Torr)	38.2± 6.4	37.0± 3.7	NS

(MEANS±SD)

Fig.4 Survival Curve of IIP and IPCTD (in all cases)

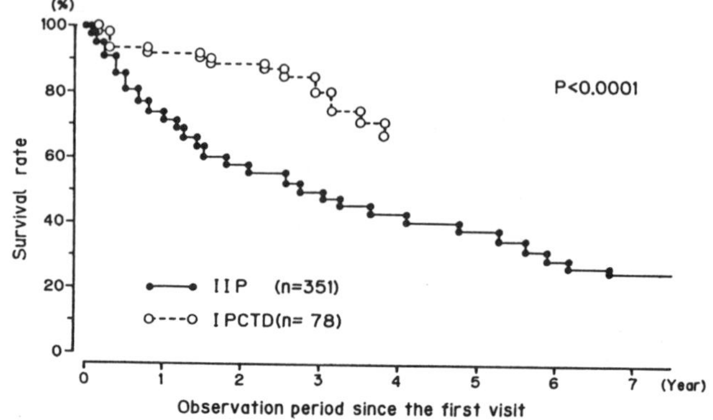

The survival for IIP was significantly worse than for IPCTD, at one year 71% vs 93% and at three year 48% vs 78%. We then had the age and pulmonary function at the time of first visit matched for this population. This has reduced the number of the subjects submitted for the analysis of survival(Table 3).

Table 3. Subjects Matched for Age, %VC and PaO2
(at the first visit)

		IIP (n=155)	IPCTD (n= 69)
AGE	(y.o.)	53.5± 8.2	52.1±1 1.1
%VC	(%)	70.6±20.2	69.3±19.6
%TLC	(%)	74.4±20.1	79.8±18.5
FEV1%	(%)	82.0± 9.9	81.4±13.5
%DLco	(%)	52.7±19.2	56.3±14.8
Pao2	(Torr)	79.5± 9.9	81.9±1 1.7
Paco2	(Torr)	38.7± 6.1	37.1± 3.6
Male		63.9%	36.2% p<0.01

(MEANS±SD)

The result of survival curve analysis is shown in Fig.5. The difference between IIP and IPCTD became smaller but it was still statistically significant. The first year survival was 85% for IIP, 97% for IPCTD ; the third year 63% for IIP and 80% for IPCTD.

Fig.5 Survival Curve of IIP and IPCTD (in cases matched for age, %VC and PaO2 at the first visit)

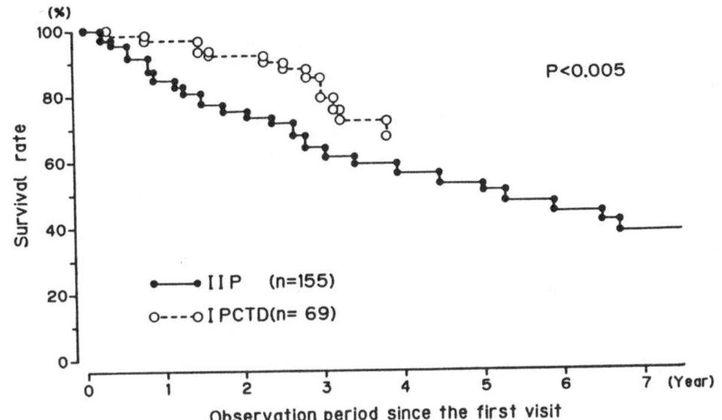

Because higher incidence of complicating lung cancer among IIP might affect the survival in adverse way, we went on to exclude those cases with bronchogenic carcinoma from subjects to calculate the survival curve for both diseases. We now were left with 187 cases of IIP and 66 cases of IPCTD. They were matched in all the relevant factors except for male predominance in IIP (Table 4)

Table 4. Subjects without complicating lung cancer matched for age and pulmonary function at first visit.

	IIP (n=137)	IPCTD (n= 66)
AGE (y.o.)	53.2± 8.0	51.7±11.0
%VC (%)	69.5±19.8	69.8±19.7
%TLC (%)	73.0±20.2	80.9±17.8
FEV₁% (%)	82.5± 9.8	81.2±13.7
%DLco(%)	51.1±19.0	56.0±15.0
Pao2 (Torr)	79.7± 9.9	82.1±11.9
Paco2 (Torr)	38.8± 6.2	36.9± 3.5
Male	61.3%	34.8% P<0.01

(MEANS±SD)

The survival curve thus derived remained to show significantly worse survival for IIP. The survival was 86% for IIP and 98% for IPCTD at one year. It was 65% for the former and 80% for the latter at three years (Fig.6).

Fig.6 Survival Curve of IIP and IPCTD (in cases without bronchogenic carcinoma, matched for age, %VC and PaO2)

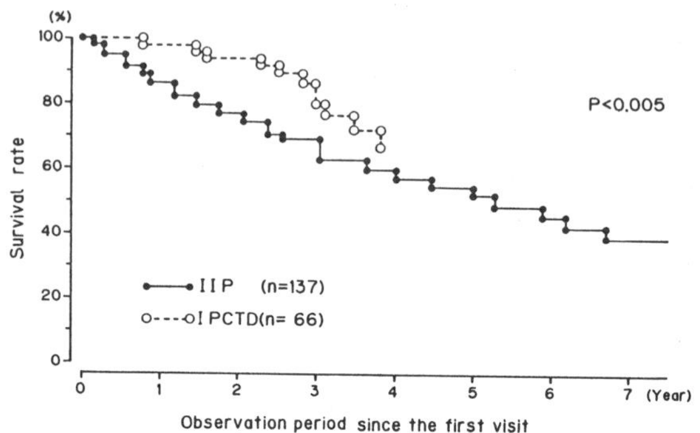

Finally, contribution of various items of symptoms, signs and laboratory findings were evaluated as a risk factor to predict poor prognosis in IIP. After categorizing each factor by degree of derangement, changes of survival curve were calculated and compared to find out significant level of causing worse survival. This procedure resulted to define the risk factors responsible for making the prognosis of IIP worse. They are as follows.
1.Higher age(particularly over 60 years of age) 2.Fever 3.Clubbed finger 4.Dyspnea greater than Grade 3 of Hugh-Jones criteria 5.Interstitial shadows on chest film more than two third of entire lung field. 6.Peripheral distribution of interstitial shadow. 7.Peripheral WBC count in excess of 9000. 8.Peripheral Lymphocyte fraction less than 25%. 9.Abnormally elevated LDH. 10.Elevated ESR. 11.%VC less than 80%. 12.FEV1% greater than 90% 13.%DLCO less than 50%. 14.PaO2 lower than 60 Torr. 15.PaCO2 less than 35 or greater than 45 Torr. 16.Complicating lung cancer.

Discussion

This study disclosed notable differences in clinical pictures which exists between IIP and and IPCTD. Most of earlier study which addressed to examine clinical features did not clearly separated IIP from IPCTD [1-4]. In these investigation, 20% [4], 20.9% [2] and 33% of the cases submitted for analysis were those with connective tissue disease. The ratio of IPCTD/IIP was 22.2% in this survey which was close to these reports. Rheumatoid arthritis was known to be most common with 47.8% [2] and 57.6% [3] of prevalence in IPCTD. Majority of histologic examination depended on TBLB rather than open lung biopsy which reflects a common practice prevailing in this country at the time of the survey. The result and its interpretation from this study should remain within this constraints of diagnostic modality.

The frequency of symptoms and signs which was found in this study are in agreement with previous reports [1,2]. Rather high prevalence of sputum in this survey (66%) was similar to other reports by Turner-Warwick (56.8%) and Mikami (57%). Though fine crackles were more common in IIP, they were not specific to this illness with 79% of patients of IPCTD also presenting them. Higher frequency of fever, arthralgia and skin eruptions among IPCTD may be related to the underlying disease.

Both IIP and IPCTD seem to share common features of interstitial shadows with diffuse, reticulonodular and multiple ring shadows. The signs of volume loss were comparable. IIP was characterized by more preferential distribution of shadows as compared to IPCTD.

It has been pointed out that IIP is associated with high incidence of bronchogenic carcinoma. The incidence reported were 4.4% [3], 5.2% [5], 9.8% [2] and 15.8% [6]. The figure of 10.7% for IIP and 2.6% observed in this survey is among higher incidence of earlier study. General incidence of bronchogenic carcinoma in Japan is less than 0.2 % and much higher incidence observed in this study warrants the need for close clinical follow-up to detect the cancer at early stage. The histologic type of these carcinoma was not much different from what one finds among general population. But relatively high frequency of alveolar cell carcinoma was also noteworthy in this analysis [5].

Mean survival time for IIP was 48.8 months from the onset of symptoms and 20.4 months from the time of first visit in this study. This survival time was shorter than that reported by Turner-Warwick (38 months from first visit). But that study included IPCTD cases into the subjects and ours did not. The survival turned out to be significantly longer in IPCTD than in IIP. This observation remained unchanged even after controlling such risk factors as age and pulmonary function at first visit [8]. In view of higher prevalence of complicating lung cancer, we eliminated cases with lung cancer from analysis. Yet the survival was still worse in IIP. This suggests that IIP patient may die of this illness in many cases before developing cancer. The risk of complicating lung cancer markedly increased in smoking population of IIP. Hence smoking cessation is mandatory in the management of IIP [9].

Reference

1.Scadding JG, Hinson KFW : Diffuse fibrosing alveolitis (diffuse interstitial fibrosis of the lung) : correlation of histology at biopsy with prognosis. Thorax 22:291-304,1967.

2.Turner-Warwick M, Burrows B, Johnson A : Cryptogenic fibrosing alveolitis : clinical features and their influence on survival. Thorax 35:171-180,1980.

3.Tukiainen P, Takinen E, Holsti P, Kohola O, Valle M : Prognosis of cryptogenic fibrosing alveolitis. Thorax 38:349-355, 1983.

4.Crystal RG, Fulmer JD, Roberts WC, Moss ML, Line BR, Reynolds HY : Idiopathic pulmonary fibrosis : clinical, histologic, radiographic, physiologic and biochemical aspects. Ann.Int.Med.85 : 769-788,1976.

5.Stack BHR, Choo-Kang YFG, Heard BE : The prognosis of cryptogenic fibrosing alveolitis. Thorax 22 : 535-542, 1972.

6.Mikami R and other members of research group :The result of the fourth nation-wide survey on pulmonary fibrosis. The report of survey and research group of the ministry of health and welfare : 49-55,1977.

7.Tamura M and other members of research group : Summary of epidemiological subcommittee--a survey on diffuse interstitial pneumonia of unknown etiology and related disease. The report of survey and research group of the ministry of health and welfare : 34-43,1978.

8.Fukuchi Y, Ishida K, Yamaoka M et al : Different prognosis in idiopathic interstitial pneumonia and pulmonary fibrosis associated with connective tissue disease. Amer.Rev.Respir.Dis. 135 : A347,1987.

9.Fukuchi Y, Matsuse T, Yamaoka M et al : Influence of smoking on the prevalence of bronchogenic carcinoma in idiopathic interstitial pneumonia. Amer.Rev.Respir.Dis. 137 : A 181,1988.

Inhaled Dust and Collagen Vascular Diseases as the Possible Causes of Idiopathic Interstitial Pneumonia (IIP)

Yukihiko Homma, Kazunori Tanimura, Hirotaka Kusaka, and Mitsuru Munakata

Department of Medeicine, Medical Center and First Department of Medicine, Hokkaido University, Sapporo, Japan

To elucidate the primary cause of IIP in the initial immune process, the clinical course, history of dust inhalation, and chest x-ray findings of 55 IIP patients were compared with those of 60 patients with interstitial pneumonia due to collagen vascular disease (CVD-IP). 1) Thirteen of the 60 CVD-IP patients were clinically and even histologically defined as having IIP 1 to 129 months before their CVD systemic symptoms appeared ('preceded form'), 2) 71.7% of IIP patients had a dust inhalation history by contrast to the 32.1% of CVD-IP, and 3) by chest x-ray examination, honeycombing or bulla were typically seen in IIP, and restricted distribution of reticulo-nodular shadows to lower lung field, discoid atelectasis, or pleural thickening in CVD-IP. These findings suggest that inhaled dust is the primary cause of IIP and immune complexes are of CVD-IP.

Introduction

The etiology of idiopathic interstitial pneumonia, IIP, is still unknown. However, a great deal is clarified about its inflammation process. Crystal et al. [1] stressed the central role of alveolar macrophages, AM,

in its immune process. Irreversible fibrotic changes in
lung parenchyma are caused by a series of immunological
reactions after the aggregation, proliferation, and
activation of AM. For successful prevention or treatment of IIP, we should know the activator of AM or the
initiator in the immune process. Crystal et al. [1]
supposed the immune complex to be its factors, and that
the immune complexes were derived from self-components
of the alveolar wall itself. We discuss the problem of
overlap among collagen vascular disease (CVD) and IIP,
and the possibility of immune complex as an initiator in
collagen vascular disease-associated interstitial pneumonia, CVD-IP. In addition to this problem, we also
discuss the relationship of inhaled dust to this disease
from clinical view points, as we previously reported [2,
8].

Method

The subjects were composed of 55 patients with IIP and
60 CVD-IP who were admitted to our hospital during the
past 10 years. IIP was defined according to the clinical criteria of IIP proposed by a Project Team for IIP
organized by the Japanese Ministry of Health and Welfare
[3]. Histological examination by open lung biopsy and/
or autopsy were performed on 17 out of 55 patients with
IIP. CVD was defined according to the criteria proposed
by the American Rheumatic Association (ARA) [4, 7].
Histological examination as above was done in 12 out of
60 patients with CVD-IP.
Chest x-ray findings were reviewed by 3 expert chest
physicians and finally judged by one of us (YH).
Histological specimens were routinely stained by Hematoxylin-Eosin, and additionally by Elastica-van Gieson
as necessary. They were histologically defined according to the criteria proposed by the Project Team [3].
Statistical analyses were done by Student's t test or X^2
test using the commercial program of SAS.

Results

1. Age, sex, and smoking habits of the subjects
As shown in Table 1, IIP patients were much older than
the CVD-IP patients with male predominance, and more
patients were smokers (each difference was statistically
significant).

Table 1   Subjects. IIP:Idiopathic interstitial pneumonia,
CVD-IP:Interstitial pneumonia associated with collagen
vascular disease

	IIP	CVD-IP	P<
N	55(17)	60(12)	
Age(m ± SD)	61 ± 9	51 ± 13	0.001(t-test)
Sex			
Male	45(14)	16(6)	
Female	10(3)	44(6)	0.001(X²-test)
Smoking habit			
Smoker	48(16)	23(6)	
Non-smoker	7(1)	37(6)	0.001(X²-test)

*Numbers in parentheses represnt the patients who were defined
by open lung biopsy and/or autopsy.

2. Cases of 'preceded form' of CVD-IP whose systemic
   symptoms appeared a certain period after the lung
   involvement

First, we present a 59-year-old housewife. On Feb.
1977 dry cough and dyspnea on exertion (DOE) appeared,
and next month abnormal shadows on chest films were
pointed out by a doctor. Fig. 1 is an x-ray film when
she was admitted to our hospital in Aug. 1977. She was
clinically defined with IIP by the above symptoms, fine
crackles heard over bilateral lower lung fields, hypoxia
with restricted and diffusion impairment in lung function tests (%VC 45%, %TLC 53%, FEV1/FVC 88%, %DLco 34%,
PO2 62.0 torr, AaDO2 54.7 torr), and typical x-ray findings to IIP. LDH was 361 unit, ESR 37mm/hr., and RA
test negative. She was orally given an initial dose of
60mg/day predonisolone, and thereafter the symptoms of
cough and DOE and abnormal chest x-ray findings showed
marked recovery (Fig. 2).

On Feb. 1979 she was histologically defined as having
IIP by open lung biopsy (Fig. 3). However, on Feb. 1983,
i.e., 6 years after the appearance of the symptoms,
morning stiffness of fingers, arthralgia and swelling of
extremity joints appeared, and the RA test became positive. She was defined as definitely having rheumatoid
arthritis (RA) according to the criteria proposed by
ARA.

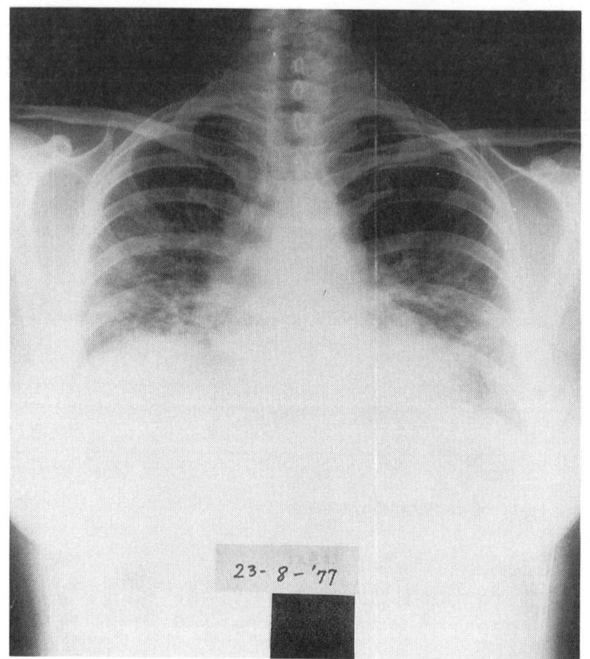

Fig. 1. An x-ray film taken at admission to our hospital
in Aug. 1977. diffuse nodular shadows consistent with
IIP are seen.

This case was thought to be a typical case of 'preceded form' of CVD-IP, and it is interesting because she
was defined as having IIP clinically and even histologically before her RA systemic symptoms appeared.
Thirteen of the 60 CVD had the 'preceded form'
(21.7%)(Table 2). They all were defined as IIP at their
first visit to our hospital. The final diagnosis of CVD
was RA in 5 patients, dermatomyositis-polymyositis
(DM.PM) in 5, systemic lupus erythematodes (SLE) in 1,
Sjögren syndrome in 1, and Overlap syndrome in 1. The
period preceded by pulmonary involvement ranged from 1
to 129 months.

3. Comparison of chest x-ray findings between 55 IIP and
   60 CVD-IP patients
   We compared the differences in 8 roentgenological
findings frequently seen in diffuse lung diseases bet-

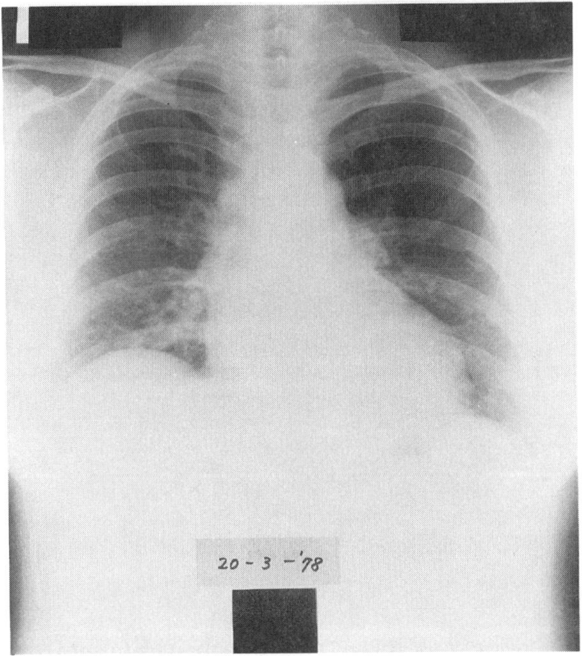

Fig. 2. X-ray findings after predonisolon treatment (in
Mar, 1978). The abnormal shadows seen in Fig. 1 are
markedly reduced.

ween the two groups (Table 3). Honeycombing or bulla
were typically seen in IIP and restricted distribution
of reticulo-nodular shadows to lower lung field, discoid
atelectasis, or pleural thickening in CVD-IP, while
volume loss of lower lung lobes and partial overinflation of the lung were evenly observed in both diseases.
  We additionally compared the differences in these 8
findings between the 17 IIP patients associated with
histological examinations and 38 IIP patients without
it, but found no significant difference in any finding.

4. Dust inhalation histories in IIP and CVD-IP patients
  Table 4 shows the different incidence of dust inhalation history in both groups. Of the IIP patients 71.7%
had an inhalation history, and this incidence was significantly predominant over 32.1% of CVD-IP. In addition,
we gave attention to 13 patients in this table who had

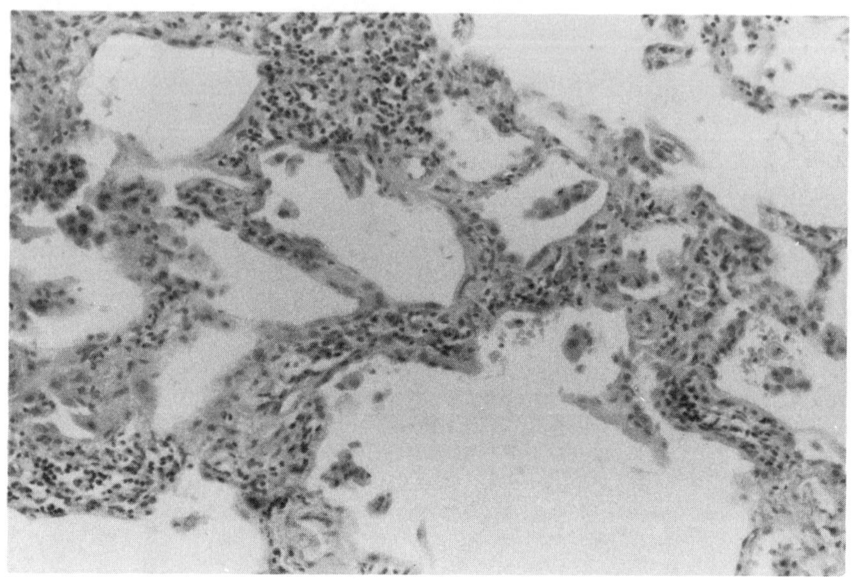

Fig. 3. Histological findings by open lung biopsy. Honeycombing and thickening of alveolar septum typical to IIP are seen.

Table 2   CVD-IP patients whose CVD symptoms were preceded by abnormal chest x-ray findings (Preceded form)

No	Age	Sex	CVD (definite)	Period preceded by pulm.changes(M)	Histology
1	52	Female	RA	71	IIP*(Open biopsy)
2	60	Female	RA	1	
3	52	Male	RA	1	
4	60	Male	RA	9	
5	74	Male	RA	129	IIP*(Autopsy)
6	68	Male	DM.PM	4	
7	49	Female	DM.PM	3	
8	57	Female	DM.PM	2	IIP*(Open biopsy)
9	41	Male	DM.PM	1	
10	62	Male	DM.PM	34	
11	37	Female	SLE	4	IIP*(Autopsy)
12	58	Female	Sjogren	59	
13	55	Female	Overlap	6	

* Histologically defined as IIP based on the criteria proposed
   by a Japanese Project Team for IIP

no dust inhalation history.

Table 5 shows the brief contents of the 13 patients. Although they had no symptoms related to CVD, some of them had positive results of immunological tests or certain x-ray findings thought typical to CVD as shown in Table 3. Moreover, females were predominant over males as seen in CVD-IP (Table 1).

Table 3 Comparison of roentgenological findings between IIP and CVD-IP patients

	IIP(%)	CVD-IP(%)	P< (X^2-test)
N	55(100.0)	60(100.0)	
Pleural thickening	15(27.3)	27(45.0)	0.05
Honeycomb lung	36(65.5)	25(41.7)	0.05
Bulla	29(52.7)	12(20.0)	0.001
Restricted distribution to lower lung fields	8(14.6)	20(33.3)	0.05
Volume loss of lower lung lobes	26(47.3)	32(53.3)	NS
Partial overinflation of the lung	3(5.5)	5(8.3)	NS
Discoid atelectasis	3(5.5)	15(25.0)	0.01

Table 4 History of environmental dust inhalation

	IIP	CVD-IP	P<
N(%)	46(100.0)*	53(100.0)*	
Dust inhalation(+)	33(71.7)	17(32.1)	
Coal miner	7(15.2)	1(1.9)	
Civil engineer	5(10.9)	2(3.8)	
Constructive worker	6(13.0)	1(1.9)	
Railroad man	2(4.3)	2(3.8)	0.001(X^2-test)
Ironworker	1(2.2)	0	
Farmer	8(17.4)	7(13.2)	
Teacher	4(8.7)	4(7.5)	
Dust inhalation(-)	13(28.3)	36(67.9)	
Housewife	7(15.2)	24(45.3)	
Clerk	6(13.1)	12(22.6)	

*History of dust inhalation was unknown in 9 out IIP and 7 out of 60 in CVD-IP, respectively.

Table 5 IIP patients (housewife & clerk) without a history of dust inhalation

N(%)	13(100.0)
Sex	
Male	6(46.1)
Female	7(53.9)
Symptoms related to CVD	
Arthralgia	0
Raynaud'phenomenon	0
Others	0
Immunological tests	
RA positive	3(23.1)
ANA positive *	4(50.0)
X-ray findings probably typical to CVD	
Discoid atelectasis	3(23.1)
Pleural thickening	5(38.5)
Without bulla	4(30.8)
Lower lung fields only	3(23.1)

*ANA tests were done in 8 out of 13 patients.

5. Histological findings of IIP and CVD-IP patients

Seventeen IIP and 12 CVD-IP patients who were histologically examined showed typical IIP findings compatible to the histological criteria proposed by the Project Team for IIP[3].

Discussion

Overlap of IIP and CVD-IP cases

Substantial histological changes of the lung were similar in IIP and CVD-IP except for the degree of the changes. Haslam et al. [5] reported no difference even in the findings of broncho-alveolar lavage (BAL) fluid.

In this series, we found 13 out of 60 cases of CVD-IP defined as IIP clinically and even histologically in some before the systemic CVD symptoms appeared (Table 1). We now conveniently call them the 'preceded form' of CVD-IP. On the other hand, IIP patients who had no dust inhalation history revealed some positive serological reactions and/or roentgenological findings supposingly related to CVD (Table 5). The possibility that some of these patients will be defined as CVD-IP 11 years after the appearance of pulmonary involvement (Case 5 in Table 2) strongly supports this possibility. We assume that the cases defined as IIP include some CVD-IP patients.

CVD has been believed to be an autoimmune disease and a disease characterized by the tissue damage of certain related organs by immune complexes. From the clinical point of view, we believe that the immune complexes are the initiator which initially stimulate AM in the course of the immune process in CVD-IP.

Dust inhalation as a cause of IIP

Most investigators do not consider the exposure to inorganic or organic dust known to induce interstitial lung disease as the cause of IIP. By contrast, Abraham et al. [6] reported that 75% of the patients with DIP had a history of dust or hume exposure, and specific types of particulate exposure were documented in 92% of cases subjected to tissue microanalysis. We also reported that inorganic particles such as silica were frequently observed in lung tissue specimens of IIP patients examined by analytical electron microscopy (AEM) and proton-induced x-ray emission (PIXE) [2], and that, moreover, 'IIP like' pulmonary changes revealed by x-ray and histological examination were frequently observed in workers in 'dust' environment [8].

In this series, 71.7% of the IIP patients had a dust inhalation history in contrast to 32.1% in CVD-IP patients (Table 4). This may suggest the different etiology between IIP and CVD-IP. We suppose that the inhaled dust activates and/or proliferates AM, and acts as the initiator of a course of immune processes in IIP.

The environment under which the person inhales dust require consideration. For example, should the environment of the farmer or teacher be included as such an environment or not, as seen in Table 4. We included them into the dust environment because we had found many dust particles by SEM and PIXE analyses in the IIP patients who were farmers or teachers. For example, many particles of chalk were observed in the lung tissue of a teacher with IIP. However, the problem for the definition of a dust environment needs further study.

Difference of chest x-ray findings between IIP and CVD-IP

By determining the differences in chest x-ray findings

between IIP and CVD-IP, we may be able to identify 'preceded form' of CVD-IP at their first visit to the hospital and to select an appropriate counterplan. The x-ray findings of honeycombing or bulla were typical in IIP and those of restricted distribution of reticulo-nodular shadows to lower lung fields, discoid atelectasis, or pleural thickening in CVD-IP, while volume loss of lower lung lobes and partial overinflation of the lung were observed similarly in both diseases (Table 3).

In the cases of IIP, the peripheral airways may be easily affected by the inhaled dust, and honeycomb- or bulla-formation may result. In the case of CVD-IP, contrary to IIP, noxae such as immune complex may be easily born to the lower lung parenchyma by blood stream. The difference in x-ray findings seen between IIP and CVD-IP may suggest the different route to bear such different noxae.

In conclusion, we speculate that inhaled dusts is the most probable initiator which stimulate alveolar macrophages in the initial immune process, and that circulating immune complexes in the cases of CVD also act as an initiator for CVD-IP.

References

1) Crystal, R.G., Bitterman, R.B., Rennard, S.I., et al. N Engl J Med 310, 154-166, 1984.
2) Inoue, M. Hokkaido Med J 61, 745-754, 1986 (with English abstract).
3) Murao, M. In: Report of the XIII World Congress on Diseases of the Chest, Japan Chapter of ACCP, Tokyo, pp. 234-246, 1978.
4) Ropes, M.W., Bennett, G.A., Caleb, S., et al. Bull Rheum Dis 9, 175, 1958.
5) Haslam, P.L., Turton, C.W.G., Lukoszek, A., et al. Thorax 35, 328-339, 1980.
6) Abraham, J.L., Hertzberg, M.A. Chest 80(suppl), 67S, 1981.
7) Arnett, F.C., Edworthy, s., Bloch, E., et al. In: 51st Annual Meeting of American Rheumatism Association, Washington DC, June, 1987.
8) Homma, Y., Inoue, M., Ogasawara, H., et al. Kokyuu To Junkan 34, 709-7201986 (in Japanese).

Acute Exacerbation in Idiopathic Interstitial Pneumonia (IIP)

Ariyoshi Kondo* and Shigeki Saiki**

* *Department of Respiratory Disease, Nishi-Niigata National Hospital, Niigata, Japan*
** *Department of Pathology, St. Luke's International Hospital, Tokyo, Japan*

Two series of 155 and 22 IIP cases with the diagnosis established by open lung biopsy or autopsy were analyzed for acute exacerbation with the following results:
1)Acute exacerbation occurred in 89(57.4%) of 155 cases and a comparison of survival curves showed that cases with acute exacerbation had a significant poorer prognosis than those without it. 2)In the vast majority of cases acute exacerbation occurred once during the entire course of disease and was associated with a fever, aggravation of shortness of breath, deterioration of chest x-ray findings, accelerated erythrocyte sedimentation rate, elevated serum LDH and decreased Pao_2. 3)In many instances, aggravation of the primary disease, infection or a reduction of corticosteroid dosage were assumed to be or identified as the direct or precipitating cause of acute exacerbation. 4)On histologic examination of the lung there have recently been noted lesions compatible with acute interstitial pneumonia, in addition to those characteristic of IIP, e.g., fibrosis of alveolar walls and honeycombing.

Introduction

Idiopathic interstitial pneumonia (IIP) is usually a

slowly progressive chronic disease with a poor prognosis
(1,2), but it may occasionally become abruptly worsened
on the course of disease to prove fatal in days or weeks
(3,4). Such an acute exacerbation may occur with or
without a corticosteroid regimen and what it really is
still remains obscure. In an effort to characterize this
phenomenon, we attempted to analyze episodes of acute
exacerbation and to explore associated histological
changes of the lung in cases of IIP proven by open lung
biopsy or autopsy.

Subjects and Methods

Subjects: Involved in this study were 155 cases
collected in a questionnaire survey by the Interstitial
Lung Diseases Research Group of the Ministry of Health &
Welfare and 22 cases collected by the IIP Study Group
during the year of 1988, with a histological diagnosis
being established by open lung biopsy or autopsy in all
cases. There were 110 males and 45 females in the former
series and 19 males and 3 females in the latter, with
mean ages at the time of first examination being 60.0 ±
12.8 and 63.3 ± 10.3 years, respectively.

Methods: In the former 155 cases acute exacerbation was
studied by a questionnaire survey, while in the latter
22 cases the diagnosis of IIP was confirmed and an investigation of acute exacerbation made by the IIP Study
Group on the basis of medical records including chest x-
ray films and pathological specimens. Pathological
examination of the lung was carried out in 4 cases with
acute exacerbation among the latter series of cases.

Statistical analysis: Data were expressed as mean ± SD
and the Student's t-test was used to test differences for
statistical significance. Survival curves were developed
by the Kaplan-Meier method, starting with first examination invariably in all cases. Statistical significance
of survival rates was tested by the log rank method and
generalized Wilcoxon test.

Results

1. Clinical features of 4 cases of acute exacerbation

collected by the IIP Study Group

Of 22 cases of IIP collected by the IIP Study Group, acute exacerbation was noted to have occurred in 4 cases. In 2 of these 4 cases dosage reduction of corticosteroid was identified as the precipitating cause, while the other 2 cases are currently under observation. Phenomena common to these 4 cases were a fever and shortness of breath of acute onset, accentuation of fine crackles, acceleration of ESR, conversion to positive of CRP, elevation of serum LDH and leukocytosis, with micro-nodular shadows (ground glass-like opacities) on chest x-ray being superimposed. The pathological findings which will be described later were apparently those of acute diffuse interstitial pneumonia.

2. Results of a questionnaire survey of acute exacerbation

Incidence of acute exacerbation: Among IIP cases collected in a questionnaire survey, there were 155 cases, 110 males and 45 females, proven by autopsy or open lung biopsy. Of these 155, acute exacerbation occurred in 63 males (57.3%) and 26 females (57.8%), totalling 89 (57.4%). These acute exacerbations occurred irrespective of whether corticosteroid was being used or not, taking place with the drug in 39 cases, without it in 40 cases and 'uncertain' in 10 cases. The time elapsed from the presumed onset of disease till acute exacerbation was 36.4 ± 37.6 months.

Age: The presumed age at disease onset was 58.3 ± 14.0 years for cases with acute exacerbation and 56.7 ± 11.9 years for those without it, with the difference being not statistically significant. The mean ages at first examination for these two groups of cases were 61.3 ± 13.5 years and 58.3 ± 11.8 years, respectively, again with no significant difference between the groups in this respect.

Frequency of episodes of acute exacerbation: The number of episodes of acute exacerbation per patient was 1 in 30 cases, 2 in 10 cases, 3 through 7 in 1 case each and 'unknown' in 44 cases, with an average of 1.52.

Precipitating cause of acute exacerbation: The precipi-tating causes of or triggering factors for acute exacer-bation, presumed or identified, were aggravation of primary disease in 35 cases, respiratory tract infections in 31 cases, dosage reduction of corticosteroid in 12 cases, lung cancer and its treatment in 5 cases, pneumo-thorax in 2 cases, open lung biopsy, TBLB, acute pancrea-

titis in 1 case each and 'unknown' in 38 cases when overlapping was admitted. A similar trend was observed in
other reported series(3). 'Unknown' as stated in the response may well be construed as meaning 'precipitating
cause unidentified or unknown (aggravation of primary
disease)'.

There were 12 cases in which acute exacerbation was induced by dosage reduction of corticosteroid. The dosage
of the corticosteroid before acute exacerbation ranged
from 15 mg to 100 mg of prednisolone, averaging 38.3 ±
25.2 mg, which was reduced to 7.5 mg - 75 mg, hence the
decrement was 5 mg to 45 mg with an average of 13.1 ±
12.4 mg (Fig.1).

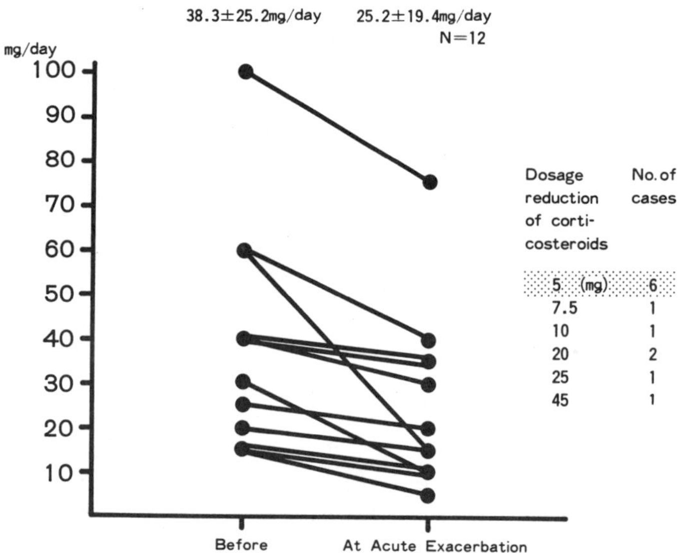

Fig. 1. Reduction of corticosteroid as a
        trigger of acute exacerbation in
        IIP.

It should be remembered that only a 5 mg reduction of
dosage was inductive to acute exacerbation in half the
cases.

Clinical symptoms before and after acute exacerbation:
A fever often accompanied an acute exacerbation. As indicated in Tab.1, 10 cases in our present series had a
fever prior to exacerbation, whereas 40 had this symptom
during an acute exacerbation. Moreover, whereas short-

ness of breath was of grade 2 to 4 according to the Hugh-Jones' classification prior to acute exacerbation in most instances, the symptom became worsened to the point of dyspnea or grade 5 during acute exacerbation.

Table I. Clinical symptoms before and after
acute exacerbation in IIP.

		Before No. of cases	After No. of cases
Fever			
	≥ 37.0 °C	10	40
	37.0 °C >	43	23
	Unknown	36	26
	Total	89	89
Dyspnea			
Hugh-Jones	I	2	0
	II	11	0
	III	21	4
	IV	16	9
	V	1	53
	Unknown	38	23
	Total	89	89

Laboratory findings before and after acute exacerbation: Significant changes in laboratory test results that occurred in association with acute exacerbation included an increase in erythrocyte sedimentation rate from a mean of 27.3 ± 21.2 mm/h prior to acute exacerbation to 51.6 ± 38.9 mm/h, elevation of serum LDH from 481.8 ± 413.6 IU/L to 814.2 ± 555.7 IU/L and a reduction of Pao_2 from 69.8 ± 13.1 torr. to 47.1 ± 13.8 torr.(Tab.2).

Table 2. Comparison of laboratory findings
before and after acute exacerbation.

Study		Before	After	
ESR (mm/h)	n=46	27.3 ± 21.2	51.6 ± 38.9	**
LDH (IU/L)	n=40	481.8 ± 413.6	814.2 ± 555.7	*
PH	n=43	7.42 ± 0.04	7.42 ± 0.08	
Pao_2 (torr)	n=48	69.8 ± 13.1	47.1 ± 13.8	**
$Paco_2$ (torr)	n=48	37.0 ± 5.5	38.9 ± 10.6	

** p<0.001
* p<0.01

As for chest x-ray findings, these were worsened in 46

cases, remained stationary in only 5 cases, aside from
38 cases from which no response was obtained.

From what has been mentioned above, it seemed plausible
to surmise that a fever, worsening of dyspnea, deterioration of chest x-ray findings, accelerated ESR, elevated
LDH and a reduction of Pao_2 could be important indices
for acute exacerbation.

Prognosis: The prognosis of IIP with acute exacerbation was found badly poor. Thus, in 85 (95.5%) of 89
such cases the disease had a fatal outcome. The direct
cause of death almost invariably was respiratory failure,
aside from 2 cases where disease of an organ other than
the lung proved fatal. Survival time as reckoned from
the first examination, as indicated in Fig.2, averaged
35.2 ± 5.5 (Mean ± SE) months for 39 cases without acute
exacerbation (with exclusion of those where the date of
first examination or disease outcome was unclear or unknown) as against a corresponding figure of 21.8 ± 3.2
months for those with acute exacerbation, with the difference being significant and in favor of those without
acute exacerbation.

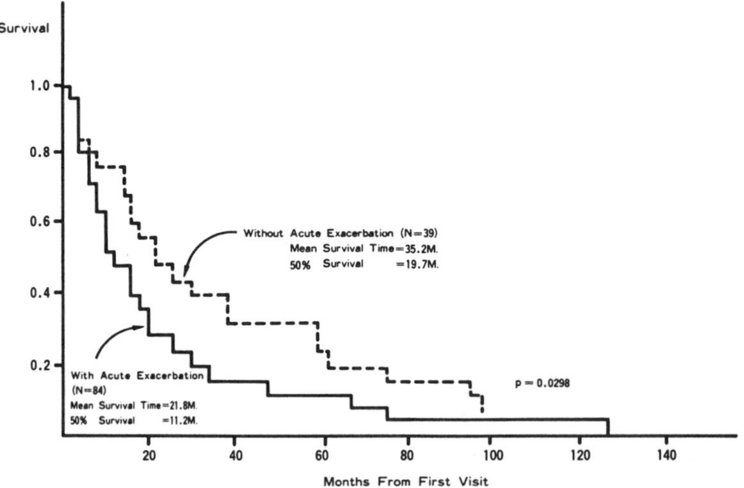

Fig. 2. Comparison of survival curves in IIP
        patients with and without acute exacer-
        bation.

While IIP itself is a disease with an ominous prognosis,
acute exacerbation can thus be said to be one of factors

that make the prognosis even more unfavorable.
3. Pathological findings of IIP with acute exacerbation
     Among 22 cases of IIP collected recently by the IIP
Study Group, there were 4 cases with acute exacerbation.
These cases were assessed histologically. As shown in
Tab.3 and 4, in addition to pathologic findings typical
of IIP including subpleural honeycombing predominantly in
the base of lungs, histopathological changes indicative
of acute interstitial pneumonia, i.e. hyaline membrane
formation and extensive alveolitis were noticeable microscopically.

Table 3. Pathological findings of IIP with
         acute exacerbation.
         - Macroscopical appearances -

	T.T	M.T	K.Y	T.M
Pleural adhesion				
r.lung	(−)	(+)	(−)	(+)
l.lung	(+)	(−)	(−)	(−)
Distribution of honeycombing	upper << lower	lower	upper < lower	upper ≦ lower
Fibrosis	(+)	(+)	(+)	(+)
Contraction of lower lobes	(+)	(±)	(+)	(±)

Table 4. Pathological findings of IIP with
         acute exacerbation.
         - Microscopical appearances -

	T.T	M.T	K.Y	T.M
Alveolitis	(+)	(+)	(+)	(+)
Hyaline membrane formation	(±)	(±)	(+)	(±)
Infiltration of histiocytes	(+)	(+)	(±)	(+)
Swelling of type II pneumocytes	(±)	(±)	(+)	(±)
Collapse of alveolar sacs	(+)	(±)	(+)	(+)
Cystic changes	2(+)	(±)	(+)	(+)
Terminal infections	(−)	2(+)	(±)	(±)

In some cases, however, there was noted localized focal
pneumonia presumed to have supervened in terminal stage.

Discussion

IIP is a disease with a poor prognosis that proves
fatal in an average of 3 to 6 years after onset (5,6),
being usually chronic and progressive in nature. In
occasional patients, however, the disease may become abruptly worsened on the course of disease and quickly
terminate in death. Such an abrupt aggravation of a
chronic primary disease from some precipitating cause(s)
is called acute exacerbation. The underlying process,
frequency, precipitating cause(s), histopathology and
prognosis of acute exacerbation in IIP are not fully
understood yet. Under such circumstances, it was felt
worthwhile to investigate into so-called acute exacerbations that occurred in a selected group of histologically
proven IIP cases.

According to our present questionnaire survey, 89 (57.
4%) of 155 patients had acute exacerbation, while 4 (18.2
%) of 22 patients in an IIP Study Group survey were found
to have experienced similar episodes. Among reported
studies available to date, Yoshimura and associates (3)
found 35 (37.2%) of 94 patients in their series to have
experienced acute exacerbation and Izumi et al. (4) noted
5 (33.3%) of 15 patients autopsied to show evidence of
acute exacerbation. It is interesting to note that half
the number of IIP patients studied had acute exacerbation,
even though acute aggravation of other diseases than the
primary disease of interest, e.g., concurrent pulmonary
infection, is very much likely to be comprised in acute
exacerbation of IIP in this type of survey.

Yoshimura et al. (3) implicated respiratory tract infection, reduction of corticosteroid dosage and thoraco-
tomy as possible precipitating causes of or triggering
factors for acute exacerbation. According to the results
of the present survey, 35 (39.3%) of patients had no
clearly identifiable precipitating causes; in 31 (34.8%)
and 12 (13.5%) patients, intercurrent respiratory tract
infection and a reduction of corticosteroid dosage, respectively, were identified as precipitating cause of
acute exacerbation. Utmost precaution should be exercised in reducing the dosage of corticosteroid, since as
small a decrement in dosage as 5 mg resulted in acute
exacerbation not infrequently.

IIP, by nature, is a disease with an ominous prognosis
and acute exacerbation makes the disease even more

miserable. Reported studies indicate that the mortality
rate of the disease after an initial episode of acute
exacerbation is 80.1% and cumulative mortality rate after
the last episode is 97.1%, with death occurring in an
average of 31.5 days after acute exacerbation (3). The
present survey disclosed that acute exacerbation proved
fatal in 85 (95.5%) of 89 cases, while in 4 cases among
the series of the IIP Study Group the disease had a fatal
outcome 3 to 31 days (12.8 days on the average) after the
onset of acute exacerbation. Comparison of survival
curves for patients with vs. without acute exacerbation
showed a definitely poorer prognosis for the former group
of patients. Acute exacerbation was thus considered one
of important determinant factors of prognosis in IIP.

Now, what is the real essence of acute exacerbation ?
Pathological findings of the lung in 4 cases (where the
examination was feasible) were those of acute interstitial pneumonia, e.g., formation of hyaline membrane in
alveolar spaces and extensive alveolitis, superimposed on
those typical of IIP, including fibrosis of alveolar
walls and honeycombing. Izumi et al. state that the
primary pathologic change underlying acute exacerbation
is diffuse alveolar damage (DAD) represented by hyaline
membrane formation (4). However, it is uncertain whether
this pathologic process is identical with or entirely
distinct from that of IIP (which essentially is chronic
in nature) and also whether they are of the same or
different etiology. These issues remain to be settled by
further studies.

References

1) Cantin,A. and Crystal,R.G. Int.Archs Allergy appl.
   Immun. 76(suppl), 83-91, 1985.
2) Hay,J.G. and Turner-Warwick,M. In: Textbook of Respiratory Medicine (J.F.Murray and J.A.Nadel eds.)
   W.B.Saunders Company, pp. 1445-1461, 1988.
3) Yoshimura,K., Nakatani,K., Nakamori,Y., Chonabayashi,
   N., Tachibana,A., Nakata,K., Okano,H. and Tanimoto,
   H. JJTD 22, 1012-1020, 1984. (written in Japanese)
4) Izumi,T., Kitaichi,M., Nishimura,K. and Nagai,S.
   medicina 24, 1688-1700, 1987. (written in Japanese)
5) Murao,M. 13th World Congress on Diseases of the Chest,
   1980.
6) Carrington,C.B., Gaensler,E.A., Coutu,R.E.,

FitzGerald,M.X. and Gupta,R.G. <u>N.Engl.J.Med.</u> 298, 801-809, 1978.

The Diagnostic and Assessment of the Course of Idiopathic Pulmonary Fibrosis

M.I. Schwarz, L.C. Watters, T.E. King, J.A. Waldron,
R.E. Stanford, and R.M. Cherniack

*National Jewish Center for Immunology and Respiratory Medicine and
University of Colorado Health Sciences Center, Denver, Colorado, USA*

ABSTRACT

In order to assess the severity, clinical course, and response to
therapy in idiopathic pulmonary fibrosis (IPF) a clinical–radiographic–
physiologic (CRP) scoring system was designed and included seven
variables: degree of dyspnea, the extent and severity of radiographic
abnormalities, and abnormalities of spirometry (FVC, FEV_1), diffusing
capacity, lung volume, resting alveolar arterial oxygen gradient,
and exercise O2 desaturation. To prove the validity of the CRP
score, the relation between it and a histopathologic scoring system
was determined. The histopathologic score was divided into a
cellular and fibrotic score and was felt to represent the overall
histologic derrangement in IPF. Twenty–six open lung biopsy
proven untreated IPF patients were included. The initial CRP score
correlated significantly with the total pathology score. The CRP
score determined after six months of treatment with prednisone
correlated significantly with the fibrotic component of the pathology
scoring system. The change in CRP score after six months of therapy
tended to reflect the cellular component of the CRP score, but this
was not significant. This data suggests that the CRP score is a
useful method for determining initial severity of the underlying
disease as well as a method for the longitudinal assessment of IPF
patients.

Supported by SCOR grant # HL–27353–04 from the
National Heart, Lung, and Blood Institute
Tables and figures reproduced by permission of the
American Review of Respiratory Disease

INTRODUCTION

Idiopathic pulmonary fibrosis (IPF) is an inflammatory fibrotic lung parenchymal disease with a generally poor prognosis. Because the agents used to treat this disorder have potentially harmful side effects. it is important to accurately assess whether these drugs have beneficial effects over a period of time. It is the purpose of this report, to evaluate a scoring system known as the clinical – radiographic–physiologic (CRP) score and to see if this system accurately reflects both changes in the clinical course of IPF as well as whether it predicts the underlying histopathologic derrangement.

METHODS

A. Patients
Twenty–six subjects (17 men, 9 women) (12 smokers, 14 non-smokers) were utilized for this study. The mean age was 57±2 years and the range was 30 to 77 months. The mean duration of symptoms was 20±5 mos and the range was 2 to 108 months. No patient was treated prior to enrollment in the study and all subjects underwent open lung biopsy to verify the diagnosis of IPF.

B. CRP Score
Prior to and six months following open lung biopsy a CRP score was determined. This score was obtained from the sum of points assigned to each of seven variables: (1) Dyspnea: Each subject was questioned as to the type and amount of exercise that would produce this system. A maximum of 20 points was assigned and awarded according to the scale in Table I.
(2) Radiography: A standard chest radiography was assigned points (maximum of 10) according to a modification of UICC scoring system [1]. Three radiographic abnormalities were assigned points (Table II); extent and severity of parenchymal infiltrates, the presence of radiographic honeycombing and the presence of pulmonary hypertension. The regional extent (number of zones involved) and severity of infiltrates in each zone was determined and this represented a parenchymal subscore. If both alveolar and reticulonodular infiltrates are present the scores are added.

Table I

Level of Dyspnea	Number of Points
None (or same as peers) even after 30 min of vigorous activity, such as running; ability to lift and carry 60 lbs for a prolonged period of time	0
After 5 flights of stairs or 10 min of vigorous activity; prolonged use of heavy tools	2
After walking more than a mile on level ground, up 3 flights of stairs, or less than 10 min of vigorous activity such as running or tennis	4
Upon walking 0.25 to 1 mile on level ground or up 2 flights of stairs; dyspnea with paper hanging	6
Upon walking 300 to 1,320 feet on level ground, bed-making	8
Upon walking 150 to 300 feet on level ground or up 1 flight of stairs; scrubbing; truck driving; assembly-line work	10
Upon walking 50 to 150 feet on level ground at approximately 3 mph, light janitorial work	12
Upon walking 20 to 50 feet on level ground, light steady work at one's own pace; seated operation of heavy equipment	14
With minor exertion, such as dressing, walking less than 20 feet, prolonged talking	16
With minimal activity such as eating, defecating, writing, sitting up	18
At rest	20

Table II

A. Parenchymal Infiltrates (Points assigned)
1. Predominantly Alveolar

Number of Zones Involved	Profusion		
	Mild	Moderate	Severe
1–2	4	5	6
3–4	7	8	9
5–6	10	11	12

2. Predominantly Reticulonodular

Number of Zones Involved	Profusion		
	Mild	Moderate	Severe
1–2	10	11	12
3–4	13	14	15
5–6	16	17	18

Parenchymal Subscore _______

B. Honeycombing
(One point for each of the 6 regions involved by radiographic honeycombing)

Honeycombing Subscore _______

C. Pulmonary Hypertension
(If present, score 6)

Pulmonary Hypertension Subscore _______

D. Radiographic score*

$$\frac{\text{Parenchymal Score + Honeycombing Score + Pulmonary Hypertension Score}}{3}$$ _______

* To determine the score from the chest radiograph, add the parenchymal, honeycombing, and pulmonary hypertension subscores and divide the sum by 3.

(3) Spirometry: The forced vital capacity (FVC) and forced expiratory volume in one second (FEV_1) were measured with either a spirometry or a pneumotachograph. The maximal value for reduction of the FVC was 12 points and that for the FEV_1 was 3 points [2] (Table III). (4) Lung Volume: The thoracic gas volume (Vtg) was measured in a constant body plethysmograph. The maximum points assigned for a reduction in Vtg were 10 [3] (Table III). (5) Diffusing Capacity: A single breath diffusing capacity was determined [4] and corrected for alveolar volume (DLCO/VA) and assigned a maximum of 10 points based on predicted values [5] (Table III). (6) Gas Exchange at Rest: The resting alveolar–arterial oxygen gradient (AaDO2) was calculated and assigned a maximum value of 10 points (Table III). (7) Gas Exchange with Exercise: Exercise was performed on a bicycle

Table III

	% Predicted	Points[*]
Spirometry		
FVC	$\geqslant 80$	0
	75–79	1
	70–74	2
	65–69	3
	60–64	5
	55–59	7
	50–54	9
	< 50	12
FEV_1	$\geqslant 80$	0
	70–79	1
	60–69	2
	< 60	3
Lung volume		
Vtg	$\geqslant 90$	0
	85–89	2
	75–84	4
	65–74	6
	60–64	8
	< 60	10
Diffusing capacity		
D_{LCO}/V_A	$\geqslant 80$	0
	70–79	1
	60–69	2
	50–59	3
	40–49	4
	< 40	5
Resting gas exchange, mmHg		
$AaPO_2$	$\leqslant 10$	0
	11–15	2
	16–20	4
	21–25	6
	26–30	8
	> 30	10
Exercise gas exchange		

$$* \text{ Points } = \frac{\Delta O_2 \text{ saturation (rest minus exercise)}}{\Delta \dot{V}O_2 \text{ (exercise minus rest)/predicted } \dot{V}O_2 max} + 3\,(FIO_2 - 0.21) \times 100.$$

ergometer and inspired and expired oxygen and carbon dioxide concentrations were measured by mass spectometry. Values for maximal oxygen consumption were obtained from the equations of Jones and Campbell [6] and a maximum of 30 points was assigned for exercise gas exchange abnormalities (Table III). If while breathing known concentrations of oxygen the number of points exceeds 30 only 30 points are assigned.

C. Histopathologic Scoring System

The open lung biopsies were obtained from two different sites, usually the upper and lower lobes. Multiple sections were stained with Massons trichrome and hematoxylin–eosin stains and independently evaluated by two pathologists. Eleven pathologic entities were graded as to the extent and severity. Five of these were felt to be reversible and termed cellular and 6 were thought to be irreversible and termed fibrotic. Table IV lists the various entities scored as well as the scoring system. As can be seen the maximum possible cellular score was 21. The maximum possible fibrotic score was 24, and the total pathology score which was felt to represent the total derrangement of the lung parenchymas is the sum of both the cellular and fibrotic scores.
Because the entities of alveolar desquamation, alveolar septal fibrosis, and honeycombing are felt to be particularly relevant in determining therapeutic responsiveness, they were given twice the value of the other entities [7,8].

Table IV

Pathologic Abnormalities	Score			
	Absent	Mild	Moderate	Severe
Cellular				
Alveolar desquamation	0	2	4	6
Alveolar septal inflammation	0	2	4	6
Inflammatory airway narrowing	0	1	2	3
Obstructive pneumonitis	0	1	2	3
Lymphoid nodules	0	1	2	3
Maximal possible cellular pathology score = 21				
Fibrotic				
Alveolar septal fibrosis	0	2	4	6
Cystic changes (pathologic honeycombing)	0	2	4	6
Obliterative airway narrowing	0	1	2	3
Smooth muscle hypertrophy	0	1	2	3
Thickened pulmonary arterioles	0	1	2	3
Cuboidalization of alveoli	0	1	2	3
Maximal possible fibrotic pathology score = 24				
Maximal possible total pathology score = 45				

D. Treatment and Follow-up

Following open lung biopsy prednisone therapy was initiated in 21 subjects according to the following treatment protocol: 1.5mgm/kgm daily (not to exceed 100mgm) for 6 weeks; then 1.0mgm/kgm daily for the next 6 weeks; then 0.5mgm/kgm for the ensuing 3 months and then a gradual taper to 0.25mgm/kgm daily. Sixteen of the 21 patients were available for follow-up after 6 months of prednisone therapy.

RESULTS

A. Histopathology and CRP Scores

Table V shows the mean cellular and fibrotic pathology scores as well as the initial and 6 month post treatment CRP scores. The initial pathology scores for the entire 26 patients as well as the 16 treated patients are shown. The mean CRP score for the 26 subjects was 53±4.2 (range 18.6 – 91.1 months). The 16 treated patients had CRP scores of 58.5±46 (range 31.5 – 87.8 months). The mean number of points assigned to clinical (subjective) and radiographic components of the CRP score are shown as well as the individual components of the physiologic score. Table V also indicates the change in CRP score following 6 months of treatment according to the protocol. The mean CRP

Table V

	All Patients Initial Evaluation (n = 26)	Treated Patients with Follow-up after 6 months Corticosteroid Therapy (n = 16)		
		Initial	6 Months	Changes
Pathology scores				
Cellular	8 ± 1	8 ± 1	—	—
Fibrotic	11 ± 1	12 ± 1	—	—
Total	18 ± 2	20 ± 1	—	—
CRP score	53.5 ± 4.2	58.5 ± 4.3	48.1 ± 5.4	− 10.4 ± 3.8
Subjective[†]	11 ± 1	10 ± 1	8 ± 1	− 2 ± 1
Chest radiograph[†]	6.1 ± 0.4	6.2 ± 0.3	5.6 ± 0.3	− 0.6 ± 0.3
FVC[‡]	67 ± 4	66 ± 5	68 ± 4	+ 2 ± 3
FEV_1[‡]	74 ± 4	75 ± 6	74 ± 4	− 1 ± 4
Vtg[‡]	85 ± 3	84 ± 3	82 ± 4	− 3 ± 3
D_{LCO}/V_A[‡]	61 ± 3	63 ± 5	71 ± 6	+ 9 ± 4
Resting $AaPO_2$	22 ± 2	23 ± 3	21 ± 2	− 2 ± 2
Exercise score[§]	23.1 ± 3.1	28.3 ± 3.9	21.6 ± 4.0	− 6.6 ± 4

* All data are expressed as mean ± SE.
† Mean scores derived from CRP scoring method.
‡ Percentage of predicted values.
§ Calculated from the equation defined in METHODS but with no upper limit of 30 for the score.

score was 48.1±5.4 indicating a 10.4±3.8 point reduction in the score and clinical improvement.

B. The Correlation of Histopathologic and CRP Data
The relationship between the pretreatment or initial CRP score and the total pathology score is depicted in Figure 1.

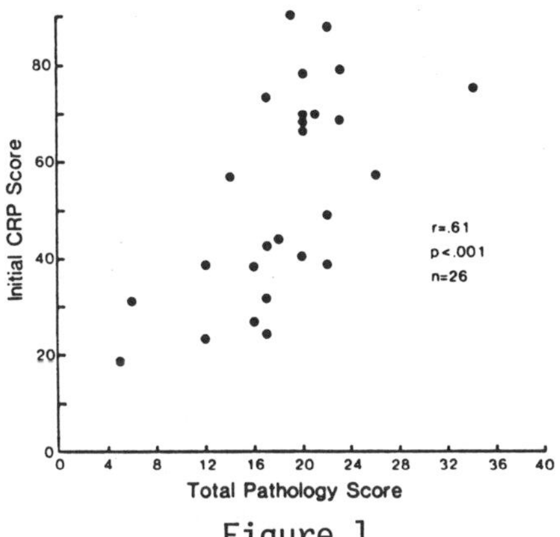

Figure 1

It is clear that the CRP score accurately reflects the overall pathologic derrangement in IPF. None of the individual components of the CRP score showed as high a correlation (data not shown). The correlation of the 6 month CRP score and the fibrotic component of the pathology score is shown in Figure 2.

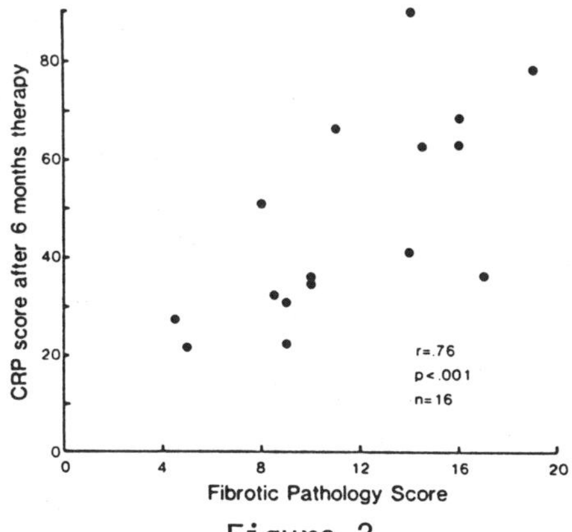

Figure 2

Figure 2 indicates that if the fibrotic component of the pathology score was high, the 6 month post treatment showed significantly greater clinical impairment. The relationship between the 6 month post treatment CRP score and the cellular component of the pathology score is shown in Figure 3.

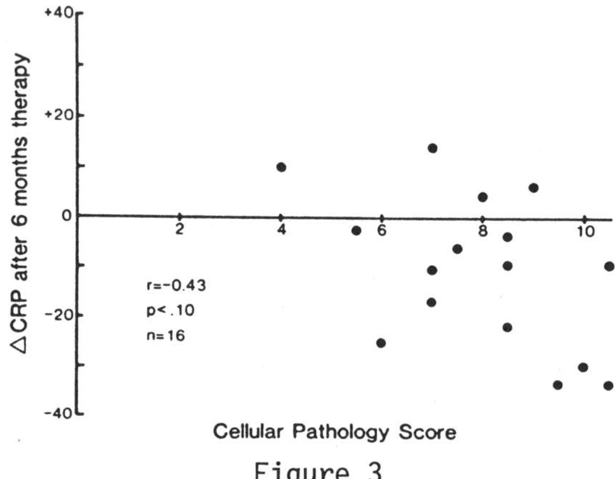

Figure 3

The apparent improvement in post treatment CRP score appears.to reflect the underlying cellular component of the pathology score. However, it only approaches statistical significance.

DISCUSSION

The potential uses of a CRP scoring system to evaluate patients with IPF and other interstitial lung diseases are several. It would provide a means for evaluating the severity of the disease as well as a response to various immunosuppressive regiments. In addition treatment trials with new therapeutic regiments and possibly modifiers are forthcoming and various centers will require a uniform method for determing improvement, stabilization or deterioration. Further, defined clinical criteria are necessary to evaluate the diagnostic and prognostic utility of newer modalities such as bronchoalveolar lavage and lung gallium scanning.

Also the individual clinical, radiographic, and physiologic components of the CRP score do not predict the severity of the underlying histopathology and have not consistently predicted therapeutic responsiveness. Although points assigned to the individual components of the CRP score were unequal, it was based on the relative value of each according to the previous literature. For example, a total of

45 points would be gained by alterations in gas exchange. These
include exercise oxygen saturation (30 points), resting alveolar
arterial oxygen gradient (10 points), and resting single breath
diffusing capacity corrected for alveolar volume. Exercise gas
exchange demonstrates the best correlation with underlying
histopathology [9,10]. Resting alveolar-arterial oxygen gradient
correlates with the severity of pulmonary hypertension as well as
fibrosis in the lung biopsy [11,12].

SUMMARY

While the CRP score does not aid in the diagnosis of IPF or reflect
the extent of the underlying lung inflammation in this disorder, it is
a quantitative means for assessing the initial clinical impairment,
and the response to present and future therapeutic modalities. In
addition it reflects the severity of the overall initial pathologic
derrangement of the lung architecture (cellularity and fibrosis) and
the persistent elevation of the score following six months of
prednisone therapy correlates with the fibrotic component of the
pathology score. While there is a trend of an improving CRP score
following treatment to reflect the cellular pathology score, this
relationship is not as strong as the previous.

REFERENCES

1. UICC/Cincinnati classification of the radiographic appearances of
    pneumoconiosis. Chest 1970;58:57-67.
2. Morris JF, Koski A, Johnson LC. Spirometric standard for healthy
    non-smoking adult. Am Rev Resp Dis 1971;163:57-67.
3. Goldman HI, Becklake MR. Respiratory function tests. Normal
    values at medium altitudes and the prediction of normal results.
    Am Rev Tuberc 1959;79:457.
4. Ogilvie CM, Forster RE, Blakemore WS, Morton JW. A standardized
    breathholding technique for the clinical measurement of the
    diffusing capacity of the lung for carbon monoxide. J Clin Invest
    1957;36:1-17.
5. Crapo RO, Morris AH. Standardized single breath normal values for
    carbon monoxide diffusing capacity. Am Rev Resp Dis 1981;123:185-
    9.
6. Jones NL, Campbell EJM. In: Clinical exercise testing. 2nd ed.
    Philadelphia: W.B. Saunders Co., 1982:249.
7. Stack BHR, Choo-Kang YFJ, Heard BE. The prognosis of cryptogenic
    fibrosing alveolitis. Thorax 1972;27:535-42.

8. Scadding JG, Hinson KFW. Diffuse fibrosing alveolitis (diffuse interstitial fibrosis of the lungs). Correlation of histology at biopsy with prognosis. Thorax 1967;22:291–304.
9. Fulmer JD, Roberts WC, VonGal ER, Crystal RG. Morphologic–physiologic correlations of the severity of fibrosis and degree of cellularity in idiopathic pulmonary fibrosis. J Clin Invest 1979;63:665–76.
10. Gaensler EA, Carrington CB, Coutu RE, Fitzgerald MX. Radiographic–physiologic–pathologic correlations in interstitial pneumonias. Prog Respir Res 1975;8:223–41.
11. McLees B, Fulmer J, Adair N, Roberts W, Crystal R. Correlative studies of pulmonary fibrosis (abstract). Am Rev Resp Dis 1977;115:354.
12. Green GM, Graham WGB, Hanson JS et al. Correlated studies of interstitial pulmonary disease. Chest 1976;69(Suppl:263).

Multiple Lung Cancers in Patients with Idiopathic Interstitial Pneumonia

Shiro Kira* and Shuichi Watanabe**

* *Department of Respiratory Medicine, Juntendo University, School of Medicine, Tokyo, Japan*
** *Fukushima Prefectural Hospital, Fukushima, Japan*

This is a study based on 140 autopsied male lung cancer patients. Double lung cancer was significantly frequent in lung cancer patients complicated with IIP in comparison with those in lung cancer patients complicated with PE, miscellaneous lung diseases or of lung cancer alone. Furthermore, the incidence of small cell carcinoma was also significantly high in IIP, and the location of the primary lesion were all in peripheral lung field in IIP. These results suggest that idiopathic interstitial pneumonia is a state of high risk for development of lung cancer.

It is widely known that the incidence of lung cancer is high in patients with idiopathic interstitial pneumonia (IIP) [1-5]. There are several papers in Japan which reported the incidence in 33-15% among IIP patients [6-9]. Based on these findings we have questioned that if pathological conditions with IIP contribute to the high incidence of the complication with lung cancer, the incidence for the multiple lung cancer would be found high in patients with IIP among the various background patients complicated with lung cancer, and studied autopsied patients with lung cancers in our department.

SUBJECTS AND METHOD

The subjects were patients with lung cancer who were diagnosed and treated on their admission to our department in Jichi Medical School in Tochigi, Japan from 1975 to 1985, and autopsied in the department of pathology of Jichi Medical School. Their pathophysiological background in the lung were studied in detail clinically and pathologically.

RESULTS

Total number of autopsied lung cancer patients were 180, composed of 140 of male and 40 of female during the study period as shown in Fig. 1. To eliminate an influence of sexual difference, we selected male patients for this study.

Fig.1; Background of the lung specially in male patients of lung cancer, autopsied

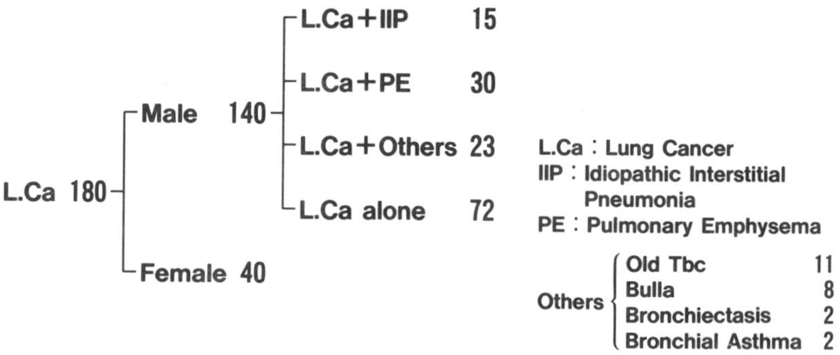

Of the 140 male patients, 72 had no particular pathological condition in the lung other than lung cancer (L.Ca alone), 30 had lung cancer complicated with pulmonary emphysema (L.Ca + PE), 15 lung cancer with IIP (L.Ca. + IIP) and 23 lung cancer with other miscellaneous pulmonary diseases (L.Ca + others) such as sequela of old pulmonary tuberculosis in 11, pulmonary bullae in 8, bronchiectasis in 2 and bronchial asthma in 2 as underlying diseases.

Table 1 gives the profile of patients regarding age
and smoking history in the respective group. There
was no significant difference in age, ratio of smoker
to nonsmoker and Brinkman Index between the groups.

TABLE 1.   PROFILE OF PATIENTS IN 4 GROUPS

	L.Ca+IIP	L.Ca+PE	L.Ca+others	L.Ca alone
No. of Case	15	30	23	72
Age	65.5+5.8	68.3+6.3	64.1+10.6	62.1+11.7
Smoker /nonsmoker	15/0	30/0	22/1	67/5
Brinkman Index	1044+552	1331+428	879+392	852+625

As shown in Fig. 2, the incidence of double cancer
was 5 in 15 patients of L.Ca+IIP (33.3%), 2 in 30
patients of L.Ca+PE (6.7%), 2 in 72 patients of L.Ca
alone (2.8%) and non in 23 patients of L.Ca+others.
The incidence in the group of IIP was significantly
high in comparison with the groups of L.Ca+PE, L.Ca+
others and L.Ca alone.

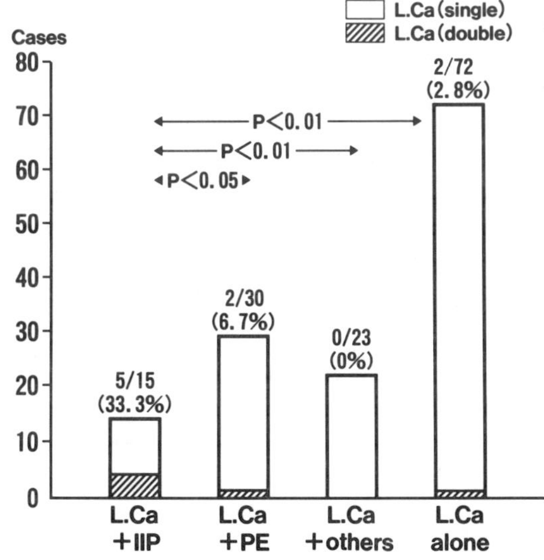

Fig. 2;
Incidence of
double lung cancer
in patients of
4 groups

5 patients of double lung cancers in the L.Ca+IIP group were composed of 2 of adenocarcinoma plus small cell carcinoma, 2 of epidermoid carcinoma plus small cell carcinoma and 1 of epidermoid carcinoma plus alveolar cell type adenocarcinoma. 2 patients of double lung cancers in L.Ca+PE were of epidermoid carcinoma plus adenocarcinoma and epidermoid carcinoma plus epidermoid carcinoma. In L.Ca alone group, there were also 2 patients of double lung cancers of epidermoid carcinoma plus adenocarcinoma and epidermoid carcinoma plus small cell carcinoma.

As described above, small cell carcinoma was so conspicuous as the cell type in double lung cancer in L.Ca+ IIP group (4/5), we analyzed a distribution of cell type of lung cancer in all subjects in these 4 groups. The total number of the primary lesion was 20 in 15 L.Ca+IIP patients including 5 double lung cancer patients, and 32 in 30 L.Ca+PE patients including 2 double lung cancer, 23 in 23 patients of L.Ca+others and 74 in 72 L.Can alone including 2 double lung cancer patients. We abbreviated adenocarcinoma, epidermoid carcinoma, small cell carcinoma, large cell carcinoma and other type as A, E, S, L and O.

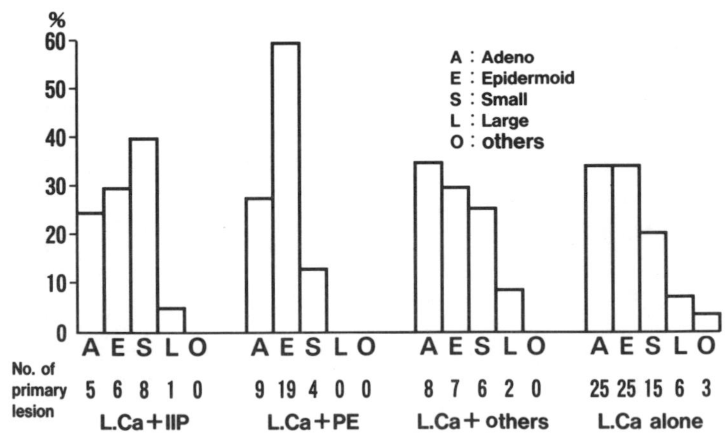

Fig. 3 ; Histological types of lung cancer in patients of 4 groups

Fig. 3 gives number of the respective primary lesion
in 4 groups in horizontal axis and % of the respective
primary lesion in each group in vertical axis.   In L.Ca+
IIP, A was 5 among 20 primary lesion and 25%, E 6 among
20 and 30%, S 8 among 20 and 40% and L 1 among 20 and
5%.   As seen in Fig. 3, S was most frequent in L.Ca+PE,
and A and E were equally frequent in L.Ca+ others and
L.Ca alone, however S was most frequent among 5 cell
types in L.Ca+IIP and its incidence was significantly
high among 4 groups (p<0.05).

The next specific feature observed in L.Ca+IIP was
the location of the primary lesion developed within
the lung.   From either chest X ray finding and bronchoscopic finding, we classified the location of primary
lesion as central when the lesion developed more oral
than in segmental branch of the bronchus and peripheral
when the lesion did more peripheral than in subsegmental
branch of the bronchus.

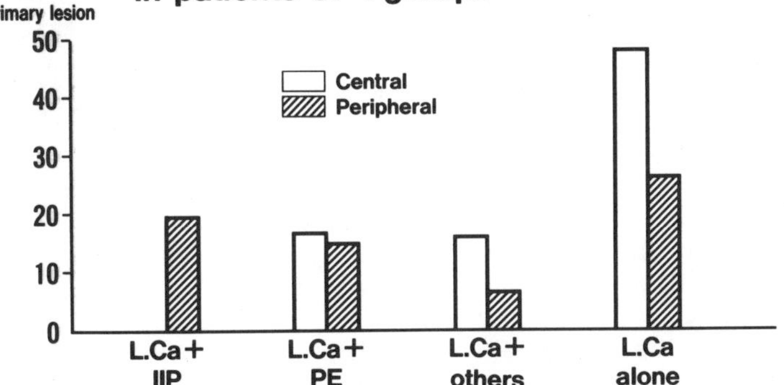

**Fig. 4; Central and peripheral type of lung cancer
in patients of 4 groups**

As shown in Fig. 4, all primary lesions were peripheral in L.Ca+IIP although the lesions were distributed
almost evenly in both central and peripheral areas in
L.Ca+PE, and rather dominantly in central area in L.Ca
alone and L.Ca+others.

As for the lung lobe in which the primary lesion
developed, there was no special tendency observed and
the lesion distributed almost evenly in every lobes
within bilateral lungs.

DISCUSSION

Since a report by Callahan in 1952 of a complication of lung cancer in a patient of acute diffuse interstitial fibrosis of lungs[1], the reports which suggested a high incidence of lung cancer complication in patients of idiopathic interstitial pneumonia have been accumulated world-widely. Turner-Warwick et al reported 20 lung cancer patients in 205 patients (9.8%) of their cryptogenic fibrosing alveolitis in 1980[5], Yoneda and Yamanaka 17 patients of lung cancer among 195 patients of idiopathic interstitial pneumonia (IIP) based on a national survey carried out by a task force study supported by Japanese Ministry of Health and Welfare in 1979[7]. We also clinically experience 20 lung cancer patients among 42 autopsied and nonautopsied IIP patients. From these evidences a view is widely held currently that the incidence of the lung cancer is high in these IIP patients.

In spite of these observation, it is true there is some bias in patient population depending on respective institution, and the number of patients in these studies are not statistically sufficient to draw a discrete conclusion that the incidence of lung cancer is truly high in patients of idiopathic interstitial pneumonia.

From these viewpoint we assumed that this was the case, the incidence for the multiple lung cancer would be found high in patients of IIP among various background patients complicated with lung cancer, and analyzed double lung cancer patients in our autopsied lung cancer patients specially paying attention to pathophysiological conditions in the background in their lung.

As described above, the incidence of double lung cancer in L.Ca+IIP was significantly higher in comparison with double lung cancer patients in L.Ca+PE, L.Ca+ others and L.Ca alone. Furthermore, there were observed another several specific features in patients of L.Ca+ IIP. There were observed all 5 types of cancer cell types, namely adenocarcinoma, epidermoid carcinoma, small cell carcinoma, large cell carcinoma and others in all 4 groups, but the incidence of small cell carcinoma was highest in 5 cancer cell types in L.Ca+IIP, and in the third in other 3 groups, and also significantly high among 4 groups. All primary lesion developed in peripheral lung field in patients of L.Ca+IIP

irrespectively with cell types, although the cancer
developed evenly in central and peripheral portions
in L.Ca+PE and rather frequently in central in other
two groups.

From these observation, it seems reasonable to conclude that the lung cancer developed in patients of
idiopathic interstitial pneumonia has several unique
features in incidence, cell types and anatomical location in the lung for their development, and their pathophysiological condition appeared in the lung may promote
development of lung cancer. From these results we would
like to propose to pay much attention to see possibili-
ties of complication of lung cancer in every patient
of IIP and complication of IIP in every patient of lung
cancer.

REFERENCES
[1] Callahan WP, Sutherland JC, Fulton JK and Kline
    JR.: Acute diffuse interstitial fibrosis of lungs.
    Arch Intern Med. 90:468-482,1952.
[2] Spain DM.: The association of terminal bronchiolar
    carcinoma with chronic interstitial inflamation
    and fibrosis of the lung. Am Rev Tuberculosis. 76:
    559-566,1957.
[3] Haddad R and Massaro D.: Idiopathic diffuse inter-
    stitial pulmonary fibrosis (Fibrosing alveolitis),
    atypical epitherial proliferation and lung cancer.
    Am J Med. 45:211-219,1968.
[4] Fraire AE and Greenberg SD.: Carcinoma and diffuse
    interstitial fibrosis of lung. Cancer 73:1078-86,
    1973.
[5] Turner-Warwick M, Lebowitz M, Burrows B and Johnson
    A.: Cryptogenic fibrosing alveolitis and lung cancer.
    Thorax 35:496-499,1980.
[6] Yoneda R and Yamanaka A.: Lung cancer complicated
    with lung fibrosis (in Japanese). Task force study
    for "Lung fibrosis in Japan" Supported by Ministry
    of Health and Welfare. The Report in 1979,37-44.
[7] Araki T, Iijima H, Nakamura T, Suzuki T, Natori H,
    Arai T, Kira S, Matsumoto S, Moriyama S, Koike M
    and Yokoyama T.: Two autopsied cases of double
    lung cancer complicated with interstitial pneumonia
    (in Japanese). Haigann 20:65-71,1980.
[8] Kohno S, Takami S, Uetsuna A, Taisei J, Yamakido M,
    Nishimoto Y and Tsukiyama F.: Clinical analysis

of patients of lung cancer complicated with lung
fibrosis (in Japanese). Jap J Int Med. 72:1731-39,
1983.

[9] Okano M, Khaled R, Takahashi Y, Inui K and Yakeuchi
Y.: 6 patients of lung cancer complicated with
idiopathic interstitial pneumonia (in Japanese).
Nihonn Kyoubu Rinshou 44:25-29,1985.

Bronchiolitis Obliterans Organizing Pneumonia (BOOP): Profile in Japan

Masahiko Yamamoto*, Yasutaka Ina*,
and Masanori Kitaichi**

 * *Second Department of Medicine, Nagoya City University Medical
   School, Nagoya, Japan*
** *Chest Disease Research Institute, Kyoto University, Kyoto, Japan*

Thirty Japanese patients with bronchiolitis obliterans organizing pneumonia (BOOP), diagnosed by the open lung biopsy were reviewed. Seventy % of the patients were idiopathic and 2/3 of the remaining were associated with connective tissue disease. BOOP can be classified into two major types, Type I and Type II, based on the chest X-ray findings. In the Type I the shadows wandered in the lung fields. In the Type II the abnormal shadows were seen in the bibasilar peripheral field with the reduction of the lung volume. Cases of Type I more frequently demonstrated inflammatory findings than cases of Type II.

INTRODUCTION

Several cases of bronchiolitis obliterans organizing pneumonia (BOOP) [1] have been reported in the Japanese literature during the past three years [2, 3]. Using these cases, we reviewed the clinical features of BOOP. Especially, we focused on the classification of BOOP using the chest X-ray findings, correlating with other major clinical findings. Here, we discussed the profile of BOOP cases in Japan.

HISTOLOGICAL DIAGNOSIS

The histopathological criteria for BOOP include the presence of 1) bronchiolitis obliterans, 2) organizing pneumonia and 3) interstitial pneumonia. Besides the criteria, there are many exclusive findings for BOOP as shown by Dr. Kitaichi [4].

MATERIALS

Among 36 cases gathered and investigated by the Research Committee for Intractable Diseases during 1986 to 1988, 20 cases were histologically diagnosed as BOOP, and the remaining 16 cases were excluded from BOOP. Ten cases of BOOP were diagnosed by the Research Group for Diffuse Pulmonary Diseases during 1985 to 1988. Thus, 30 cases of BOOP were reviewed in the present study. All cases were histologically diagnosed as BOOP by Dr. Kitaichi. Among the excluded 16 cases, 5 were diagnosed as eosinophilic pneumonia, 5 were lymphoproliferative disorders, 2 were diffuse alveolar damage and the remaining four included each one case of hypersensitivity pneumonitis, eosinophilic granuloma, bronchiectasis and necrotizing pneumonia.

UNDERLYING DISEASES

As shown in Table 1, 21 of 30 cases of BOOP were idiopathic and 6 were associated with collagen vascular disease (CVD), 2 with chronic thyroiditis and one with alcoholic liver cirrhosis. Among 6 BOOP cases associated with CVD, 2 had been treated with gold.

Table 1. Underlying Diseases

None (idiopathic)	21
Collagen Vascular Disease	6
Rheumatoid Arthritis	4*
Dermatomyositis	1
Behçet	1
Chronic Thyroiditis	2
Alcoholic Liver Cirrhosis	1

*2 treated with gold

SEX AND AGE

Table 2 shows the sex and age distribution of BOOP patients. The idiopathic cases consisted of 10 males and 11 females with an average age of 58.8 years old. The CVD accompanying cases consisted of 3 males and 3 females with an average age of 49.8 years old.   The chronic thyroiditis accompanying BOOP cases consisted of 2 females aged 60 and 61 years old.   One case associated with alcoholic liver cirrhosis was a 64 year old male patient.   There are no sex predominance among the groups, although BOOP patients associated with CVD were slightly younger than the others.

Table 2.   Sex and Age

	Male	Female	Age (y/o)
Idiopathic	10	11	58.8
Collagen Vascular Disease	3	3	49.8
Chronic Thyroiditis	0	2	60.5
Alcoholic Liver Cirrhosis	1	0	64
Total	14	16	57.3

CLASSIFICATION OF BOOP BASED ON CHEST X-RAY FINDINGS

All patients showed bilateral, multiple abnormal shadows on the chest X-rays.   These findings could be classified into 2 major groups; Type I or wandering type and Type II or not wandering type.

Type I was defined as showing bilateral patchy densities which wandered throughout the lung fields.   In contrast, Type II was defined as showing bilateral basilar abnormal shadows, predominantly distributed in the peripheral lung fields, with reduction of volume.   The shadows seen in Type II patients resemble those seen in idiopathic pulmonary fibrosis (IPF) patients.

CASE PRESENTATION-TYPE I BOOP

In April 1985, a 57 year old male noticed chest pain and subsequently developed general fatigue, fever, cough and dyspnea.   On May 16, he was admitted to a local hospital.   His chest X-ray on admission showed infiltrative shadows in the left lung field (Fig. 1).   He was transfered to the Chest Disease Research Institute Hospital of Kyoto University because of new infiltrative shadows in the right lung field, although abnormal shadows in the left upper lung field almost disappeared at that time (Fig. 2).

On July 16, new infiltrative shadows appeared in both lower lung fields, and the abnormal shadow in the right upper lung field disappeared (Fig. 3).

On September 2, almost all abnormal shadows disappeared except for

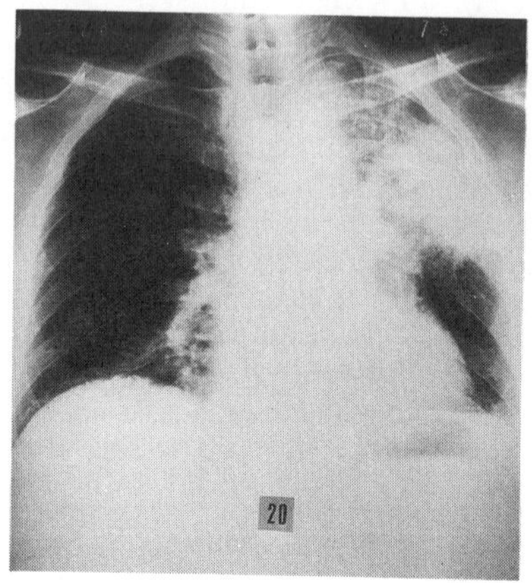

Fig. 1   Chest X-ray on
May 19, 1985

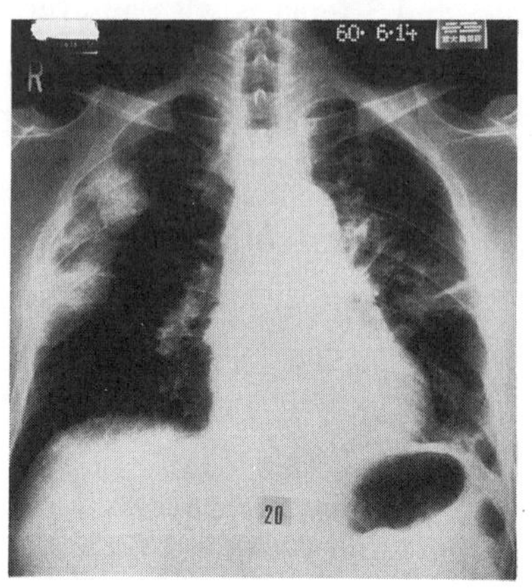

Fig. 2   Chest X-ray on
June 14, 1985

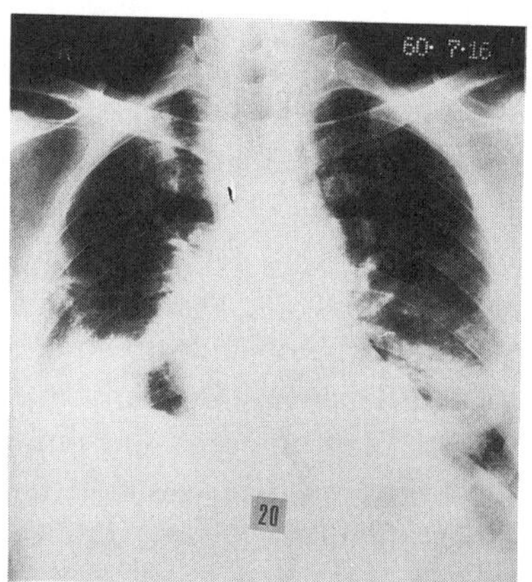

Fig. 3   Chest X-ray on
July 16, 1985

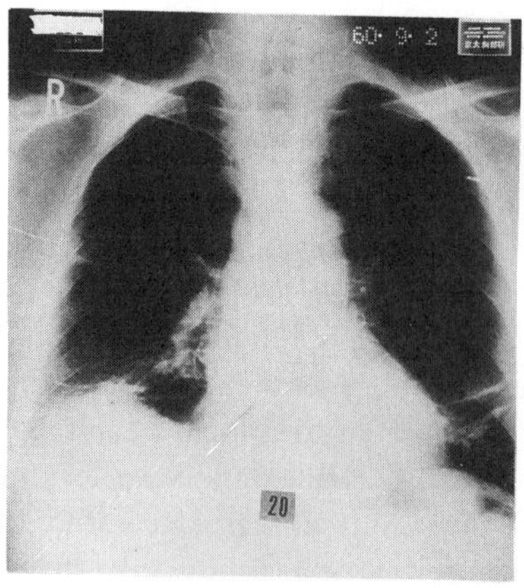

Fig. 4   Chest X-ray on
Sept. 2, 1985

minor shadows in both lower lung fields (Fig. 4). Fig. 5 shows a microscopic view of the biopsied sample taken from the 6th segment of the right lung. A bronchiole is filled with granulation tissue in the lumen. Adjacent alveolar walls show mild fibrous thickening with infiltration of lymphoid cells.

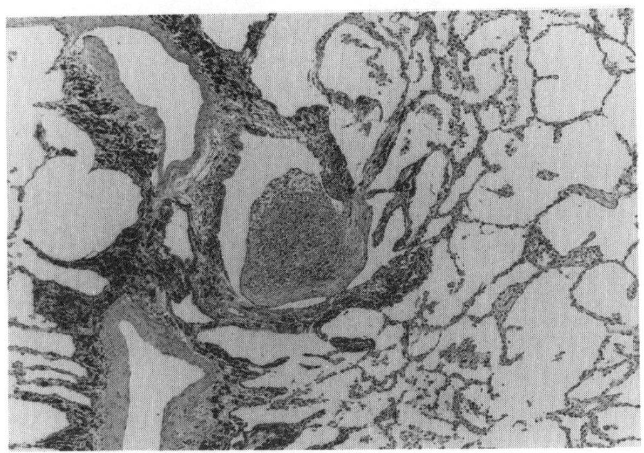

Fig. 5   A microscopic view of the biopsied lung
(rtS$_6$, HE stain   × 40)

CASE PRESENTATION-TYPE II BOOP

In June 1984, a 57 year old male noticed to have dry cough and dyspnea. In July 1984, he was pointed out as having abnormal shadows on his chest X-ray during a routine check up and was admitted to the Kyoto Mitsubishi Hospital.

Chest X-ray on admission shows bibasilar micronodular shadows, predominantly located in the peripheral lung fields with volume loss of the lungs (Fig. 6).

A microscopic view of the biopsied sample taken from the 8th segment of the left lung reveals granulation tissues in a respiratory bronchiole, alveolar ducts and alveolar spaces with moderate fibrous thickening of alveolar walls (Fig. 7).

CHEST X-RAY

The chest X-ray findings of each case are listed in Table 3. A summary of the chest X-ray findings of BOOP is shown in Table 4.

In the idiopathic group, 11, 6 and 4 cases are in Type I, Type II and Unclassified type, respectively.

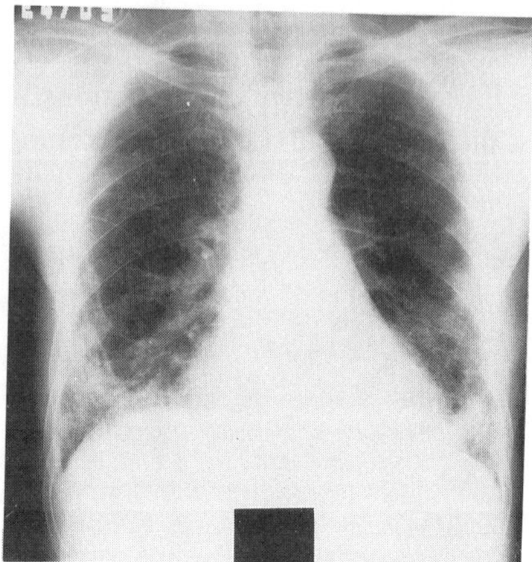

Fig. 6   Chest X-ray on admission

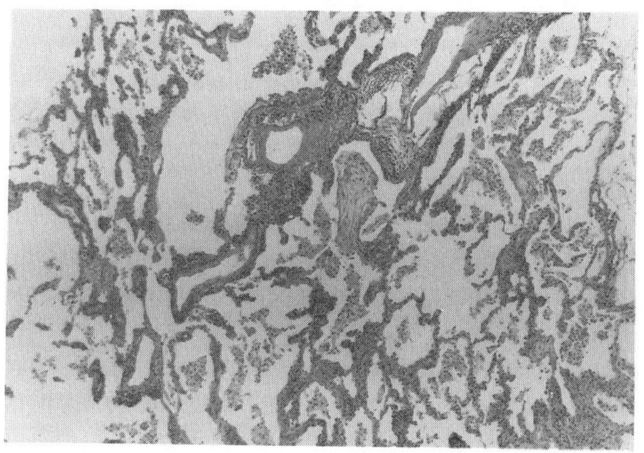

Fig. 7   A microscopic view of the biopsied lung
(ltS$_8$,   EVG stain   ×40)

In the CVD accompanying group, only 1 case is in Type I, while the other 5 cases were Unclassified.

In the chronic thyroidifis accompanying cases, 1 is in Type I and the other is Unclassified.   The alcoholic liver cirrhosis accompanying case is Type I.

Thus, Type I cases are mainly seen in the idiopathic cases. In the group with extrapulmonary disease, unclassified type is more frequently observed.

CLINICAL SYMPTOMS

Table 5 shows the presenting symptoms. Dyspnea and cough are seen in 83% and 87% of the patients. Sputum and fever are seen in 57% and 53% of the patients. In the idiopathic group, Type I cases more frequently present sputum and fever than Type II cases.

LABORATORY FINDINGS

As shown in Table 6, leukocytosis, eosinophilia, accelerated ESR (more than 50 mm/hr), positive CRP (more than 2 positive) and elevated LDH values are seen in 40%, 17%, 44%, 62% and 48%, respectively.

Type I patients more frequently show leukocytosis, accelerated ESR, positive CRP than Type II patients.

PULMONARY FUNCTION TESTS

The results of pulmonary function tests are shown in Table 7. Hypoxemia, reduced vital capacity and reduced DLco are seen in 80%, 79% and 94% of the patients, respectively. In contrast, reduced $FEV_1\%$ was seen only in 11%.

In the idiopathic group, there is no difference in pulmonary function tests between Type I and Type II patients.

COMPARISON BETWEEN TYPE I AND TYPE II

Fig. 8 shows the clinical features of Type I patients in comparison with those of Type II patients in the idiopathic group.

Type I cases more frequently demonstrate fever, leukocytosis, accelerated ESR, and positive CRP than Type II cases. Therefore, Type I appeared to be very different from Type II in terms of clinical features.

CLINICAL COURSE AND PROGNOSIS

Table 8 summarizes the clinical course and prognosis of BOOP. All patients show recovery. Twenty-seven % of them recover without corticosteroid therapy and the remaining of 73% recover with the therapy. But 2 cases associated with CVD have relapses despite the

Table 3 Pattern of Chest X-ray shadows

Case No	Underlying disease	Patchy density	Micronodular density	Basilar dominant	Peripheral dominant	Reduction of volume	Wandering of shadow	Type
1	Idiopathic	O	X	X	X	X	O	I
2	Idiopathic	O	X	X	X	X	O	I
3	Idiopathic	O	X	X	X	X	O	I
4	Idiopathic	O	X	X	X	X	O	I
5	Idiopathic	O	X	X	X	X	O	I
6	Idiopathic	O	X	X	X	X	O	I
7	Idiopathic	O	O	X	X	X	O	I
8	Idiopathic	O	O	X	X	X	O	I
9	Idiopathic	O	O	X	X	X	O	I
10	Idiopathic	O	O	X	X	X	O	I
11	Idiopathic	O	O	X	X	X	O	I
12	Idiopathic	X	O	O	O	O	X	II
13	Idiopathic	X	O	O	O	O	X	II
14	Idiopathic	X	O	O	O	O	X	II
15	Idiopathic	X	O	O	O	O	X	II
16	Idiopathic	X	O	O	O	O	X	II
17	Idiopathic	X	O	O	O	O	X	II
18	Idiopathic	O	O	X	O	X	O	Unclassified
19	Idiopathic	O	O	X	X	O	O	Unclassified
20	Idiopathic	O	O	X	O	X	X	Unclassified
21	Idiopathic	O	O	O	O	O	X	Unclassified
22	RA	O	O	X	X	X	X	Unclassified
23	RA	O	O	X	X	X	X	Unclassified
24	RA	O	O	X	X	O	X	Unclassified
25	RA	X	O	X	X	X	X	Unclassified
26	Behçet	O	O	X	X	O	O	Unclassified
27	DM	X	O	O	O	O	X	II
28	Chr. Thyroid.	O	O	X	X	O	X	Unclassified
29	Chr. Thyroid.	X	O	O	O	O	X	II
30	Alcoholic LC	O	O	X	X	X	O	I

Table 4 Summary of the Types of Chest X-ray Findings

	I	II	Unclassified
Idiopathic	11 (52%)	6 (29%)	4 (19%)
Collagen Vascular Disease	0	1 (17%)	5 (83%)
Chronic Thyroiditis	0	1	1
Alcoholic Liver Cirrhosis	1	0	0

steroid therapy, and 1 of them die of subsequent acute respiratory failure.

Table 5   Symptoms

	No of Case	Dyspnea	Cough	Sputum	Fever
Idiopathic	21	86%	90%	57%	48%
I	11	91%	91%	64%	64%
II	6	83%	100%	33%	17%
Unclassified	4	75%	75%	75%	50%
CVD	6	83%	83%	67%	67%
Others	3	67%	67%	33%	67%
Total	30	83%	87%	57%	53%

Table 6   Laboratory Findings

	No of Case	W B C >9000	Eosino >400	E S R >50	C R P >+2	L D H
Idiopathic	21	29%	14%	65%	60%	33%
I	11	27%	9%	70%	90%	27%
II	6	0%	17%	17%	0%	33%
Unclassified	4	75%	25%	25%	75%	50%
CVD	6	83%	33%	50%	67%	83%
Others	3	50%	0%	50%	67%	67%
Total	30	40%	17%	44%	62%	48%

Table 7   Pulmonary Function Tests

	No of Case	PaO2 <80torr	% VC <80%	FEV 1% <70%	% DLCO <70%
Idiopathic	21	76%	76%	14%	92%
I	11	73%	67%	9%	86%
II	6	67%	83%	0%	100%
Unclassified	4	100%	83%	50%	100%
CVD	6	83%	75%	0%	100%
Others	3	100%	100%	0%	–
Total	30	80%	79%	11%	94%

Table 8   Course and Prognosis

	No of Case	Remission Spontaneous	Remission With steroid	Remission Total	Relapse	Death
Idiopathic	21	24%	76%	100%	0%	0%
I	11	18%	82%	100%	0%	0%
II	6	33%	67%	100%	0%	0%
Unclassified	4	25%	75%	100%	0%	0%
CVD	6	17%	83%	100%	33%	17%
Others	3	67%	33%	100%	0%	0%
Total	30	27%	73%	100%	6%	3%

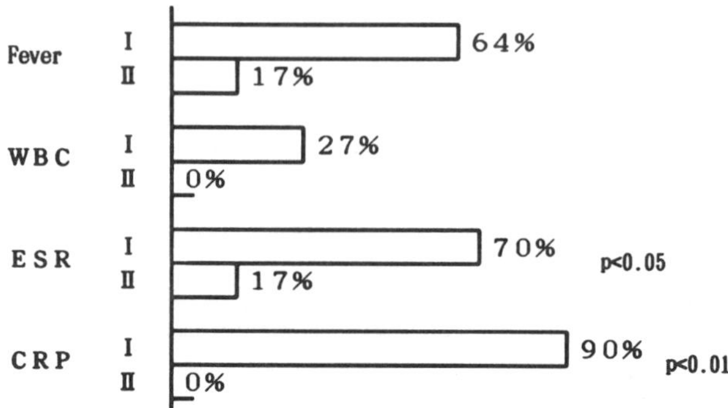

Fig. 8   Comparison between Type I and Type II Cases
in Idiopathic BOOP

In our investigations, the idiopathic BOOP patients seem to have a better clinical course than patients associated with CVD. This finding is similar as in the report by Epler et al.[1].

CONCLUSION

The profile of BOOP in Japan are summarized as follows.

1) Seventy% of BOOP patients in Japan are idiopathic. Two-thirds of the remaining cases are CVD accompanying patients.

2) BOOP can be classified into two major types; Type I and Type II. In the Type I, the abnormal shadows on chest X-rays wander throughout the lung fields. On the other hand, in the Type II, the abnormal shadows are seen in the bibasilar peripheral fields with the reduction of the lung volume.

3) Type I more frequently demonstrates fever, leukocytosis, accelerated ESR, and positive CRP, indicating more severe inflammatory processes, than Type II does.

REFERENCES

1) Epler, G.R., Colby, T.V., Mcloud, T.C., et al. N Engl J Med 312, 152−8, 1985.
2) Konishi, H. Nippon Kyobu Shikkan Gakkai Zasshi, 26 (9), 1005− 9, 1988.
3) Ohno, S., Nakahahsi, Y., Kuriyama, T., et al. Nippon Kyobu Shikkan Gakkai Zasshi 26(8), 904−10, 1988.
4) Kitaichi, M. and Izumi, T. Respiration and Circulation 36(10), 1075−81, 1988.

Interstitial Pneumonias Associated with Human Immunodeficiency Virus Infection

John F. Murray

Chest Service, San Francisco General Hospital Medical Center, and Department of Medicine and Cardiovascular Research Institute, University of California, San Francisco, California, USA

Interstitial pneumonias are being recognized with increased frequency as complications of infection with human immunodeficiency virus (HIV). These disorders include cytomegalovirus (CMV) pneumonia, reactions to cytotoxic and other drugs (trimethoprim-sulfamethoxazole), lymphocytic interstitial pneumonitis (LIP), and nonspecific interstitial pneumonitis (NIP). Cough and dyspnea are the most common presenting complaints. Chest x-rays may show diffuse reticulonodular densities or be normal. Gallium scans are often positive. Diagnosis may be difficult and usually requires histologic confirmation; finding a marked lymphocytosis in bronchoalveolar lavage liquid is strongly suggestive of LIP. CMV pneumonia responds poorly to available drugs. Withdrawing the offending agent helps drug-induced pneumonitis. The natural history need for and response to treatment of LIP and NIP are unknown.

INTRODUCTION

A bewildering variety of pulmonary diseases may complicate infection with the human immunodeficiency virus (HIV) (1). Of these, Pneumocystis carinii pneumonia and pulmonary infection with other opportunistic microorganisms are by far the most common, but pyogenic bacterial pneumonias and involvement by Kaposi's sarcoma and other HIV-related malignancies are also important. To this long list must now be added those types of HIV-associated interstitial pneumonias shown in the following table.

Types of Interstitial Pneumonias Associated with Human
Immunodeficiency Virus Infection

    Infections of the Lung Parenchyma
        Cytomegalovirus Virus
        Herpes Simplex Virus
    Drug-Induced Reactions
        Trimethoprim-Sulfamethoxazole
        Cytotoxic Drugs
    Unknown Causes
        Lymphocytic Interstitial Pneumonitis*
        Nonspecific Interstitial Pneumonitis

*May be related to infection of the lung with either human
immunodeficiency virus or Epstein-Barr virus (see text).

The term _interstitial pneumonia_ has been used to describe
several different pathologic processes. Some authors include all
parenchymal inflammatory disorders in the classification of interstitial
pneumonias (or pneumonitis); others reserve the term for non-
bacterial infection; and still others use it solely for those cases in
which no specific diagnosis is available (2). In this report, interstitial
pneumonia is used as a generic term to refer to certain pneumonias
that are characterized by an inflammatory process, which may vary
from an acute cellular infiltration to chronic fibrosis, that is mainly
situated in the interstitial space of the interalveolar septum. There
may be some "spill-over" of the commonly associated alveolitis into
the alveolar space (hence the diagnostic utility of bronchoalveolar
lavage), but frank alveolar consolidation is not a prominent feature.

According to this terminology, pneumonias with consolidation
of alveoli as their pathologic hallmark, such as pneumococcal or
Pneumocystis carinii pneumonia, are not interstitial pneumonias,
even though interstitial inflammation may be found in these
conditions. The distinction between interstitial pneumonias on the
one hand and "classic" consolidative pneumonias on the other, is
made on the basis of the relative amounts of inflammation present in
the interstitial and alveolar spaces. It should be acknowledged,
however, that _Pneumocystis_ and other pneumonias with alveolar
consolidation are far more common complications of HIV infection
than interstitial pneumonias, and therefore, are important
considerations in the differential diagnosis of infiltrative pulmonary
disorders in patients suspected of having HIV-related disease.

TYPES OF INTERSTITIAL PNEUMONIAS

As shown in Table 1, there are three generic types of interstitial pneumonias in patients with HIV infection: those caused by viruses, those related to the administration of certain drugs, and those of uncertain origin. Each category has two subtypes that will be briefly discussed.

Cytomegalovirus: In the report of the first National Heart, Lung and Blood Institute (NHLBI) Workshop on the pulmonary complications of AIDS, pulmonary infection with cytomegalovirus (CMV) was common; the diagnosis was made either by culture or on the basis of characteristic cytopathic changes, in specimens obtained by fiberoptic bronchoscopy in 74 of 441 patients (17%). An equal number of patients had M. avium complex cultured from bronchoscopic or sputum specimens, which made infection with CMV and M. avium complex second only to P. carinii among the pulmonary complications of AIDS in adults (1). These observations were reaffirmed at the second NHLBI Workshop, which also noted the difficulty in distinguishing between infection (the mere presence of the virus) and disease (the clinical abnormalities caused by the organism) (3). This presents a problem that is still not easily solved, because CMV often coexists with other respiratory pathogens, particularly P. carinii, or with other causes of pulmonary involvement, particularly Kaposi's sarcoma, making it virtually impossible to establish whether the CMV or the other process is responsible for whatever respiratory symptoms, signs, radiographic abnormalities or pulmonary function disturbances may be present. At San Francisco General Hospital, the survival of patients with P. carinii pneumonia who also had CMV recovered from the same bronchoscopic specimens was similar to that in patients with P. carinii pneumonia who did not have identifiable CMV. Because the CMV was not treated in those in whom it was isolated, these results indicate that the virus, by itself, was not producing significant clinical disease.

But it is clear that CMV, from time to time, can cause serious interstitial pneumonias in patients with HIV infection, and when it does so it establishes (or confirms) the diagnosis of AIDS. Histologic findings include interstitial pneumonia that may be focal or diffuse and associated with varying amounts of alveolar damage. Cytomegalic cells with typical intranuclear and intracytoplasmic inclusion bodies are usually plentiful (4).

The diagnosis of CMV pneumonia is difficult to make during life; neither culturing the organism, recognizing its presence by monoclonal antibodies or CMV-specific DNA probes, nor even finding cytopathic changes in cells obtained by BAL reliably establishes that clinically significant lung disease exists. The diagnosis of CMV pneumonia is most easily made in the setting of disseminated disease with retinitis, gastrointestinal or other demonstrable organ involvement. Treatment of CMV interstitial pneumonia in patients with AIDS with the only drug available, dihydroxymethyl propoxymethylguanine (DHPG), produces at best modest and transient improvement (5).

Herpes Simplex Virus: Both type 1 and type 2 herpes simplex viruses (HSV) can produce serious disease in immunocompromised patients. Presumably for this reason, the latest (1987) CDC case definition of AIDS includes "herpes simplex virus infection causing a mucocutaneous ulcer that persists longer than 1 month; or bronchitis, pneumonitis, or esophagitis for any duration affecting a patient >1 month of age" (6). HSV has been identified as a cause of pulmonary disease in patients with AIDS (1), but the association is rare. At San Francisco General Hospital where we have diagnosed and treated more than 1000 cases of AIDS, we have not made a diagnosis of HSV bronchitis or pneumonitis during life or at autopsy in a single one of these patients. The virtual absence of HSV involvement of the lungs in patients with HIV infection is surprising because HSV is a recognized cause of mucocutaneous ulcers (7) and of esophagitis (8), and because of the frequency with which HSV causes pulmonary complications in other (nonAIDS) patients with immune deficiency. For example, in recipients of bone marrow transplants, HSV infection accounted for 5% of all cases of interstitial pneumonia confirmed by biopsy or autopsy. Two mechanisms of pulmonary inoculation with HSV are postulated: direct spread from the upper respiratory tract, which presumably is how esophagitis develops, and hematogenous dissemination from distant mucocutaneous lesions. Because HSV esophagitis and mucocutaneous ulcers certainly exist in AIDS, HSV interstitial pneumonia should also occur; why it is so uncommon is a

Antineoplastic Agents: The relationship between cytotoxic drugs and interstitial pneumonia was considered a medical curiosity for many years after it was first described in 1961. During the last decade, however, cytotoxic drug-induced lung disease has become a major problem. Bleomycin, methotrexate, and cyclophosphamide are the drugs most frequently involved, but scattered reports implicate a large number of other agents. Radiation in sufficient doses also causes interstitial pneumonia, and the injurious effects on lung tissue of cytotoxic drugs and radiation are synergistic.

A definitive diagnosis of cytotoxic drug-induced interstitial pneumonia depends on 1) a history of drug exposure, 2) compatible histologic findings, and 3) exclusion of other causes of similar lung disease. The differential diagnosis of new-onset pulmonary infiltrations, usually with fever, in HIV-infected patients includes opportunistic and other pulmonary infections, pulmonary involvement by the neoplasm (e.g., Kaposi's sarcoma or lymphoma) for which the cytotoxic drug was being administered, nonspecific interstitial pneumonias, and other conditions (e.g., fat embolism, cardiogenic pulmonary edema, adult respiratory distress syndrome).

The presentation of patients with cytotoxic drug-induced lung disease who also have AIDS is seldom straightforward, owing to the complicating features of the underlying disorder. The symptoms may be acute or chronic in onset, fever and cough are usually prominent, and weight loss is common. The chest radiograph may be normal early in the course of the disease and, when abnormal, shows a diffuse pattern of parenchymal infiltrations that mimics many opportunistic pulmonary infections, especially pneumocystis pneumonia. Gallium uptake and the results of pulmonary function tests are similar to other interstitial pneumonias. Thus, the diagnosis of drug-induced lung disease is one of exclusion, and is made by eliminating other possible causes of the same clinical-radiographic-pathologic findings. Drugs should always be considered in the differential diagnosis of new-onset diffuse lung disease and, when in doubt, should be discontinued to prevent further worsening and the prospects of irreversible changes.

Trimethoprim-Sulfamethoxazole: Adverse reactions to trimethoprim-sulfamethoxazole (TMP-SMX), one of the drugs of choice for the treatment of P. carinii pneumonia, are common, and typically consist of fever, rash and/or neutropenia. In addition, new pulmonary infiltrations and hypoxemia, often associated with fever and hypotension, related to TMP-SMX administration have been described in five patients (9). In four of these the reaction occurred upon re-exposure to the drug. No pathologic specimens are available but the pulmonary lesions have been attributed to interstitial pneumonia.

Lymphocytic Interstitial Pneumonitis: Practically from the time it was first described in 1966, there has been debate about whether or not lymphocytic interstitial pneumonitis (LIP) is a pathogenetically distinct pulmonary disorder. The fact that LIP has been recognized in a high percentage of infants and children with AIDS supports the argument that this is a disorder of multiple etiologies that all cause a similar pulmonary pathologic process.   (The reliable diagnosis of LIP in a child less than 13 years of age who also has serologic or cultural evidence of HIV infection is diagnostic of AIDS.) Non-HIV-related cases have been associated with dysproteinemias and several different autoimmune diseases. Data in reports from three different centers indicated that 18 of 36 (50%) infants with AIDS had biopsy or autopsy evidence of LIP (10,11,12); the high prevalence in children greatly exceeds that which we have observed in adults (only one case of LIP in more than 1000 cases of AIDS in adults) and which can be inferred from the scattered case reports in the literature (13,14,15). The explanation for this striking age difference is unknown.

LIP is characterized by a histologic pattern of diffuse infiltration of the alveolar walls and peribronchiolar areas by non-neoplastic mature lymphocytes, plasma cells with Russell bodies, plasmacytoid lymphocytes and immunoblasts as well as by nodular aggregates of lymphoid cells with or without germinal centers (16). An apparently related disorder has also been described called pulmonary lymphoid hyperplasia (PLH) that consists of peribronchiolar nodular lymphoid aggregates with or without germinal centers. More recent data suggest there is a continuum of benign lymphoid infiltrative disorders of the lung that includes LIP at one end and PLH on the other, with overlapping varieties in between (17). Joshi also proposed that the LIP/PLH complex is part of a systemic polymorphic, polyclonal B-cell lymphoid hyperplasia that may progress to a lymphoproliferative disorder. This theory, however, is inconsistent with the fact that the infiltrating lymphocytes derive from the T-cell not the B-cell series (13).

The cause of LIP in AIDS is unknown. Even before the HIV was discovered, it was suggested that Epstein-Barr virus might be involved, a theory that subsequently was supported by the finding of Epstein-Barr virus DNA in 8 of 10 lung biopsy specimens from infants and children with LIP (18). However, HIV itself has been recovered from BAL fluid from a child with LIP and, more recently, highly sensitive _in situ_ hybridization techniques have identified HIV RNA in the lung of another infant with LIP; accordingly, the authors proposed that HIV may play a direct causal role in the development of LIP. Recently, this suggestion was supported by Resnick (19) who detected both HIV antigen and specific IgG antibody in BAL fluid from two adults with LIP.

There are two ways to make the diagnosis of HIV-related LIP. Both require proof of HIV infection, either by demonstrating the virus in blood or tissues or by finding a positive HIV antibody test. In this setting LIP may be diagnosed 1) either from its typical histologic findings on biopsy (or autopsy) specimens of lung tissue, 2) or, in the absence of a histologic diagnosis, from the presence of a chronic pneumonitis - characterized by bilateral reticulonodular interstitial infiltrates with or without hilar adenopathy - present on chest x-ray for a period of at least 2 months and unresponsive to appropriate antimicrobial therapy for likely pathogens. Other causes of interstitial infiltrates should be excluded, and for this to be done reliably, BAL should be performed. Finding a marked BAL lymphocytosis provides additional confirmatory evidence.

The natural history of LIP associated with HIV infection is not completely known but it is clear that the prognosis is better than when opportunistic infections supervene, both in children and adults. Anecdotal evidence suggests that prednisone may be beneficial (13). Azidothymidine has also been used with possibly favorable results in two adults, but not in a third. It is also clear that some patients with LIP have progressed to develop one or more of the opportunistic infections or malignancies that are characteristic of AIDS and that have caused death. It is beginning to appear that LIP may be misclassified as an indicator disease of AIDS (i.e., Stage IV of HIV infection, which is regarded as uniformly fatal), and should be considered, much like generalized lymphadenopathy, as a manifestation of Stage III (pre-AIDS) in the evolution of HIV-related disease.

Nonspecific Interstitial Pneumonitis: The pulmonary disorder called nonspecific interstitial pneumonitis (NIP) has been described in patients with many kinds of immunosuppressive diseases, and has been attributed to drug toxicity, radiation effects, oxygen toxicity, occult viral infection, or to the immunosuppressive disease itself. Thus, it is not surprising that NIP has also been reported in patients with immunosuppression from HIV infection, and is believed to be immunologically mediated (20), perhaps from increased levels of circulating immune complexes or antigen overload, which may play a pathogenetic role. It is of interest that NIP was considered part of the spectrum of the pulmonary complications of HIV infection by the authors of two large series of patients (21,22), but was considered a "nondiagnostic" finding by the authors of another report (23).

The latter author's position is justified up to a point, because it is true that when transbronchial biopsy specimens reveal only variable amounts of inflammatory cells within the interstitium or alveolar spaces (i.e., nonspecific interstitial pneumonitis), one always must be concerned that there was a sampling error and that a specific diagnosis such as an infection, a granulomatous process or a malignancy was missed. Sampling error from transbronchial biopsy was persuasively demonstrated in the work up of non-HIV-related infiltrative lung diseases,   but it appears to be infrequent in HIV-associated pulmonary complications. Indeed, the burden of evidence obtained from postmortem studies indicates not only that NIP exists (20), but that it is also encountered in routine clinical conditions and can be diagnosed by transbronchial biopsy. (One reason for the reliability of transbronchial biopsy in diagnosing HIV-associated NIP is because the results of examination of induced sputum and BAL will identify nearly all patients with infections complications leaving mainly those with malignancies and noninfections pneumonitides for biopsy diagnosis.) However, neither the prevalance of HIV-related NIP is known with certainty, although it was noted in 7 of 130 patients reported by Stover (4) and in 41 of 110 patients reported by Suffredini (3), nor is it known where to place NIP in the progressive continuum of HIV-associated disease, although it does not warrant the diagnosis of AIDS and carries a better prognosis than most other pulmonary complications, with the possible exception of LIP.

Given the lack of knowledge at present about the clinical importance and natural history of HIV-related NIP, it is impossible to define the need for and response to therapy. For the most part the disease is a "self-limited cause of pulmonary dysfunction" (3), and the "prognosis is good with or without treatment" (4).

SUMMARY

Interstitial pneumonias are encountered for less often than ordinary pneumonias with alveolar consolidation, such as those caused by pyogenic bacteria and P. carinii, in patients with HIV infection. Nevertheless, interstitial pneumonias as a group are an important category in the spectrum of pulmonary complications of HIV infection. Some interstitial disorders, such as CMV pneumonia or LIP in a child with HIV infection less than 13 years of age, establish a diagnosis of AIDS; others, such as drug-induced interstitial pneumonias, require revision of on-going therapy; and still others, such as LIP and NIP, have a better prognosis than most HIV-associated pulmonary diseases. However, experience with the interstitial pneumonias is still limited, and much more needs to be learned about their causes, natural history and specific treatment.

REFERENCES

1.   Murray JF, Felton CP, Garay S, Gottlieb MS, Hopewell PC, Stover DE, Teirstein AS. Pulmonary complications of the acquired immunodeficiency syndrome. Report of a National Heart, Lung, and Blood Institute Workshop. New Engl. J. Med. 1984; 310:1682-1688.

2.   Rosenow EC,III, Wilson WR, Cockerill FR III. Pulmonary disease in the immunocompromised host (First of two parts). Mayo Clin. Proc. 1985; 60:473- 487.

3.   Murray JF, Garay SM, Hopewell PC, Mills J, Snider GL, Stover DE. Pulmonary complications of the acquired immunodeficiency syndrome: An update. Am. Rev. Respir. Dis. 1987; 135:504-509.

4.   Wallace JM, Hannah J. Cytomegalovirus pneumonitis in patients with AIDS. Findings in an autopsy series. Chest 1987; 92:198-203.

5.   Jacobson MA, Mills J. Serious cytomegalovirus disease in the acquired immunodeficiency syndrome (AIDS). Clinical findings, diagnosis and treatment. Ann. Int. Med. 1988; 108:585-594.

6.   CDC. Revision of the CDC surveillance case definition for acquired immunodeficiency syndrome. MMWR 1987; 36suppl:3s-15s.

7.   Siegal FP, Lopez C, Hammer GS, Brown AE, Kornfeld SJ, Gold J, Hassett J, Hirochman SZ. Severe acquiredimmunodeficiency in male homosexuals, manifested by chronic perianal ulcerative herpes simplex lesions. New Engl. J. Med. 1981; 305:1439-1444.

8.   Gold JWM. Clinical spectrum of infections in patients with HTLV-III associated diseases. Cancer Res. 1985; 45:4652s-4654s.

9.   Silvestri RC, Jensen WA, Zibrak JD, Alexander RC, Rose RM. Pulmonary infiltrates and hypoxemia in patients with the acquired immunodeficiency syndrome re-exposed to trimethoprim- sulfamethoxasole. Am. Rev.Respir. Dis 1987; 136:1003-1004.

10.   Scott GB, Buck BE, Leterman JG, Bloom FL, Parks WP. Acquired immunodeficiency syndrome in infants. N. Engl. J. Med. 1984; 310:76-81.

11.   Oleske J, Minnefor A, Cooper Jr, R, Thomas K, de la Crug A, Ahdieh H, Guerrero I. Immune deficiency syndrome in children. JAMA 1983; 249:2345- 2349.

12.   Pahwa S, Kaplan M, Fikrig S, Pahwa R, Sarngadharan MG, Popovic M, Gallo RC. Spectrum of human T-cell lymphotropic virus type III infection in children. Recognition of symptomatic, asymptomatic and seronegative patients. JAMA 1986; 255:2299-2305.

13.   Morris JC, Rosen MJ, Marchevsky A, Teirstein AS. Lymphocytic interstitial pneumonia in patients at risk for the acquired immune deficiency syndrome. Chest 1987; 91:63-67.

14.   Solal-Celigny P, Couderc LJ, Herman D, Herve P, Schaffar-Deshayes L, Brun- Vezinet F, Tricot G, Clauvel JP. Lymphoid interstitial pneumonitis in acquired immunodeficiency syndrome-related complex. Am. Rev. Respir. Dis. 1985; 131:956-960.

15.   Grieco MH, Chinoy-Acharya P. Lymphocytic interstitial pneumonia associated with the acquired immune deficiency syndrome. Am. Rev. Respir. Dis. 1985; 131:952-955.

16.   Joshi VV, Oleske JM, Minnefor AB, Singh R, Bokhari T, Rapkin RH. Pathologic pulmonary findings in children with the acquired immune deficiency syndrome. Pediatr. Pathol. 1984; 2:71-87.

17.   Joshi VV, JM Oleske. Pulmonary lesions in children with the acquired immunodeficiency syndrome: A reappraisal based on data in additional cases and follow-up study of previously reported cases. Hum. Pathol. 1986; 17: 641-642.

18.   Andiman WA, Martin K, Rubinstein A, Pahwa S, Eastman R, Katz BZ, Pitt J, Miller G. Opportunistic lymphoproliferations associated with the Epstein- Barr viral DNA in infants and children with AIDS. Lancet 1985; 2:1390-1393.

19.   Resnick L, Pitchenik AE, Fisher E, Croney R. Detection of HTLV-III/LAV- specific IgG and antigen in bronchoalveolar lavage fluid from two patients with lymphocytic interstitial pneumonitis associated with AIDS-related complex. Am. J. Med. 1987; 82:553-556.

20.   Ramaswamy G, Jagadha V, V Tchertkoff. Diffuse alveolar damage and interstitial fibrosis in acquired immunodeficiency syndrome patients without concurrent pulmonary infection. Arch. Pathol. Lab. Med. 1985; 109: 408-412.

21.   Suffredini AF, Ognibene FP, Lack EE, Simmons JT, Brenner M, Gill VJ, Lane HC, Fauci AS. Nonspecific interstitial pneumonitis: A common cause of pulmonary disease in the acquired immunodeficiency syndrome. Ann. Int. Med. 1987; 107:7-13.

22.   Stover DE, White DA, Romano PA, Gellene RA, Robeson WA. Spectrum of pulmonary diseases associated with the acquired immune deficiency syndrome. Am. J. Med. 1985; 78:429-437.

23.   Barrio JI, Harcup C, Baier HJ, Pitchenik AE. Value of repeat fiberoptic bronchoscopies and significance of nondiagnostic bronchoscopic results in patients with the acquired immunodeficiency syndrome. Am. Rev. Respir. Dis. 1987; 135:422-425.

II
PATHOPHYSIOLOGY

Mechanical Aspects of Idiopathic Pulmonary Fibrosis (IPF)

Wataru Hida and Tamotsu Takishima

First Department of Internal Medicine, Tohoku University School of Medicine, Sendai, Japan

We studied pulmonary function and respiratory muscle function in 30 patients with idiopathic pulmonary fibrosis (IPF), and compared pulmonary function between infiltrative (group I) and fibrotic type (group F) divided by lung biopsy and among ground glass pattern (group A), reticulonodular pattern (group B) and ground glass, reticulonodular and honeycombing pattern (group AB) divided by chest X-rays. Group I showed a significant decrease in lung volume and increase in maximal esophageal pressure (Pes max), compared to group F. Group B also showed a significant increase in the coefficient of retraction (Pes max/TLC), compared to group A. Furthermore, patients with bad prognosis had decrease in lung volume and increase in Pes max. Thus decrease in lung volume and pulmonary stiffness may be key points in the pathophysiology and prognosis of IPF.

Introduction

Idiopathic pulmonary fibrosis (IPF) is a fatal disorder characterized by interstitial and intra-alveolar infiltrates and progress to interstitial fibrosis. Pulmonary function test of IPF is improtant to know pathophysiology, clinical stage or clinical course of IPF. However, the correlation between the pulmonary function and pathological findings is still unclear. In the present study, we examined from mechanical aspects 30 patients with IPF diagnosed by clinical, roentgenographic and histologic criteria described by Cristal et al. (1).

Subjects and Method

Subjects: We studied 30 IPF patiernts who were diagnosed by clinical, roentgenographic and physiological criteria (1). These patients had no history of inhalation of inorganic or organic dusts and showed negative precipitating antibodies using 11 major commercially available antigens (Hollister-Stier Labs., WA, USA). Informed consent was obtained from each subject for this study.

Pulmonary function test: Slow vital capacity (VC) and forced expiratory volume in one second (FEV_1) were measured using the 13.5L Benedict-Roth type spirometer and the ratio of FEV_1 for VC (FEV_1%) was calculated. Functional residual capacity (FRC) was obtained with He-gas dilution method using water-sealed spirometer, and total lung capacity (TLC) and residual volume (RV) were also obtained. %VC, %TLC, %FRC and %RV were calculated by Cotes' predicted formula (2). Static pressure-volume curves were obtianed by the esophageal balloon catheter system and body plethysmography according to standard technique (3), and Pes max and static lung compliance (Cst) were also obtained. Diffusing capacity for carbon monoxide (DLCO) was measured with the single breath method, and diffusing capacity per unit volume (DLCO/VA) was calculated. Two ml of arterial blood was sampled anaerobically from brachial artery while the patients breathed room air, and the blood was soon analyzed to obtain arterial oxygen tension (PaO_2), arterial carbon dioxide tension ($PaCO_2$) and pH by pH blood gas analyzer (Model 213, Instrumentation Laboratories, Lexington, MA).

Muscle power measurement: Maximal static inspiratory and expiratory mouth pressure were measured according to the technique of Black and Hyatt (4) using the device developed by us (VITALOPOWER KH101, Chest Corporation, Tokyo, Japan). The device for measurement of mouth pressure was consisted of two parts; a plastic cylinder and a calculator. The cylinder had a closed end with strain gauge pressure sensor and a pin side hole which minimized oral pressure artifacts. The other end was fitted with a mouth piece. Time-pressure curve was displayed on the chart. Maximal inspiratory mouth pressure was measured at levels of RV and·FRC (PImax and

PI$_{FRC}$, respectively) and maximal expiratory mouth pressure
was obtained at levels of TLC and FRC (PEmax and PE$_{FRC}$,
respectively). Patients performed maximal inspiratory and
expiratory efforts against an obstructed mouth piece at
least three times at each lung volume and we adopted the
mean value obtained from two reproducible values for
analysis. The predicted values for correction of age and
sex were obtained from Black and Hyatt's formula (4),
and percentage of PImax and PEmax for predicted values
(%PImax and %PEmax, respectively) were calculated.

Classification based on chest X-rays: Anteroposterior
chest X-ray was taken within one week before bronchoscopic
examination. Three groups were divided based on chest
X-rays. Patients with a ground glass pattern were
assigned to group A, those with a reticulonodular pattern
to group B and those with ground glass, reticulonodular
and honeycombing pattern to group AB.

Bronchoalveolar lavage (BAL): After medication with
atropine sulphate (0.5 mg/50 kg of body weight) and
pentazocine (15 mg/50 kg), a fiberoptic bronchoscope
(RBS-6T, Machida Co., Tokyo) was introduced and wedged
into a segmental or subsegmental bronchus of the middle or
lingual lobe under local anesthesia with lidocaine. Then,
20 ml of 0.9% sterile saline was infused and immediately
aspirated by a low negative pressure (-100 mmHg) to
prevent collapse of the bronchus. This procedure was
repeated five times. The fluids obtained were strained
through one layer of surgical gauze and centrified for 8
minutes at 180xg. The pellet of cells was used to count
the total cell number and then smeared to determine the
differential cell count by means of Wright-Giemsa and
nonspecific esterase stains. BAL fluids were examined at
the same time lung biopsies were performed on the opposite
lung.

Transbronchial lung biopsy (TBLB): Using a fiberoptic
bronchoscope, two to four specimens from the peripheral
regions of different unilateral lobes were obtained from
each patient. The specimens were embedded in paraffin,
sectined (4 um thickness) and stained with hematoxylin –
eosin, elastica-masson and periodic acid-Schiff. Samples
of about 3x3 to 5x5 mm in size from alveolar region of
different lobes were obtained.

Classification based on TBLB: Based on histology from
TBLB, IPF patients divided into infiltrative and fibrotic
types. When we observed mainly desquamation cells in
alveoli or mononuclear cell infiltration, this patient was

thought as infiltrative type, whereas when we observed massive fibrosis in alveolar regions, this patient was thought as fibrotic type.

Results

Pulmonary function: %VC and %TLC of IPF decreased compared with those of systemic lupus erythematosus (SLE) (n=8), other collagen disease (n=12) and sarcoidosis (n=42) which were within normal values. Progressive systemic sclerosis (PSS)(n=7) and chronic bronchiolitis (n=16) also showed decrease in %VC. PSS showed slight increase in %RV and chronic bronchiolitis showed decrease in FEV_1% and increase in %RV. Cst and Pes max of IPF decreased and increased, respectively, compared with other fibrosing lung diseases. %DLCO, DLCO/VA and PaO_2 of IPF decreased. Decrease in %DLCO, DLCO/VA and PaO_2 were also observed in PSS, other collagen disease and chronic bronchiolitis. From these results, characteristics of pulmonary function of IPF would be a decrease in lung volume and in Cst with increase in Pes max.

Pulmonary function and muscle power: Relationships between %PImax and %RV or %TLC were significant, however, relationships between %PImax and other parameters (FEV_1%, Pes max, Cst, DLCO/VA and PaO_2) of pulmonary function were not significant. %PEmax did not have significant correlation with lung function. Fig.1 shows the relationship between %PImax and %RV. Reduced lung volume had increased %PImax. This may suggest that stiffness of the lung causes decrease in lung volume and increase in elastic loading on respiratory muscles.

Pulmonary function and chest X-rays: Fig.2 shows the relationship between pulmonary function (%VC, %DLCO, PaO_2 and Pes max/TLC) and subgroup of IPF divided by chest X-rays. Group B showed a significant increase in the coefficient of retraction

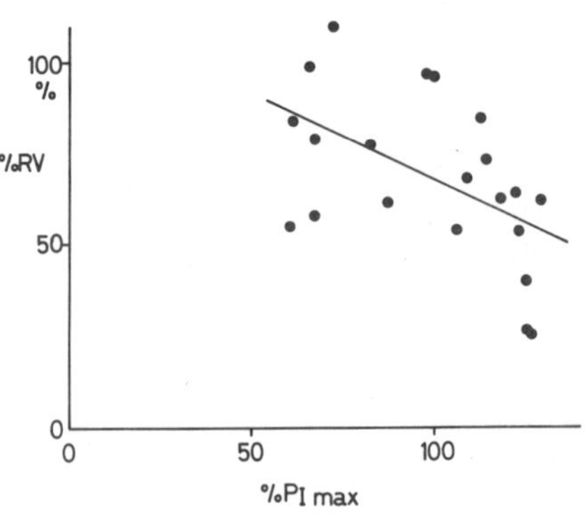

Fig. 1. Relationship between %PImax and %RV.

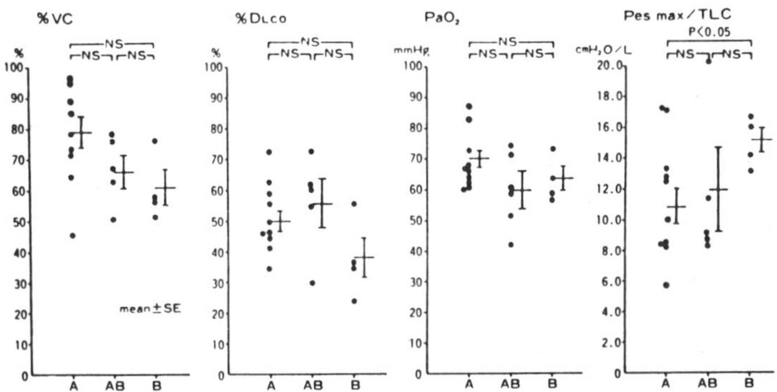

Fig.2.   Relationship between pulmonary function
     and subgroup of IPF based on chest X-rays.
(Pes max/TLC) compared with the group A.   %VC,
%DLCO and PaO$_2$ were not significantly different among
group A, B and AB.

Pulmonary function and lung biopsy: Fig.3 shows the
relationship betweem pulmonary function and the subgroup
divided by histology from TBLB.   Fibrotic patients showed
a significant decrease in %VC and a significant increase
in the coefficinet of retraction (Pes max/TLC), compared
to infiltrative patients.   However, %DLCO and PaO$_2$ did not
differ between the two groups.   Furthermore, examination
of BAL fluid showed that the percentage of lymphocytes to
total cells was greater in infiltrative than in fibrotic
patients.   Neutrophil, eosinophil and macrophage

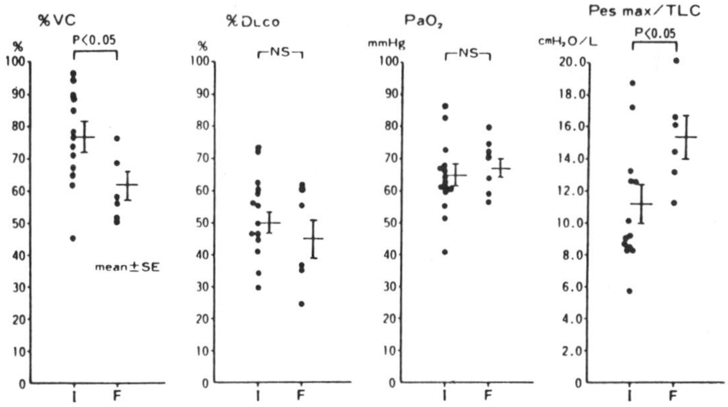

Fig.3.   Relationship between pulmonary function
and subgroup divided by histology from TBLB.

populations did not differ between the two groups.

Pulmonary function and prognosis: As shown in Fig.4, patients who had died while undergoing steroid therapy (group C) showed significant decreases in %TLC and Cst, and an increase in Pes max, compared with living patients with (group B) or without (group A) steroid therapy, even if %VC and PaO_2 among these three groups were not significantly different.

Discussion

The characteristics of pulmonary function of IPF showed a decrease in lung volume and static lung compliance, and an increase in maximal esophageal pressure. These results confirmed Cristal et al. (1). This tendency was stronger in fibrotic type than in infitrative type based on histology of TBLB, or in reticulonodular type than in type with ground glass, reticulonodular and honeycombing patterns based on chest X-rays. Particularly the coefficient of retraction differentiates subgroups. Thus, this parameter is usefull to estimate the clinical stage of IPF.

Infiltrative type or ground glass pattern on chest X-ray seemed to be in early stage, because these findings were observed in patients who had a duration within one year

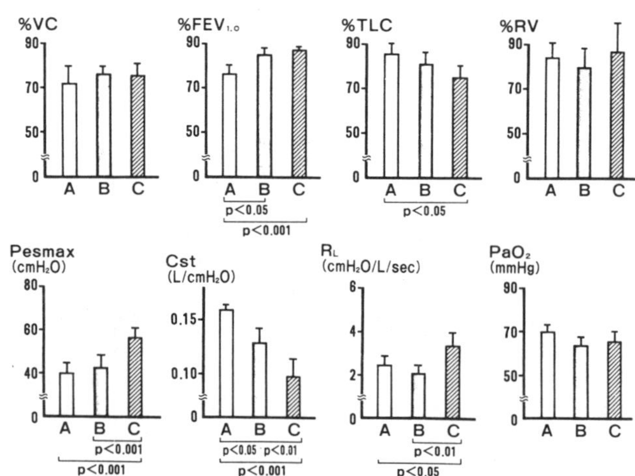

Fig.4. Pulmonary function and prognosis.

from onset of dyspnea or cough compared to patients who had
a duration over one year from onset of the symptoms. We
observed a remarkable increase in lymphocyte in BAL fluid
in infiltrative type of IPF. On the contrary, in fibrotic
type, increase in neutrophil was observed compared with
control values from the additional patients who complained
hemoptysis and/or contralateral localized abnormal shadow.
These findings suggest that the lymphocyte play an important tole in the pathogenesis of the early stage of IPF,
whereas neutrophil in the advanced stage of IPF. These
findings may be compatible with the findings in
bleomycin induced fibrosis in rats by Thrall et al (5),
who found a sinificant increase in lymphocytes shortly
after a single intratracheal injection of bleomycin.
On the other hand, Crystal et al. (1) reported that
increase in neutrophils in BAL fluid of IPF. We did not
know the reasons for the discrepancy between ours and
theirs.

In IPF, %VC and %TLC had a significant reverse correlation with %PImax. Decrease in lung volume induces
decrease in radius of curvature of diaphragm. Therefore,
increase in transdiaphragmatic pressure would be explic-
able by Laplace's law. IPF had a remarkable stiffness
in the lung, causing an intrinsic elastic loading on
respiratory muscles. Even though the resting PaO_2 can be
normal in IPF, PaO_2 and $AaDO_2$ during exercise decreased
and increased, respectively. These findings are universal
in IPF. However, the mechanisms of the change of gas exchange during exercise in IPF is still unknown. We have
hypothesis that elastic loading on respiraotry muscles
itself may affect the gas exchange during exercise
through hemodynamic and ventilatory change. We studied
the effect of inspiratory elastic loading on pulmonary
gas exchange with and without electrically induced
hindlimb exercise in anesthetized dogs with normal lung,
and found that small elastic loading during exercise
showed greater increase in $AaDO_2$ compared with large
elastic loading only, although the inspiratory pleural
pressures between two conditions were not different (6).
Therefore, increased elastic load on respiratory muscles
could cause abnormality of pulmonary gas exchange during
exercise. This may explain that high cardiac output
combined with low ventilation-perfusion ratio may have
increased the shunt in normal lungs.

It is important to know the prognosis from pulmonary
function. We found that patients with unhappy prognosis

had a decrease in TLC and Cst, and an increase in Pes max, although they had similar vital capacity and PaO_2 to patients with good prognosis. Therefore, decrease in lung volume and pulmonary stiffness are key points in the pathophysiology and prognosis of IPF.

References

1)   Crystal,R.G., Fulmer,J.D., Roberts,W.C., Moss,M.L., Line, B.R., and Reynolds,H.Y. Ann. Intern. Med., 85, 769-788, 1976.

2)   Cotes,J.E. In: Lung function edited by J.E.Cotes, Blackwell Scientific Publication, London, pp329-387, 1979.

3)   Macklem,P.T., Leith,D.E., and Mead,J. In: Procedures for standardized measurement of lung mechanics. National heart and lung institute, Bethesda, MS, 1974.

4)   Black,L.F., and Hyatt,R.E. Am. Rev. Respir. Dis. 99, 696-702, 1969.

5)   Thrall,R.S., and Barton,R.W. Am. Rev. Respir. Dis. 129, 279-283, 1984.

6)   Chonan,T., Hida,W., Kikuchi,Y., Shindoh,C., Taguchi,O., Miki,H., and Takishima,T. J. Appl. Physiol. (In submission).

Impaired Alveolar Gas Exchange in Interstitial Pneumonia

Tetsuro Yokoyama, Fumihiro Yamasawa,
and Kazuhiro Yamaguchi

Department of Medicine, School of Medicine, Keio University, Tokyo, Japan

Significant arterial hypoxemia associated with abnormally increased $AaDO_2$ and $aADN_2$ were noted. The cases with interstitial pneumonia of unknown etiology did not show any consistent difference of impaired alveolar gas exchange from those in other interstitial pneumonia. The patients demonstrated significant $\dot{V}_A/\dot{Q}$ uneveness on the multiple inert gas elimination study. Some cases revealed accessory peak at $\dot{V}_A/\dot{Q}$ of 30-100 with their major peak, which appeared near $\dot{V}_A/\dot{Q}$ of 1.0. The authors described possible contribution of impaired diffusivity.

Cases with interstitial pneumonia accompany significant arterial hypoxemia. This paper discusses the impaired alveolar gas exchange. The authors placed their emphasis upon the significance of ventilation-perfusion ratio distribution and impaired diffusivity.

SUBJECTS AND METHODS:

Thirty-six patients with interstitial pneumonia diagnosed on clinical basis were studied. They categorized their subjects into two groups, namely 25 patients whose etiology was not identified after intensive clinical study (the group A) and 11 patients with interstitial pneumonia of any identified etiology (the group B). The Group A is compatible to the interstitial pneumonia of unknown etiology. To assess impaired alveolar gas exchange the authors conducted (1) the arterial blood gas analysis, (2) the simultaneous measurements of alveolar-arterial O_2 tension difference ($AaDO_2$) and of arterial-alveolar N_2 tension difference ($aADN_2$), and (3) the multiple inert gas elimination study to evaluate uneven distribution of alveolar ventilation and pulmonary blood flow in terms for $\dot{V}_A/\dot{Q}$. The authors measured $AaDO_2$ and of $aADN_2$ under the steady state on supine position breathing room air. During withdrawal of arterial blood specimen they collected expired air simultaneously. N_2 content in the specimen was measured with the Farhi's gas chromatographic system.

On the multiple inert gas elimination study the authors used gas mixture containing six inert gases, i.e. SF_6, ethane, cyclopropane, halothane, diethyl-ether and acetone, for indicator. A cardiac catheter was inserted under steady state to collect specimen of mixed venous blood and to measure cardiac output. The arterial- and the mixed venous specimens as well as expired gas sample were analyzed with the gas chromatographic system. To assess uneven distribution of alveolar ventilation and of pulmonary blood flow in terms for $\dot{V}_A/\dot{Q}$ the authors assumed the lung model of 50 parallel compartments, each of which had different $\dot{V}_A/\dot{Q}$. The authors made calculation using the enforced smoothing technique with modification [1,2,4,6,7,8].

RESULTS AND DISCUSSION:

1) Impaired alveolar gas exchange in cases with interstitial pneumonia of various causes:

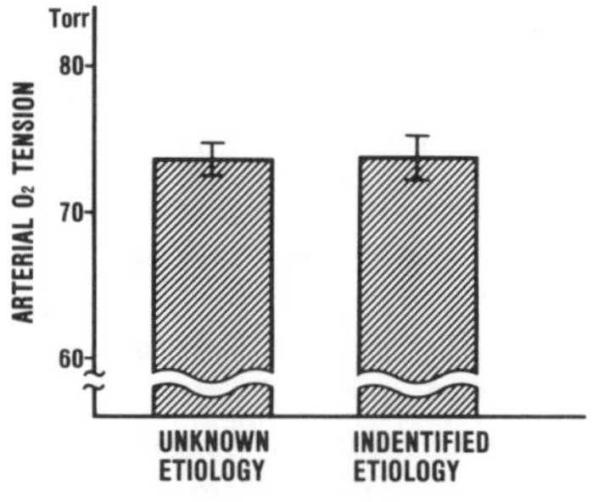

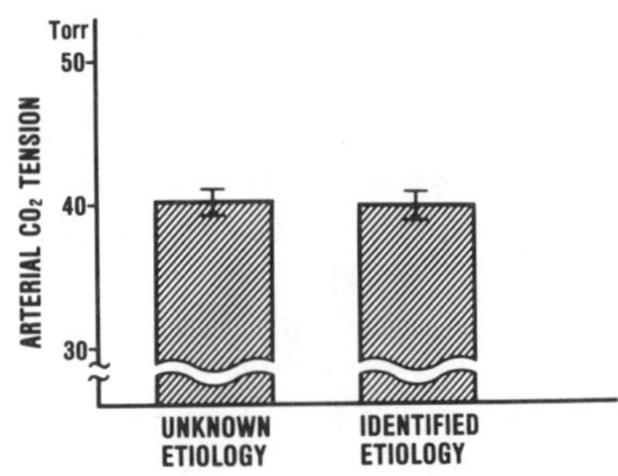

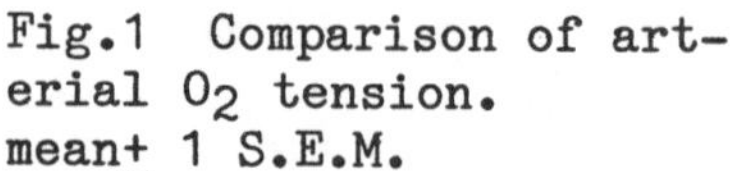

Fig.1 Comparison of arterial O_2 tension. mean$\pm$ 1 S.E.M.

Fig.2 Comparison of arterial CO_2 tension. mean$\pm$ 1 S.E.M.

The mean for arterial O_2 tension obtained for the group (A) was 73.64 ± 1.11 Torr while that for group (B) was 72.93 ± 1.42 Torr(Fig.1). These means demonstrated no consistent difference. Arterial CO_2 tension, $AaDO_2$ or

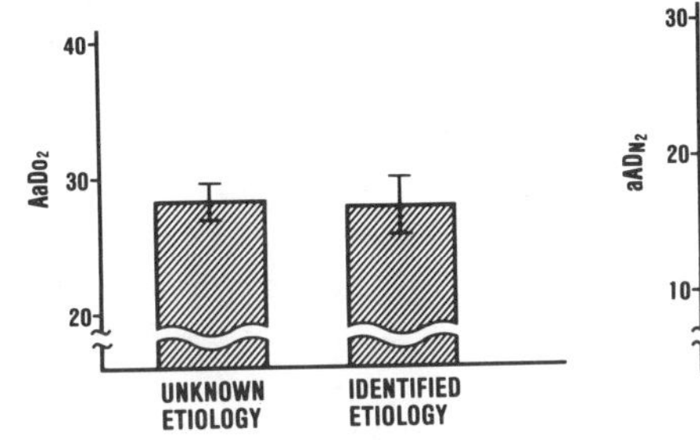

Fig.3 Comparison of $AaDO_2$. mean$\pm$ 1 S.E.M.

Fig.4 Comparison of $aADN_2$. mean$\pm$1 S.E.M.

$aADN_2$ for group (A) were not consistently different from those for group (B), respectively (Fig.2,3 and 4). **2)Alveolar ventilation and pulmonary blood flow in terms for ventilation-perfusion ratio distribution:**

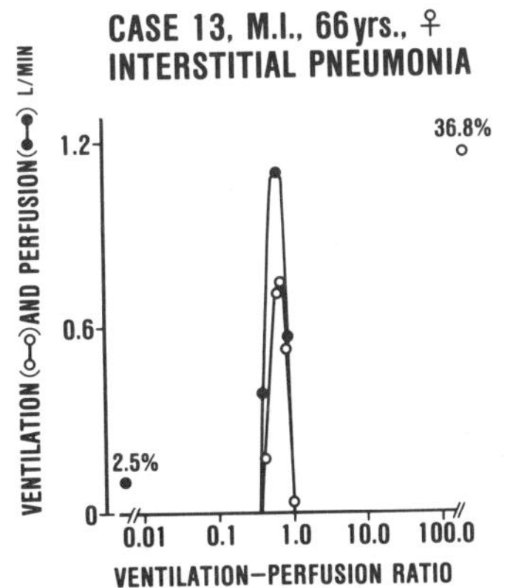

Fig.5 $\dot{V}_A/\dot{Q}$ distribution. An example of single-peaked distribution.

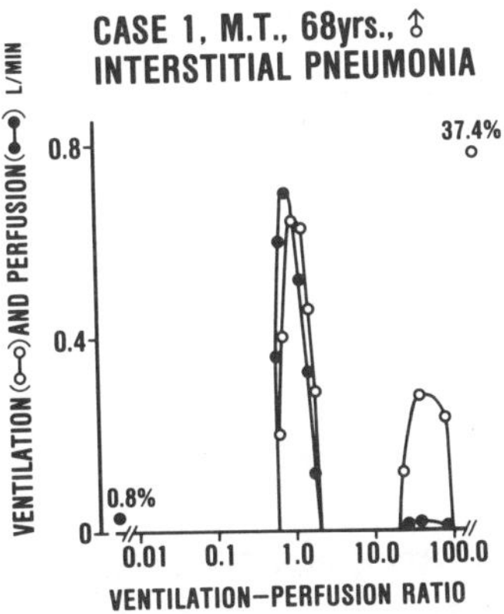

Fig.6 $\dot{V}_A/\dot{Q}$ distribution. An example of dual-peaked distribution.

The authors studied $\dot{V}_A/\dot{Q}$ distribution with the multiple inert gas elimination technique on 18 cases of the group A. Fig.5 exhibits a typical single-peaked distribution of alveolar ventilation and pulmonary blood flow (Fig.5). Fig.6 indicates a dual-peaked distribution pattern (Fig.6). The dual-peaked cases, in addition to the major peak locating at $\dot{V}_A/\dot{Q}$ of approximately 1.0, demonstrated another accessory peak at $\dot{V}_A/\dot{Q}$ between 30 and 100. 10 cases revealed single-peaked distribution and 8 cases revealed dual-peaked distribution (Fig.7).

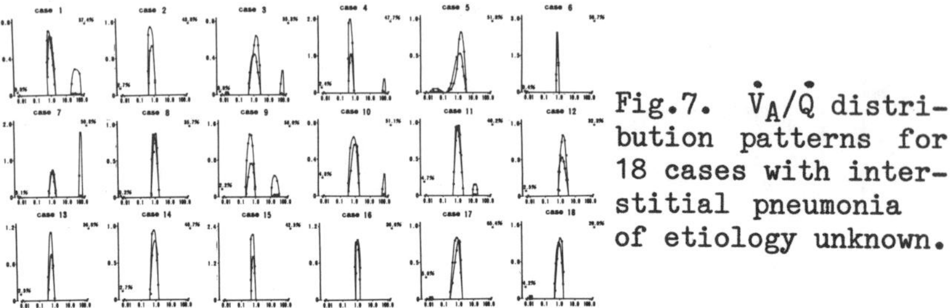

Fig.7. $\dot{V}_A/\dot{Q}$ distribution patterns for 18 cases with interstitial pneumonia of etiology unknown.

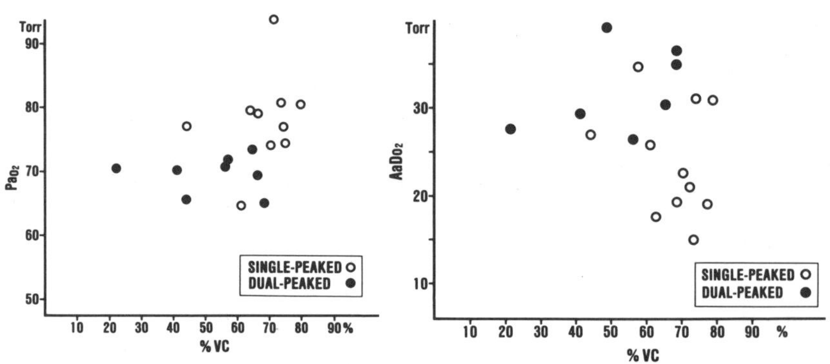

Fig.8 Relation of % vital capacity vs.arterial O_2 tension.

Fig.9 Relation of % vital capacity vs.AaDO$_2$.

3) Alveolar gas exchange and ventilatory capacity:

FEV$_1$% for the single-peaked cases was not different from those for the dual-peaked cases. Mean of % vital capacity for the dual-peaked cases was consistently smaller than that for the single-peaked cases. S.E.M. of % vital capacity for the dual-peaked cases was larger than that for the single-peaked cases.

The dual-peaked cases revealed relatively smaller % vital capacity compared with the single-peaked cases (Fig.8). They demonstrated larger AaDO$_2$ compared with the single-peaked cases (Fig.9,10).

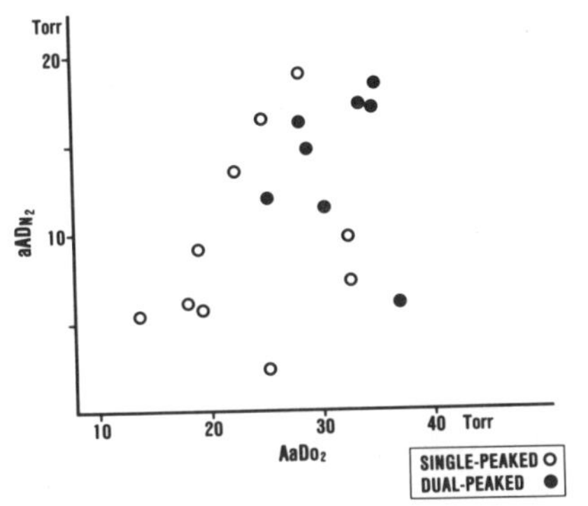

Fig.10   Relation of %vital capacity vs.aADN$_2$.

4) Arterial blood gases and alveolar-arterial gas tension differences:

Hypoxemia accompanied by these dual-peaked cases was much significant than that seen on the single-peaked cases (Table 1). The arterial CO_2 tension between these two groups was not consistently different (Table

SINGLE-PEAKED CASES

	MEASURED VALUES	CALCULATED VALUES	STATISTICAL SIGNIFICANCE
Pao$_2$	77.5±3.2	81.9±3.7	n.s.
Paco$_2$	39.9±1.3	41.2±1.4	n.s.
AaDo$_2$	22.7±2.4	11.5±2.3	P<0.05
aADN$_2$	9.3±2.1	3.7±0.8	P<0.05

FIGURES INDICATE MEAN±1S.E.M.
UNIT : Torr

Table 1 Arterial blood gases and AaD on the single-peaked cases.

DUAL-PEAKED CASES

	MEASURED VALUES	CALCULATED VALUES	STATISTICAL SIGNIFICANCE
Pao$_2$	69.8±0.9	78.6±3.2	P<0.05
Paco$_2$	40.7±1.0	41.0±1.5	n.s.
AaDo$_2$	32.9±1.8	27.5±2.2	P<0.05
aADN$_2$	14.0±1.2	9.9±1.1	n.s.

FIGURES INDICATE MEAN±1S.E.M.
UNIT : Torr

Table 2 Arterial blood gases and AaD on the dual peaked cases.

1). $AaDO_2$ for the dual-peaked cases was larger than that for the single-peaked cases (Table 1). $aADN_2$ for these two groups was not consistently different. Such pattern of dual-peaked distribution was somewhat contradictory to explain severe hypoxemia. When the subject breathing room air lung compartments with high $\dot{V}_A/\dot{Q}$ theoretically demonstrate high alveolar O_2 tension and thus lungs accompanying $\dot{V}_A/\dot{Q}$ peaks at about 1.0 and larger do not accompany hypoxemia if the subject does not accompany any impairment other than uneven $\dot{V}_A/\dot{Q}$ distribution. To explain arterial hypoxemia in relation to uneven $\dot{V}_A/\dot{Q}$ distribution subjects have to have increased pulmonary blood flow in the low $\dot{V}_A/\dot{Q}$ space and/or increased shunt. Using the mixing equation the authors calculated, based upon the data obtained on the multiple inert gas elimination study, fractional pulmonary blood flow in lung compartments with $\dot{V}_A/\dot{Q}$ lower than 0.2. They made the same calculation on the fractional blood flow for the lung compartments of $\dot{V}_A/\dot{Q}$ lower than 0.5 or 0.8 (Table 2). There was no consistent difference between the single-peaked cases

$\dot{V}_A/\dot{Q}$	SINGLE-PEAKED	DUAL-PEAKED	STATISTICAL SIGNIFICANCE
"SHUNT"	2.08±0.58	2.00±0.63	n.s.
<0.2	2.33±0.70	3.24±0.75	n.s.
<0.5	8.15±2.76	15.24±5.43	n.s.
<0.8	58.01±9.10	55.63±8.97	n.s.

UNIT : %. FIGURES INDICATE MEAN±1S.E.M.

Table 3 % fractional pulmonary blood flow in the lung compartments less than $\dot{V}_A/\dot{Q}$ of 0.2, 0.5 or 0.8.

and the dual-peaked in percent blood flow for the lung compartments of lower $\dot{V}_A/\dot{Q}$. The pulmonary blood flow for higher $\dot{V}_A/\dot{Q}$ compartments cannot explain severe arterial hypoxemia found on the dual-peaked cases. Since the authors knew the fractional pulmonary blood flow perfusing lung compartments of different $\dot{V}_A/\dot{Q}$, and since the authors had mixed venous O_2- and CO_2 tensions they were able to calculate end-capillary O_2- and CO_2 tensions for each compartment. Based on the end-capillary gas tensions and the pulmonary blood flow they calculated arterial O_2- and CO_2 tensions using the mixing equation. The arterial gas tensions obtained by calculation were assigned to the "calculated arterial O_2- and CO_2 tensions" while the arterial gas tensions obtained on the measurements were referred to the "measured arterial O_2- and CO_2 tensions". If the subject maintains a certain level of her alveolar O_2 tension the measured arterial gas tensions describe the $\dot{V}_A/\dot{Q}$ uneveness, the shunt in addition to any impaired diffusivity. The calculated gas tensions represent the $\dot{V}_A/\dot{Q}$ distribution and the shunt and they are not related to the impaired diffusivity. Consistent differences between the measured arterial gas tensions and the corresponding calculated arterial gas tensions indicate detectable impairment of diffusivity.

Table 3 shows measured- and calculated- arterial O_2 tensions (Table 3). On the single-peaked cases difference for these O_2 tensions was not consistent while on the dual-peaked cases the calculated arterial O_2 tension was higher than the measured arterial O_2 tension. This suggests that the dual-peaked cases accompany significant impaired diffusivity. Table 4 indicates the measured- and the calculated $AaDO_2$ (Table 4). The measured $AaDO_2$ was larger than the calculated $AaDO_2$. The measured $aADN_2$ was not different from the corresponding calculated $aADN_2$ both for the single-

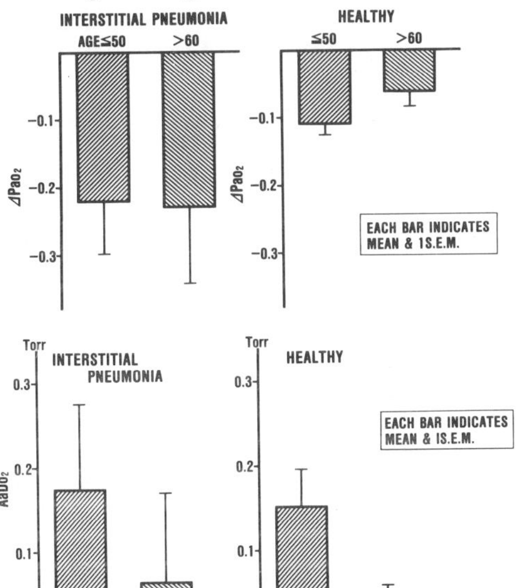

Fig.11 Change in arterial O_2 tension per annum obtained on the followed-up cases.

Fig.12 Change in $AaDO_2$ per annum obtained on the followed-up cases.

peaked cases and for the dual-peaked cases. These data suggest the significance of impaired diffusivity in addition to the $\dot{V}_A/\dot{Q}$ uneveness and/or the shunt on the dual-peaked cases to cause severe arterial hypoxemia.

5) Alveolar gas exchange on acute excerbation:

A followed-up case with interstitial pneumonia demonstrated changing arterial O_2 tension along her time-course, during which this particular caserepeatedly suffered from acute excerbation. Upon acute excerbation the case demonstrated depressed arterial O_2 tension. The depressed arterial O_2 tension elevated toits original baseline level upon recovery from the episode. Fig.11 represents the annual decline of arterial O_2 tension for the cases with interstitial pneumonia under stable condition compared with those for the healthy cases (Fig.11 and 12). Each group was divided into two separate age-groups, i.e. the subjects of age less than 50 years old and the subjects of age over 60 years old. The authors did not find any consistent difference of the change in O_2 tension per annum (delta arterial O_2 tension) between these two age groups either in cases with interstitial pneumonia or in healthy subjects. Delta arterial O_2 tension for interstitial pneumonia was -0.21 Torr/yr. while that for healthy subjects was -0.11 Torr/yr showing consistent difference.

The authors studied alveolar gas exchange upon an acute excerbation as well as under stable condition on the same cases (Fig.13 and 14). One of these cases under chronic stable condition demonstrated arterial O_2 tension of 84 Torr, CO_2 tension of 38 Torr, $AaDO_2$ of 17

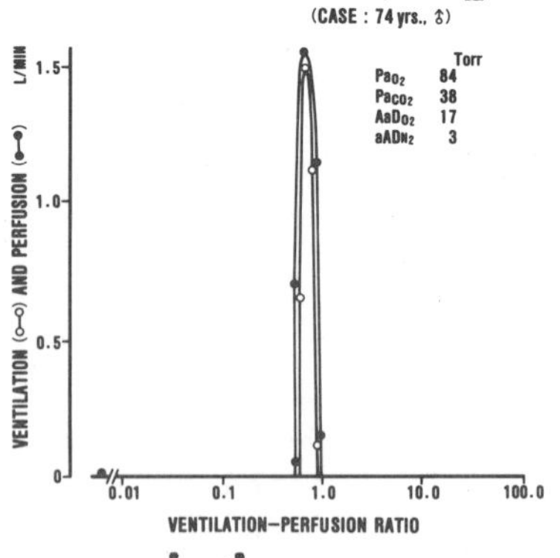

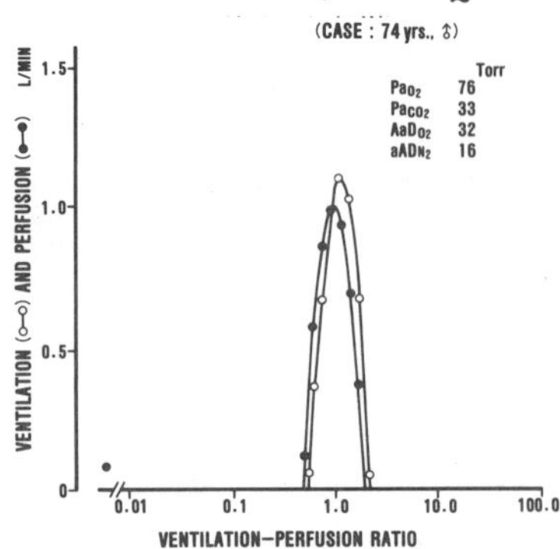

Fig.13 $\dot{V}_A/\dot{Q}$ distribution under stable condition.

Fig.14 $\dot{V}_A/\dot{Q}$ distribution on acute excerbation.

Torr and $aADN_2$ of 3 Torr. This particular case revealed sharp single-peaked $\dot{V}_A/\dot{Q}$ distribution. On acute excerbation this patient demonstrated arterial O_2 tension of 76 Torr, arterial CO_2 tension of 33 Torr, $AaDO_2$ of 32 Torr and $aADN_2$ of 16 Torr showing a single-peaked $\dot{V}_A/\dot{Q}$ distribution.

The authors repeated the inert gas elimination study on three cases with interstitial pneumonia during and after an acute excerbation. All these cases demonstrated single-peaked $\dot{V}_A/\dot{Q}$ distribution under stable condition. During acute excerbation none out of these three cases demonstrated multi-peaked $\dot{V}_A/\dot{Q}$ distribution, but they demonstrated single-peaked $\dot{V}_A/\dot{Q}$ distribution although the width of the peak was wider.

The authors analyzed the uneven distribution of diffusivity in the lungs in terms of $\dot{V}_A/\dot{Q}$ distribution. The technique was a modification of the multiple inert gas elimination technique. In addition to the six inert gases used for the indicators to study $\dot{V}_A/\dot{Q}$ distribution the authors used two additional diffusion dependent gases, oxygen and carbon monoxide, to collect information on the distribution of uneven diffusivity. Finally the authors obtained information to construct the three dimensional diagram (Fig.15). This three-dimensional diagram indicates the pulmonary blood flow in terms for $\dot{V}_A/\dot{Q}$ and $G/\dot{Q}$. The cases with interstitial pneumonia demonstrated uneven distribution of $G/\dot{Q}$ as one of the important factor to cause arterial hypoxemia.

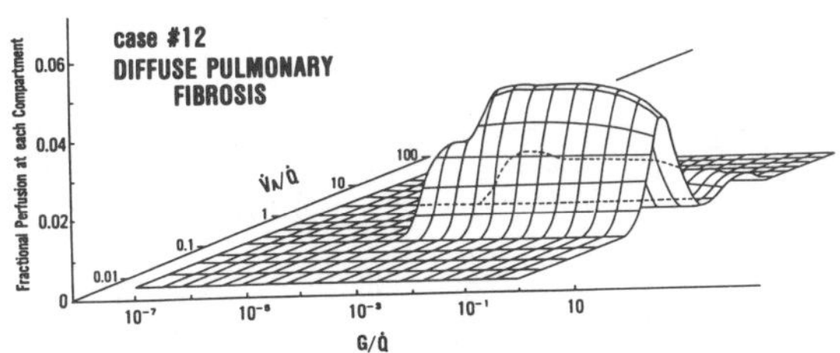

Fig.15   Three-dimensional diagram showing fractional perfusion in terms for $\dot{V}_A/\dot{Q}$ and $G/\dot{Q}$.

CONCLUSION:

The authors described impaired alveolar gas exchange in cases with interstitial pneumonia associated with arterial hypoxemia, abnormally increased $AaDO_2$ and $aADN_2$. They did not find any specific difference of impaired alveolar gas exchange in cases with interstitial pneumonia of unknown etiology compared with those with interstitial pneumonia of any identified etiology. Some cases with interstitial pneumonia of unknown etiology demonstrated the dual-peaked distribution of $\dot{V}_A/\dot{Q}$ on the multiple inert gas elimination study. The dual-peaked cases revealed much significant arterial hypoxemia as compared with the single-peaked cases. The $\dot{V}_A/\dot{Q}$ distribution pattern did not sufficiently explained significant arterial hypoxemia found in the dual-peaked cases. Since the blood perfused through compartments with higher $\dot{V}_A/\dot{Q}$ does not cause arterial hypoxemia the authors conducted on such cases further assessment to demonstrate the possible role of diffusion impairment. The data obtained by the modified multiple indicator gas elimination study suggested the uneven distribution of diffusivity in addition to the uneven $\dot{V}_A/\dot{Q}$ distribution to explain arterial hypoxemia.

REFERRENCES

1)Dantzig,G.B.: Linear programming and extensions. New Jersey: Princeton,pp94-108,1963

2)Evans, J.W.,Wagner,P.D.:Limits on $\dot{V}_A/\dot{Q}$ distributions from analysis of experimental inert gas elimination. J Appl Physiol 42:889-898,1977

3)Farhi,L.E.,Yokoyama,T.: Effect of ventilation-perfusion inequality on elimination of inert gases. Respir Physiol 3:12-20,1967

4)Hoerl A.E.,Kennard, R.W.: Ridge regression: biased estimation for nonothogonal problems. Technometrics 12:55-67,1970

5)Jernudd-Wilhelmsson Y., Hornblad,Y, Hedenstierna,G.: Ventilation-perfusion relationships in interstitial lung disease. Eur J Respir Dis 68:39-49,1986

6)Kapitan,K.S.,Wagner,P.D.: Linear programming analysis of $\dot{V}_A/\dot{Q}$ distributions: Limits on central moments. J Appl Physiol 60:1772-1781,1986

7)Wagner,R.P.,Saltzman,H.A.,West,J.B.: Measurement of continuous distributions of ventilation-perfusion ratios: theory. J.Appl Physiol 36:588-599,1974

8)Wagner,P.D.,Dantzker,D.R.,Dueck,R.,de Polo, J.L., Wasserman,K.,and West,J.B.: Distribution of ventilation-perfusion ratios in patients with interstitial lung disease. Chest 69(suppl.):256-257,1976

9)Yokoyama,T.,Farhi,L.E.: Study of ventilation-perfusion. ratio distribution in the anesthetized dog by multiple inert gas washout. Respir Physiol 3:166-176,1967

Pathophysiology Based on BAL Findings

J. Chretien, A. Venet, D. Israel-Biet, B. Herer, and C. Danel

Laennec Hospital, Clinique de Pneumo-phtisiologie, INSERM, Paris, France

ABSTRACT

A review of BAL findings in interstitial pneumonia of unknown etiology (IPUE) based on a personal experience of 2366 patients with complete documentation and follow-up has helped to delineate the place of BAL for a patho physiological approach. In an overview of the main data given by BAL, we successively analyse information on fixed lung structures and those related to the sequence of events (from alveolitis to the fibrosis). Critical evaluation of the method is presented. The exact place of BAL in the understanding of the mechanisms and in the course of IPUE is discussed.

Bronchoalveolar lavage (BAL) is now a current procedure in clinical practice for the diagnosis of various pulmonary disorders and for the patient follow-up. The technics of <u>recovering, the handling of samples and the expression of results are now well codified</u>. (1)
Our own experience now concerns more than 4.000 BAL in 2.366 patients with a complete case-history including clinical findings and clinical follow-up (at least 2 years after the 1st BAL). A great majority of these patients

presents with pulmonary interstitial disorders (ILD) which are clinically, radiologically and functionally documented (n=1324). Whatever the type of interstitial involvement, the disorder may result in activation, multiplication and functional differenciation of lung fibroblasts which represent 36% of the total alveolar parenchymal cells. This phenomenon induces collagen hypertrophy and imbalance in collagen type ratio, altering the lung function.(2,3)

If we exclude ARDS which is a particular feature owing to its mechanism and its occurences, ILD, whether subacute or chronic, may be classified (Table 1) in diseases of identified etiology and diseases of unknown etiology (IPUE) (4). Among the latter, some are nosologically defined on biological and clinical bases. For others, nosology has not been defined or is still debated (5).The second group will be given special attention. Many methods can be used routinely or optionally to investigate ILD, namely in IPUE. Most of them may be applied in clinical practice, but the question is : **Can BAL provide information on the triggering factors, the unfolding and the sequence of local events in IPUE which would help understand the mechanisms and pathophysiology of the disease ?** That is the question we have to assess in a brief critical overview based on our current experience of this procedure.

To try and answer this question, we must first clearly delineate the place of BAL. The following diagram helps understand its contribution as regards two components.
One is the interstitial lung structures which are the ground of the disease initiated by an "X" agent. The other is the reflection of inflammatory events, so-called <u>alveolitis</u>, expressed by blood-dependent cells transiently resident in lung. BAL directly informs on the latter and only indirectly on the former, in terms of types and degree of inflammatory process and of mediators.

The pathophysiological approach through BAL in
IPUE involves 2 types of information:

1. The alteration of pulmonary structures
2. The sequence of events and determinants.

1. ALTERATION OF PULMONARY STRUCTURES

1.1. Early damages of anatomical structures.

One of the earliest consequence of cell damage on
lung structures, namely in endothelial or
pneumocyte type I cell, is an increase of
permeability changes leading to an influx between
interstitial and blood cell compartments.
Chemo-attraction may contribute to the cell
transfer. Increase of permeability may result in
an increase in BAL of plasma proteins of low
molecular weight (such as albumin -67.000
daltons- which is the reference in biochemical
evaluation in BAL) (6,7) or may result in the
presence of large size proteins such as IgM
(about 900.000 daltons). Indirect information
may also be given by Surfactant composition in
BAL, reflecting type II cells damage.
Simultaneously, in alveolar lumen, the transfer
of marginated and circulating leucocytes (PMN,
lymphocytes and monocytes) from blood
capillaries, into alveolar lumen is also a good
indicator of early damage of blood-air membrane.

The presence of erythrocytes may be another good
indicator but of less reliable interpretation.
In fact these data are schematic in chronic
conditions and do not allow a precise analysis of
early lung alteration conversely to experimental
models or to ARDS in man.

1.2. Types of elementary lesions (granulomatous and non-granulomatous interstitial disorders).

I.L.D. are generally divided into granulomatous
and non-granulomatous diseases (8). The term
"granuloma" may in fact concern various types of
inflammatory cell clusters, bearing different
meanings.

* The most common in IPUE is <u>the sarcoid or sarcoid-like granuloma</u> (syn. tuberculoid granuloma) which can be observed in sarcoidosis, but also in various conditions ranging from genetic immune depletion (e.g. granulomatous familial disease) to excessive immune response (e.g. hypersensitivity to various agents).
This type of granuloma formation generally implies a strong activation of lymphocyte CD4 (T-Helper-inducer) and a strong cell-to-cell interaction. Epithelioid cell and giant cell result from macrophage activation and transformation but accompanied by phagocyte dysfunction (9).
Whether the cell analysis of BAL gives clear guidance in identifying this type of granuloma is questionable. Studies of epithelioid and giant cells by Electron microscopy (E.M) have demonstrated particular features in various sarcoid or sarcoid-like granulomas.

Is it possible to find this pattern in cells recovered by broncho-alveolar lavage ? This problem cas reviewed in collaboration with the Brompton Group. Lavages were performed in 28 sarcoïd patients and lavage cells were studied by transmission electron microscopy and compared with lavage cells from 17 control subjects and with lung tissue granulomas from 5 sarcoid patients (IO).

Subplasmalemmal linear densities were never observed in control lavage specimens. Fully developed epithelioid cells were not identified in lavage specimens but differences were nevertheless found between the lavage cells from sarcoid patients and from control subjects: in sarcoidosis alveolar macrophages were larger, with better developed pseudopodia and clearer polarity. Less nuclear heterochromatin was observed with larger but less electron-dense lysosomes. In sarcoidosis a variable proportion of 10 to 70% of the lavage macrophages show morphologic features of activation.

* In <u>histiocytosis X</u>, BAL is much more informative on the nature and type of lung anatomical changes. Eosinophilic granuloma comprises an increase in the total number of phagocytic cells and a significant percentage of dendritic cells (Langerhans cells): identification of these cells can be performed by E.M. analysis evidencing characteristic cytoplasmic organelles (X bodies or Langerhans cell granules). Techniques using monoclonal antibodies to Langerhans cells (OKT6) may afford a more rapid and sensitive analysis. Nevertheless, recent studies have shown that Langerhans cells could be found in the lower respiratory tract and even in the lung parenchyma in normal subjects (11). Furthermore, alteration in the epithelium of the lower respiratory tract and distal lung seems to be an important stimulus in attracting Langerhans cells to the lung. Thus two distinct conditions known to produce epithelial abnormalities in the lower respiratory tract (cigarette smoking and fibrosing alveolitis) are associated with the presence of increased numbers of Langerhans cells: up to 7% of the cells recovered by bronchoalveolar lavage. Consequently presence of Langerhans cells in BAL detected either by OKT6 monoclonal antibodies or by ultrastructural analysis must be interpreted carefully on the basis of clinical and radiological data, since the incidence of smoking is very high among those patients (90%) (12).

* For other types of granuloma involving interstitial structures (in lymphomatoid disorders or in vasculitis), BAL does not reflect with reliable or constant accuracy the exact profile of pulmonary rearrangements. It cannot give a correct classification, nor does it provide through this classification a better approach of the disorders. The same holds for the non-granulomatous types of interstitial involvement, particularly for idiopathic pulmonary fibrosis.

1.3.   The paucity of the BAL data yield is also usual in respect of <u>topography and distribution</u> of the alterations in different anatomical areas of the lung.
BAL in different sites may bring information on diffuse interstitial processes when there is a patchy   distribution,   but   it   is   of   little theoretical value.

In   terms   of   specific   localisation   (to discriminate bronchial, vascular or alveolar wall lesions)   BAL   findings   are   generally disappointing.   Vascular lesions (angeitis) may be   suggested by the number of siderophages in BAL,   but the source of alveolar bleeding cannot be   ascertained (13,14).   Red blood cells alone (without   siderophages) in BAL cannot warrant any conclusions.

More   interesting   could   be   an   approach   of <u>bronchiolitis obliterans organizing pneumonia</u> (15).   Besides the various mechanisms and agents likely   to   cause   such a   form   of   interstitial disease (e.g.   toxic fumes or vapor, drugs as well as connective tissue disorders or viral infections), there are idiopathic forms and numerous   apparently idiopathic   cases   have recently been collected in Japan. The presence of vacuolated histiocytes in BAL and even of numerous giant cells - related to bronchial destruction- might guide the diagnosis of the disease.   In fact this aspect is absolutely not specific in our experience and does not eliminate the possibility of lung thesaurismosis. It does not   exclude   other   causes   of   interstitial disorders   particularly   in   tracheobronchial aspiration due to permanent or subpermanent gastrooesophageal reflux with or without hiatal hernia. We have had a typical example of this in our series.

2. SEQUENCE OF EVENTS AND DETERMINANTS

2.1.   On the basis of the BAL data, it is now usual   to   consider   that   initial   phenomenon, whatever the cause of IPUE is represented by an alveolar inflammation ("alveolitis") (2,5) but the meaning of such a word in term of interstitial inflammatory process is not always clear. French authors usually separate <u>luminal</u> alveolitis from <u>parietal</u> alveolitis. The former is characterized by inflammatory cells in alveolar lumen and this feature may lead to a modification of the global bronchoalveolar cell number and of their distribution. But, the latter predominantly affects alveolar walls and may not be expressed by BAL data.

However a classification of various types of alveolitis has been set out on the basis of BAL. For various IPUE, it has been considered as giving informations on the mechanisms implied in the disease. According to the predominance of a given cell type (namely one of the 3 keys cells of lung immune response: alveolar macrophages, lymphocytes, neutrophils) and also according to the abnormal presence of unfrequent or unusual cell types , various interpretations and meanings of alveolitis have been put forward in IPUE. The various interpretations are related to the relevant cell functions. For instance, lymphocytic alveolitis historically has been considered important in sarcoidosis (8,9) for the mechanisms of the disease, and for the degree of activity and prognosis.

In fact, lymphocytic alveolitis is free from all specificity and may be found in many clinical occurences (9), with various lymphocytic phenotypes ratio and degree of activation to be clearly defined. Most of them are common to the state of lymphocytic activation in any immune process and few are specific to a particular antigenic situation.

In fact, lymphocytic alveolitis is a notion which may require an exact knowledge of:
- the clinical context when the alveolitis appeared,
- the associated cytological context (macrophages

+),
- the main phenotypes involved (CD4, CD8),
- the activation phenotypes (HLADR+, IL2+ receptors, etc...),
- the functional phenotypes (T8, leu15-, cytotoxic etc...).
- the capacity of proliferation and/or of IL2 secretion induced by antigens possibly responsible, etc..
- the evaluation of evidencing of a true cytotoxicity to a relevant antigen (HIV in LIP/HIV), corroborating the cytotoxic phenotype.

* The increase in number <u>of macrophages</u> is also not specific. It may result from various endogenous and exogenous lung aggressions (16). Increase in number of macrophages is common in sarcoidosis and idiopathic pulmonary fibrosis as well. The content of macrophages is more important for any etiological approach. Determination of subpopulations (17)according to various procedures (e.g. monoclonal antibodies; albumin density gradient) could be useful but their exact value is not yet clearly assessed.

* More interesting could be <u>the increase of neutrophils</u> in BAL which is usually considered as symptomatic of an evolution towards fibrosis in sarcoidosis and sometimes as characteristic of idiopathic pulmonary fibrosis (2,8,9).

In fact, the neutrophils alveolitis must be interpreted according to the clinical context, number of neutrophils and cytological environment. A high percentage of PMM suggests only an infectious process. A low increase of PMM may suggest an increasing permeability of the alveolar-capillary membrane. It may precede alterations of the lung structures, and by enzymatic activity may lead to some alterations of these structures (18).
If a moderate increase (<20%) may suggest on the one hand an evolution towards fibrosis, on the other, it provides no etiological information on the initiators of the fibrotic process.

This may be observed in idiopathic pulmonary fibrosis, sarcoidosis and collagen vascular disease as well. It does not exclude a hypersensitivity phenomenon at the onset, where it is often accompanied by red blood cells in BAL, before occurrence of predominant lymphocytosis.

* Other unusual types of cells may be observed in BAL in IPUE such as eosinophils , mast cells, dendritic cells, or siderophages (1). <u>Eosinophils</u> may suggest a hypersensitivity phenomenon and may be observed in histiocytosis X with dendritic cells. In fact, it is common to all the varieties of interstitial fibrosis, including idiopathic and collagen vascular disease. <u>Siderophages</u> in BAL fluid may be observed in small quantities in normals. But, large amounts of siderophages may be seen in connective tissue disease or in granulomatosis angeitis (13,14). Such lesions have been related to be induced by immune complexes (I.C). IC have been detected in BAL particularly in idiopathic pulmonary fibrosis, and considered as significant of local auto-immune disease. It may accompany renal disorders, suggesting a Goodpasture's syndrome and leading to advocate special therapy.

In fact, even when immune complex are isolated in BAL, the meaning of their presence is debatable and we currently lack comparative and large-scale studies on their place and role as well as on complement system in BAL.

2.2. <u>BAL and disease activity and evolutivity in IPUE.</u>

As reported in litterature, there has been considerable enthusiasm about the use of BAL in assessing disease activity, prognosis and therapeutic management. In various forms of IPUE for instance in sarcoidosis, or idiopathic pulmonary fibrosis or broncholitis obliterans, the degree of inflammatory process apparently reflected by BAL has seemed to provide information for instance on the degree of lymphocytosis in sarcoidosis or the degree of neutrophils content as indirect index of fibrogenesis. Comparative studies for various interstitial disorders but particularly for sarcoidosis or idiopathic pulmonary fibrosis (4,7,8,9) did not yield significant informations in terms of sensitivity and specificity of such particularly various markers in BAL for collagen dysfunction and/or inflammatory cell activities.

2.3 BAL and fibrogenesis

Besides neutrophils control and on the basis of BAL data, is it possible to approach the imbalance in collagen structure or metabolism in man and to follow-up sequential events toward interstitial fibrogenesis in IPUE? This approach may be performed by direct biochemical evaluation in BAL and/or by in vitro studies.

* Biochemical evaluation in BAL may inform on the different components of lung matrix composed predominantly of collagen, elastin, glycosamino-glycans and fibronectin and giving an insight into injury and repair of this matrix (19).

Alveolar macrophages play a major role in the increase, activation and differenciation of fibroblasts. Fibronectin and macrophage-derived growth factor are two mediators which can modulate the expansion of fibroblast numbers. Fibronectin , a 440,000 dalton glycoprotein is both a potent chemotactic factor of recruitment and a factor of attachment for fibroblasts.

The alveolar macrophage-derived growth factor is a I8.000 dalton protein growth factor which helps stimulation and replication of fibroblasts (20).

In interstitial lung fibrogenesis there is an increase of the respective amounts of the two mediators in BAL. Glucocorticoid therapy in idiopathic IPUE does not suppress their release (21). Their secretion may be regulated by other

AM secretions such as PGE2. Nevertheless, due to the non specificity of such mediators we cannot only obtain informations on   the nature   of alveolar macrophage dysfunction in early stages.

* Cell cultures of BAL may provide interesting data on fibrotic processes in ILD. Cultures of BAL in ILD may show presence of fibroblasts and as demonstrated it is possible with a long term cultures (8-IO weeks) to select fibroblasts among the other cells.

Presence of fibroblasts-often in large quantities may   be interpreted as   the   expression   of interstitial cell migration into alveolar spaces through gaps in the epithelial basement membrane, but may correspond to an intraalveolar fibrosis which has been considered as an essential factor in the remodeled lung, resulting namely from fibronectin activity of AM.Squamous epithelial cells from alveolar epithelium may be observed in such cases symptomatic of intraalveolar fibrosis (22). This type of fibrosis represents a variety of fibrosis in the interstitial lung disorders close   to   endobronchial   proliferation   of obliterans bronchiolitis.

In our protocole, the fibroblast proliferation in long-term   cultured   BAL   from   interstitial processes is correlated with the lymphocytosis and/or the number of neutrophils in the initial lavage.   A nodular growth with cell fibroblasts and macrophages rearrangement mimiking granuloma is obtained in cultures from BAL of sarcoid patients.

2.4 <u>BAL and unexpected events.</u>

* In the course of the IPUE, BAL may inform on unexpected events distinct from the conditions of occurence and activity of the alveolitis as well as from fibrotic process. It concerns the place and nature of surinfections in the course of the disease and other intercurrent events such as the development of cancer from pulmonary interstitial inflammation and fibrosis.

A local immune depletion often facilitated by immuno-suppressiv drugs (steroids or azathioprine) may explain the frequency of surinfection of various types and of inequal severity during the course of the IPUE. It plays a role in the prognosis of the disease inducing an evolutive process. Various types of microorganisms of common type (e.g streptococcus pneumoniae, Hemophilus influenzae or others) may be involved but opportunistic infections are possible including mycobacteriae (Tuberculosis and atypical mycobacteriae). Such opportunistic infections are rare in Sarcoidosis, frequent in Histiocytosis X and even more frequent in Chronic idiopathic interstitial pneumonia. They may be a source of misinterpretation leading to their incrimination in inducing the interstitial disease.

Conversely, non specific interstitial pneumonitis may occur in HIV infection in the absence of any identifiable infectious pulmonary pathogens. Their mechanism is still debated: masked opportunistic infection, use of chemotherapy for Kaposi sarcome, drug induced interstitial pneumonitis, lymphoid interstitial pneumonia are most commonly given as interpretation.

* The changes of immune response in IPUE and consequently the decrease of lung clearance against pollutants (infecting or not)) is of great theoretical importance. In Sarcoidosis and in idiopathic IPUE, mineral analysis with various procedure may identify particle deposition in small amount within the lung which could be the source of misinterpretation with pneumoconiosis.

Animal models of experimental fibrosis using various procedures (Bleomycine injury, paraquat ingestion, external lung irradiation or inhalation of radio-activ material) have demonstrated the failure of pulmonary clearance during the development of a fibrotic process. A personnal experimental model using complete Freund adjuvant for inducing sarcoid granulomatosis in animals has confirmed this notion of failure in eliminating dust particles from the lung when chronic interstitial inflammatory process is engaged.

* * *

Finally, the place of BAL in a pathophysiological approach of IPUE nosologically defined or not appears to be better defined after ten years of use and proves disappointing to some extent. But certain aspects have so far probably not been sufficiently prospected by BAL and could provide useful informations. These aspects concern various points , for instance:

. The precise role of blood platelets and derived factors, so important in acute lung-injury and involved in cell activation of endothelium and in immune competent cells as well, was not thouroughly approached in chronic conditions.

. The place of mast cells which interact with T-Lymphocytes and fibroblasts for abnormal collagen deposition (e.g. graft versus host disease) (23,24).

. The dendritic cells which appear as a specific and particular system in lung immune response. .

. Also, the recent progress in the knowledge on eosinophils function should lead to a better study of their subsets and of their meaning in various interstitial disorders.

. The place of genetic factors in occurence and development of IPUE, suggested by many familial cases (25,26) and assessed by experimental interstitial lung disorders (27) and heritable disease of collagen (28) merits large prospections.

What is the place of BAl material in such a

genetic approach through molecular biology, and what is the future of collagen synthesis control and the place of BAL in qualitative and quantitative determination for the enzymatic systems implied? Prospective studies are needed in this way.

Nevertheless despite these considerations, BAL cannot answer certain questions which require other types of approach. For instance: direct study of lung structures by lung cell cultures; studies on animal models with the help of molecular biology. In that way, pneumocytes type II and endothelial cells are surely the key cells in lung homeostasis but they are virtually beyond the scope of BAL. Advances in virology may also suggest a more precise approach of etiology. Attempts have been made in this field for Sarcoidosis or Histiocytosis X, but with no success. Models with lentivirus in animals for so-called idiopathic fibrosis seem to offer a promising approach but need further researchs.

REFERENCES

1.   Chrétien, J., Iraqui, G., Venet, A., Isarel-Biet, D., Laval, A.M., Danel,C. Contibution of bronchoalveolar lavage of diagnosis in pneumology: a study of 3110 BAL performed over 10 years. Bull Int Union Tuberc 62:54-58, I987.

2.   Crystal, R.G., Bitterman, P.B., Rennard, S.I., Hance, A.J., Keogh, B.A. Interstitial lung diseases of unknown cause disorders charectized by chronic inflammation of the lower respiratory tract. New Engl J Med, 1st of 2 parts, 310:154-166,1984.   2nd of 2 parts, 310:235-244,1984.

3.   Laurent, G.J. Lung collagen: more than Scaffolding. Thorax 4:418-428,1986.

4.   Chrétien, J. Interstitial lung disease.

Clinical presentation. Postgraduate medical journal (suppl 4) to be published, 1988.

5. Hance, A.J., Crystal, R.G. Idiopathic pulmonary fibrosis. In: Recent advances in respiratory medicine. Flenley, D.C., Petty, J. edit. 1 Vol. Churchill Livingstone publ. Edinburgh, London, Melbourne, N.York, 249-287, 1983.

6. Stockley, R.A. Measurement of soluble proteins in lung secretions. Thorax, 39:241.247, 1984.

7. Reynolds, H.V., Chretien,J. Respiratory tract fluids: analysis of content and contemporary use in understanding lung diseases. In: Disease a month, 1 vol. Year book medical publ. INC Chicago, Vol XXX,5,1984.

8. Chretien, J., Danel, C. Assessment of disease activity in granulomatous and non granulomatous interstitial lung disease. Therapeutic implication. In: Alveolitis (Blom-Bülow, B., Mossberg, B., Nikander, K., Selroos, O., edit, 1 vol, SLMF-Draco publ, Lund, 93-111, 1986.

9. Chrétien, J., Venet,A., Danel, C., Israel-Biet,D., Sandron, D., Arnoux, A. Broncho-alveolar lavage in Sarcoidosis. Respiration, 48,222-230, 1985.

10. Danel, C., Dewar, A., Corrin, B., Turner-Warwick, M., Chrétien, J. Ultrastructural changes in bronchoalveolar lavage cells in sarcoidosis and comparison with the tissue granuloma. Am J Pathol,112, 7-17, 1983.

11. Hance, A., Basset, F., Saumon, G., Danel, C., Valeyre, D., Battesti, J.P., Chrétien, J., Georges, P. Smoking and interstitial lung disease. The effect of cigarette smoking on the incidence of pulmonary Histiocytosis X and Sarcoidosis. Ann NY Acad Sci, 288,643-656, 1983.

12. Soler, P., Valeyre, D., Georges, R., Battesti, J.P., Basset, F., Hance, A. The role of epithelial abnormalities in recruiting Langerhans cells to the lower respiratory tract. Am Rev Resp Dis, 133, A.243, 1986.

13. Alveolar haemorrhage. Lancet, 1, 853-854,1985.

14. Thomas, H.M, Irwin, R.S. Classification of diffuse intrapulmonary hemorrhage. Chest, 68, 483-484, 1975.

15. Scully, R.E., Mark, E.J., Mc Neely, B.U. Case records of the Massachusetts general hospital. New Engl J of Med, 314, 1627-1635, 1986.

16. Dubois, R.M. The alveolar macrophage. Thorax, 40,321-327,1985.

17. Campbell, D.A., Poulter, L.W., Dubois, R.M. Phenotypic analysis of alveolar macrophages in normal subjects and in patients with interstitial lung disease. Thorax, 41,429-434,1986.

18. Parson, P.E., Sugahara, K., Cott, G.R., Mason, R.J., Henson, P.M. The effect of neutrophil migration and prolonged neutrophil contact on epithelial permeability. Amer J Path, 129,302-32,1987.

19. Turino, G.M. The lung parenchyma. A dynamic matrix. Am Rev Resp Dis, 132,1324-1334,1985.

20. Rennard, S.I., Bitterman, P.B., Crystal, R.G. Response of the lower respiratory tract to injury-mechanisms of repair of the parenchymal cells of the alveolar wall. Chest, 84,735.739,1983.

21. Lacronique, J.G., Rennard, S.I., Bitterman, P.B., Ozaki,T., Crystal,R.G. Alveolar macrophages in idiopathic pulmonary fibrosis have

glucocorticoid receptors, but glucocortid therapy does not suppress alveolar macrophage release of fibronectin and alveolar macrophage derived growth factor. Am Revv Resp dis, 130,450-456,1984.

22.   Fukuda, Y., Ishizaki, M., Masuda,Y., Kimura, G., Kawanami, O., Masugi, Y. The role of intraalveolar fibrosis in the process of pulmonary structural remodeling in patients with diffuse alveolar damage. Am J Pathol, 126,171-182,1987.

23.   Claman, H.N. Mast cells, T.cells and abnormal fibrosis. Immunology today, 6,192-195,1985.

24.   Flint, K.C., Leung, K.B.P., Hudspith, B.N., Pearce, F.L., Geraint-James, D., Johnson, N.Mcl. Bronchoalveolar mast cells in sarcoidosis: increased numbers and accentuation of mediator release. Thorax, 41, 94-99,1986.

25.   Sansonetti, M., Sandron, D., Pin, I., Labrune, S., Vervloet, D., Dumur, J.P., Charpin, J., Chrétien, J. Fibrose pulmonaire intersititielle diffuse familiale. Etude d'une famille. Rev Mal Resp, 2,75-81,1985.

26.   Bitterman, P.B., Crystal, R.G. Is there a fibrotic gene ? Chest, 78,549-550, 1980.

27.   Rossi, G.A., Szapiel, S., Ferrans, V.J., Crystal, R.G. Susceptibility to experimental interstitial lung disease is modified by immune and non-immune-related genes. Am Rev Resp Dis, 135,448-455,1987.

28.   Prockop, D.J., Kivirikko, K.I., Heritable diseases of collagen. New Eng J Med, 311,376-386,1984.

Surfactant Analysis in Cryptogenic Fibrosing Alveolitis

Patricia L. Haslam and David A. Hughes

Cell Biology Unit, Department of Cardiothoracic Surgery, National Heart and Lung Institute, London, UK

SUMMARY

We have recently demonstrated that many untreated patients with idiopathic pulmonary fibrosis/cryptogenic fibrosing alveolitis (CFA) have abnormally reduced proportions of the phosphatidylglycerol (PG) component of the pulmonary surfactant system in bronchoalveolar lavage fluids. Reductions in PG have also been reported in an experimental model of pulmonary fibrosis induced by bleomycin coinciding with alterations in lung compliance. A relationship with clinical progress is also suggested in CFA from our observation that PG levels increase to normal in patients responding to corticosteroids, while in non-responders PG levels fall or remain abnormally low. Percentages of inflammatory cells and sphingomyelin also fall in responders suggesting improvement is linked with suppression of inflammatory tissue damage. The major components of surfactant, including PG, have marked immunosuppressive properties which may help to protect normal lungs by preventing uncontrolled immune reactions to the numerous agents we inhale with each breath. Whether the reductions in PG in lung lining fluid of patients with CFA predispose to inflammation, and whether functional deficiency of the surfactant system is a contributory factor in this disease, are aspects of the pathogenesis of CFA which need to be investigated.

BACKGROUND

The 'pulmonary surfactant system' is the term given to
the fluid which lines the epithelial surfaces of the
lungs. It contains highly surface-active components,
which form a monomolecular film at the air-liquid
interface, capable of generating a film pressure when
the molecules are compressed which opposes the
increasing forces of surface tension thus preventing
alveolar collapse at low lung volumes. The system is
mainly composed of lipids (approximately 90%) with some
proteins and carbohydrates (1). The lipids are mainly
phospholipids, and dipalmitoylphosphatidylcholine is
the major surface active component.
Phosphatidylglycerol (PG) is the second major
phospholipid component and there are a number of minor
components (1). These lipid components of surfactant
are synthesised and secreted by the type II alveolar
epithelial cells and are stored within lamellar bodies
in the cytoplasm prior to release into the alveoli.
Adsorption of molecules to the surface film from the
subphase then takes place in a process which appears to
be in a state of continuous regeneration.

The clinical consequences of defects in the pulmonary
surfactant system were first demonstrated by Avery and
Mead (2), who showed that infants with respiratory
distress syndrome of the newborn (IRDS) had
functionally deficient pulmonary surfactant due to
immaturity in the alveolar epithelium. During foetal
development, surfactant is produced which contains no
PG, but very high levels of phosphatidylinositol (PI).
At final maturation, there is a switch from PI to PG
production, and deficiency of PG has proved a reliable
predictor of IRDS (3). PG- deficient surfactant has
also been reported in patients with adult respiratory
distress syndrome (4), where it appears to be a
secondary consequence of lung injury, rather than due
to a defect of maturation. Changes in lung surfactant
have been reported in a number of other pulmonary
diseases but their role in pathogenesis has been
relatively little explored.

The aim of our study was to explore whether changes in
the surfactant system also occur in patients with
interstitial pulmonary fibrosis of unknown cause. These

patients invariably have severe damage to the alveolar
epithelium with loss of type I cells, and many patients
have evidence of type II cell proliferation indicating
regeneration and repair of the alveolar epithelium (5).
Patients with interstitial pulmonary fibrosis also
demonstrate an increased rate of clearance of
aerosolised Tc-DTPA from the lungs indicating an
abnormal increase in epithelial permeability (6).
Changes in surfactant phospholipids, in particular
increases in PC and PI with consequent qualitative
reductions in PG have recently been reported following
induction of lung damage in an experimental model of
pulmonary fibrosis induced by bleomycin (7). We have,
therefore, examined the phospholipid composition of
lung lining fluid obtained by bronchoalveolar lavage
(BAL) from patients with cryptogenic fibrosing
alveolitis (synonym idiopathic pulmonary fibrosis); and
have also investigated patients before and after
treatment with corticosteroids to explore whether
changes in surfactant might be a contributory factor in
disease progression.

CHANGES IN PHOSPHATIDYLGLYCEROL IN LUNG LINING FLUID FROM PATIENTS WITH CFA

We have investigated the phospholipid composition of
pulmonary surfactant from patients with CFA by
analysing bronchoalveolar lavage samples from a group
of 32 patients, all having lone lung disease and all
with a biopsy confirmed diagnosis. There were 25 males
and 7 females, the mean age was 23 ± 12 years and the
majority (29) were current or ex-smokers.

Bronchoalveolar lavage (BAL) samples were obtained from
the lateral segment of the right lower lobe of the lung
of each patient via a fibreoptic bronchoscope using a
standard technique (8). 240 mls of pre-warmed (37 °C)
buffered saline was introduced in 60 ml installations,
and the aspirated fluid pooled and centrifuged at a low
speed of 300g for 10 minutes at 4 °C to remove cells.
The supernatant fluid was recovered and stored at − 70
°C prior to analysis. This separation procedure was
completed within 20 minutes of lavage to avoid any
contamination of the fluid with lipids from the
membranes of cells _in vitro_. Phospholipid analysis was
achieved by thawing and extracting the total lipids

from the supernatants using the methanol-chloroform
extraction procedure of Bligh and Dyer (9).   After
extraction, the lipids were evaporated to dryness under
reduced pressure at 20 °C in a rotary evaporator, and
re-suspended in chloroform-methanol (9:1 v/v) to 40 mg
lipid/ml under nitrogen at -40 °C.   The phospholipids
present in each sample were determined using the TLC
system developed by Gilfillan et al (10) to provide
clear separation of lung phospholipids, employing
silica gel plates (20 cm + 20 cm) and chloroform-
methanol-petroleum ether (BP 35-60 °C) - acetic acid -
boric acid (40:20:30:10:1.8 vol/vol/vol/vol/wt) as the
developing solvent.   The lavage extracts were run
simultaneously alongside known amounts of eight
standard preparations of purified phospholipids and,
after the plates were dried, the lipids were visualised
by charring at 180 °C for 10 minutes using the method
of Bitmen and Wood (11).   The plates were read using a
Shimazu scanner, and the amount of each phospholipid
present and its proportion of the total phospholipid
content was calculated for each sample by comparison
with the reference standards.   The total phospholipid
yield was calculated by relating the sum of the amounts
of the individual phospholipids present to the amount
of the total lipid applied to the TLC plate.

A control group of 17 patient volunteers without
evidence of parenchymal lung disease was also studied.
These individuals were undergoing routine bronchoscopy
for investigation of persistent cough or minor
haemoptysis.   There were 11 males and 6 females, the
mean age was 45 ± 16 years and 16 were current or ex-
smokers.   Ethics approval was obtained for the study
and all subjects gave their informed consent.

The results of the BAL fluid phospholipid analysis
showed that, before treatment, the CFA patients had
significantly reduced proportions of PG (Figure 1) but
higher proportions of sphingomyelin (Figure 2) compared
with the control subjects ($p < 0.01$).   There was no
significant difference in the total phospholipid
level/ml of lavage fluid compared with the controls,
but there is recognised difficulty in interpreting
quantitative results because of the unknown dilution
factor during the lavage procedure.   For this reason,
we have focused on evaluating the relative proportions

of each of the major surfactant phospholipid classes in
BAL fluids in our study. This approach seems
justifiable since proportionate changes in the relative
amounts of surface-active to non-surface active
components are known to be capable of resulting in
deficiency of surfactant function.

In total, 15 (47%) of the patients with CFA had PG
levels below the range of the control subjects, and 9
(28%) had increases in SM. We have reported these
findings in preliminary form (12) and in detail (13)
and Robinson PC et al (14) have obtained independent
confirmation.

Figure 1   Figure 2

% PHOSPHATIDYLGLYCEROL   % SPHINGOMYELIN

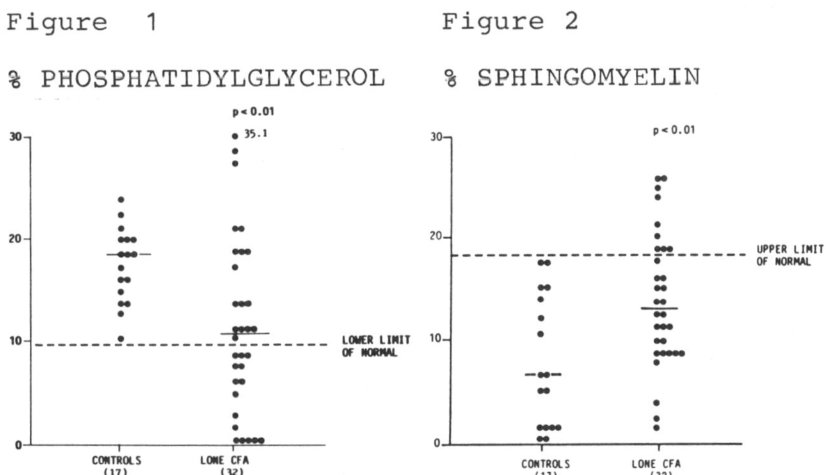

EFFECT OF CORTICOSTEROID THERAPY

In view of the need for better prognostic markers in
CFA, we explored whether the pre-treatment changes in
PG and SM in these patients might be of value in
predicting subsequent response of the patients to
corticosteroid treatment. However, no significant
differences were observed between the initial values of
either PG or SM for patients who subsequently showed
maintained improvement following one-year treatment
with prednisolone compared to patients who either
remained clinically stable, or who deteriorated over
the same follow-up period. The initial dosage of

prednisolone was 60 mg/day, continued for 4 weeks, then reduced following a standardised regimen over the next 12 weeks to a maintenance dose of not below 20 mg alternate days. Response was defined as maintained objective improvement in percent normal predicted FVC of greater than 10%, and in the radiographic profusion score of at least 4 on the modified UC/ILO point scheme.

To evaluate whether changes in PG and SM might reflect, rather than predict, clinical disease progression a different approach was used. This involved obtaining follow-up lavage samples from 14 of the patients in the study group (total 2 or 3 lavages) over a mean period of 14 ± 12 months. Five of the 14 patients responded to prednisolone treatment, but 9 were non-responders (4 stable and 5 deteriorated). The 5 responders all had a significant increase in %PG to within the normal range by their second lavage (p < 0.005) (mean duration of treatment 8.2 ± 2.5 months), and this trend was continued or maintained in those who had a third lavage. In contrast, the 9 non-responders showed either a relative decrease in %PG at second lavage or levels which remained below the lower limit of the control range (mean duration of treatment 6 ± 2.9 months). The responders also showed a trend of fall in %SM by the second lavage. These observations suggest that changes in these phospholipid components may provide some indication of the extent of alveolar epithelial damage and repair in CFA patients.

WHY DO THESE CHANGES OCCUR?

At this stage in our knowledge, explanations for the mechanisms leading to these changes in surfactant in CFA patients can only be speculative. The low levels of PG in infant respiratory distress syndrome are due to imbalance in the synthetic pathways of PG relative to PI which share a common precursor, CDP-diacylglycerol. The evidence suggests this is due to high levels of plasma myo-inositol which favour the synthesis of PI and suppress synthesis of PG (15,16). However, it is unlikely that such a mechanism is operative in CFA because our evidence does not suggest that the falls in PG are accompanied by a compensatory increase in PI in this disease.

A more likely explanation for the changes in surfactant composition in CFA is that they may be a consequence of damage to the alveolar epithelium. In this respect, it is of interest that regenerating type II cells have been reported to produce surfactant which is deficient in phosphatidylglycerol (17,18). Tissue damage could also be a possible explanation for the increased proportions of SM in lavage fluids from CFA patients, since SM is present in significantly higher levels in tissue and plasma than in lung lining fluid (10,7). Proportions of PG are also lower in tissue and plasma compared with lung lavage. Increased permeability and leakage of plasma components from the capillaries to alveolar spaces in CFA is indicated by significantly increased levels of albumin in the lavage fluids of these patients (19), and in the present study we have observed significant correlation between the levels of albumin (μg/ml) and sphingomyelin (μg/ml) in our CFA patients who failed to respond to steroids ($r_S = 0.77$, $p < 0.005$).

Finally, the possibility that the surfactant changes in CFA may be a consequence of the increased numbers of inflammatory cells in the lungs of these patients must also be considered. Lung biopsies demonstrate marked lymphocytic infiltrates in the interstitial tissues and accumulations of alveolar macrophages in the air spaces of CFA patients, while bronchoalveolar lavage samples generally contain increased numbers of neutrophils and also eosinophils in some cases (20). Enzymes and oxidants released from activated granulocytes and macrophages could either directly damage the surfactant system, or have an indirect effect by damaging the alveolar epithelium. In the serial lavage studies we conducted in 14 of our CFA patients, we observed that the percentages of inflammatory cells fell to within the normal range in the responders, but remained elevated in the non-responders. In addition, there was an overall inverse correlation between higher percentages of inflammatory cells and lower levels of PG in this patient group ($r_S = -0.49$, $p < 0.01$). We conclude that clinical improvement in CFA and the return towards normal of PG and SM levels are associated with suppression of inflammatory tissue damage.

WHAT MIGHT BE THE POSSIBLE CONSEQUENCES?

It is unclear whether the observed alterations in the
pulmonary surfactant system contribute to the
mechanisms of progression in CFA, or are merely a
consequence of the underlying disease without
functional effects. The functional importance of PG in
the surfactant system is still debated, and animal
studies have revealed that PG-deficient surfactant does
not appear to adversely affect lung function (21).
However, there is evidence suggesting that PG may be of
greatest importance in establishing the surfactant
layer at the alveolar air interface at the time of
birth (16). It has also been reported that PG modifies
the physical properties of surfactant to improve its
efficiency (22)   and that, in the presence of PG and
calcium, lipoprotein complexes are more readily
adsorbed from the subphase and spread at the air-liquid
interface (23). On the other hand, increases in the
proportions of SM relative to diphosphatidyl in
amniotic fluid PC are known to predict functional
deficiency of surfactant leading to IRDS (24).

An alternative possible consequence of reductions in PG
and increases in SM in CFA, is that this may provide an
environment within the alveolar spaces which is more
conducive to the development of inflammation. This is
suggested by our recent studies showing that normal
pulmonary surfactant from humans, pigs and rabbits can
markedly suppress the induction of lymphocyte
proliferative responses to mitogens and alloantigens
(25) supporting the earlier findings of Ansfield et al
(26) using canine pulmonary surfactant. We have
further shown that while the major phospholipid
components of surfactant, including PG are
immunosuppressive, other minor components including SM
are immunostimulatory (27). This has led us to
propose the hypothesis that alterations in surfactant
in CFA may result in inefficient immunoregulation and
be a pro-inflammatory factor.

Our observations that proportions of PG and SM return
towards normal in CFA patients responding to
corticosteroids suggests that improvement may to some
extent relate to an influence of steroids on surfactant
synthesis. The ability of corticosteroids to stimulate

PC synthesis has been demonstrated in cultured foetal
rabbit lung (28) and the therapeutic benefits of using
Betamethasone during pregnancy to stimulate synthesis
of foetal pulmonary surfactant to reduce the risk of
IRDS has been demonstrated (29). The failure of
corticosteroid therapy to elevate PG in non-responding
patients with CFA may reflect the extent of damage to
the type II surfactant-producing alveolar epithelial
cells at the time of commencement of therapy. The more
favourable response of younger CFA patients with
shorter duration of disease to corticosteroids would be
in keeping with this suggestion (30).

CONCLUSION

In conclusion, we report that reduced proportions of
PG frequently occur in lavage samples of
untreated patients with CFA and may reflect the extent of
damage to the alveolar epithelium. Damage to the
alveolar epithelium, resulting in leakage of plasma
components and contaminants from damaged tissue cells
into the lung lining fluid, may also explain the
elevated levels of SM we have observed. Our observation
that proportions of these components return to
normal in patients responding to prednisolone
emphasises that further investigations are needed to
establish whether alterations to the surfactant system
may play a role in the pathogenesis of CFA.

REFERENCES

1. Rooney SA. _Am Rev Respir Dis_ 131, 439-460, 1985.
2. Avery ME & Mead J. _Am J Dis Child_ 97, 517-23,
    1959.
3. Hallman M, Kulovich M, Kirkpatrick E, Sugarman GR,
    Gluck L. _Am J Obstet Gynecol_ 125, 613-617, 1976.
4. Hallman M, Spragg R, Harrell JH, Moser KM, Gluck L.
    J Clin Invest 70, 673-83, 1982.
5. Corrin B, Dewar A, Rodriguez-Roisin R, Turner-
    Warwick M. _J Pathol_ 147, 107-19, 1985.
6. Dusser D, Mordelet-Dambrine M, Collignon MA,
    Barritault L Chretien J Huchon GJ. _Am Rev Respir
    Dis_ 129, A65, 1984.
7. Thrall RS, Sendsen CL, Shannon TH, Kennedy CA,
    Frederick DS, Grunze MF, _et al_. _Am Rev Respir Dis_
    136, 113-18, 1987.

8. Dhillon DP, Haslam PL, Townsend PJ, Primett Z, Collins JV, Turner-Warwick M. _Eur J Respir Dis_ 68, 342-50, 1986.

9. Bligh EG, Dyer WJ. _Can J Biochem Physiol_ 37, 911-17, 1959.

10. Gilfillan AM, Chu AJ, Smart DA, Rooney SA. _J Lipid Res_ 24, 1651-56, 1983.

11. Bitman J, Wood DL. _J Liq Chromatog_ 5, 1155-62, 1982.

12. Hughes DA, Haslam PL. _Am Rev Respir Dis_ 135, A30, 1987.

13. Hughes DA, Haslam PL. _Chest_ 95, 82-89, 1989.

14. Robinson PC, Watters LC, King TE & Mason RJ. _Am Rev Respir Dis_ 137, 585-591, 1988.

15. Hallman M, Enhorning G, Possmayer F. _Paediatr Res_ 19, 286-92, 1985.

16. Bourbon JR, Doucet E, Rieutort M, Pignol B, Tordet C. _Exp Lung Res_ 11, 195-207, 1986.

17. Baker G, Duck-Chong C, Cleland K, Berend N. _Chest_ 89 (suppl), 126-27, 1985.

18. Liau DF, Barrett CR, Bell ALL, Ryan SF. _J Lipid Res_ 26, 1338-44, 1985.

19. Haslam PL, Cromwell O, Dewar A & Turner-Warwick M. _Clin exp Immunol_ 44, 587-593, 1981.

20. Haslam PL, Turton CWG, Heard B, Lukoszek A, Collins JV, Salsbury AJ _et al_. _Thorax_ 35, 9-18, 1980.

21. Beppu OS, Clements JA, Goerke J. _J Appl Physiol_ 55, 496-502, 1983.

22. Hallman M, Gluck L. _J Lipid Res_ 17, 257-62, 1976.

23. King RJ, Macbeth MC. _Biochim Biophys Acta_ 647, 159-68, 1981,

24. Gluck L, Kulovich MV, Borer RC Jnr, Brenner PH, Anderson GC, Spellacy WN. _Am J Obstet Gynecol_ 109, 440 1971.

25. Wilsher ML, Hughes DA, Haslam PL. _Thorax_ 43, 354-59, 1988.

26. Ansfield MJ, Kaltreider HB, Benson BJ. Caldwell JL. _J Immunol_ 122, 1062-66, 1979.

27. Wilsher Ml, Hughes DA, Haslam PL. _Clin Exp Immunol_ 73, 117-22, 1988.

28. Gross I, Ballard PL, Ballard RA, Jones CR, Wilson CM. Endocrinology 112, 829-37, 1983.

29. Collaberative group on antenatal steroid therapy. _Am J Obstet Gynecol_ 141, 276-86, 1981.

30. Turner-Warwick M, Burrows B, Johnson A. _Thorax_ 35, 539-49, 1980.

The Value of BALF Cell Findings for Differentiation of Idiopathic UIP, BOOP, and Interstitial Pneumonia Associated with Collagen Vascular Diseases

Sonoko Nagai

Chest Disease Research Institute, Kyoto University, Kyoto, Japan

We examined bronchoalveolar lavage fluids (BALF) cell findings in patients with idiopathic usual interstitial pneumonia (UIP), idiopathic bronchiolitis obliterans organizing pneumonia (BOOP), and interstitial pneumonia associated with collagen vascular diseases (IP-CVD) and healthy individuals as controls, in terms of clinical usefulness in differentiation of these diseases. From the findings of both the increase of lymphocytes, and decrease of $CD4^+/CD8^+$ ratio in patients with BOOP, BOOP could be differentiated from UIP. The BALF cell findings in patients with IP-CVD were heterogenous: PSS was similar to UIP and others were different from UIP. No correlation was observed between BALF cell % and the degree of alveolar septal inflammation in open lung biopsy specimens in patients with UIP, BOOP, and IP-CVD.

INTRODUCTION

It is sometimes difficult to differentiate UIP, BOOP, and IP-CVD. We evaluataed the clinical usefulness of BALF cell findings in the differentiation of these diseases, and the correlation between BALF cell findings and the histopathologically observed increases of inflammatory cells in the open lung biopsy specimens.

SUBJECTS AND METHODS

SUBJECTS; Healthy individuals (n=150), were divided into three groups: nonsmokers (NS, n=64), exsmokers (EX, n=24), and smokers (S, n=62).   Exsmokers means those who have stopped smoking for at least 6 months prior to the study.   Smokers smoked more than one pack a day on the average.   Healthy individuals were further divided into male noncurrent smokers (NCS, n=55), male S (n=62), and female NS (n=33).   Each group was further divided according to age into four subgroups: 20-29, 30-39, 40-49, and 50-59 years old.   32 cases of UIP (Carrington 1978(1)) and 8 cases of BOOP (Epler, Colby 1985(2)) were diagnosed by open lung biopsy.   No treatment with corticosteroids was done to these pataients at the time lavage was performed.   No signs of infection were observed when lavaged.   All BAL were carried out within 1 month before open lung biopsy.   Patients with RA (n=12), SLE (n=5), MCTD (n=4), Sjögren's syndrome (n=5), DM-PM (n=12), and PSS (n=9) were examined.   All cases were NCS. Some of these patients were diagnosed by open lung biopsy in terms of lung lesions.   When lavaged corticosteroid and other immunosuppressive drugs were not used, and no signs of infection could be detected.

METHODS: BAL was performed by using Olympus P10 bronchofiberscope (size 4 mm).   As the site of lavage right middle lobe was usually selected, and washed by warm sterile saline (aliquat of 50 ml x 6 times).   After filtering BALF with sterile gauzes and centrifuging, the numbers of BALF recovered cells were counted.   Cell populations were counted following May-Giemsa stain. $CD4^+/CD8^+$ ratio in T cell subsets was examined by using Ortho Spectrum Type III Cytoflowmetry.

RESULTS

I. BALF CELL FINDINGS IN HEALTHY INDIVIDUALS
Effects of smoking status (Table 1): Current smoking resulted in a significant decrease of both lymphocytes % and $CD4^+/CD8^+$ ratio compared to NS and EX.   No significant difference was observed between NS and EX and so, we combined NS and EX together as NCS.

Table 1. Effects of smoking on the BALF cell findings in healthy individuals

n	Recovered cells x 10^5/ml	L %	N %	E %	OKT4$^+$/OKT8$^+$
NS 64	0.62±0.39*	12.5±1.0	0.68±0.94	0.31±0.72	2.80±1.73
S 62	2.43±1.60**	4.0±3.3**	0.84±2.00	0.17±0.44	0.97±0.68**
EX 24	0.82±0.63	12.3±11.1	1.11±3.97	0.17±0.30	2.93±2.12

L : lymphocytes, N: neutrophils, E: eosinophils
* : mean ± SD
**: Significant difference compared to NS (p<0.05)

<u>Influences of age</u> (Table 2): CD4$^+$/CD8$^+$ ratios in groups over 40 years old tended to be higher compared to younger groups. Frequency of CD4$^+$/CD8$^+$ with a ratio of more than 3.00 increased significantly in female NCS over 40 years old. A similar finding was shown in male NCS but not to a statistically significant degree. None of S showed a CD4$^+$/CD8$^+$ ratio of more than 3.00, even among those over 40 years old. From these results, it was shown that age matched control data are required for the evaluation of BALF cell findings obtained from diseased individuals. In the evaluation of BALF cell findings in UIP, BOOP, and IP-CVD we used data of BALF cell findings obtained from healthy individuals of 48-66 years old whose ages matched the ages of patients with UIP, BOOP and IP-CVD.

Table 2. Influences of age groups on the CD4$^+$/CD8$^+$ ratio in the BALF cells from healthy NCS

Ages	Males		Females		
20-29	2.09±1.04	12%* (17)**	2.32±0.89	25%	(12)
30-39	2.05±1.19	14% (14)	1.87±0.90	20%	(5)
40-49	2.85±1.96	33% (12)	4.46±1.73	75%***	(8)
50-59	3.37±2.30	42% (12)	4.56±2.69	75%***	(8)

*   Frequency of high value individuals (≧3.00)
** No. of individuals
*** Significant high frequency compared to 20-29 group

II.   BALF CELL FINDINGS IN IDIOPATHIC UIP AND BOOP (Table 3)

In patients with BOOP, 75% of them showed lymphocytosis and 63% showed a $CD4^+/CD8^+$ ratio under 1.00. In patients with UIP, 6% of them showed lymphocytosis and 35% showed lower $CD4^+/CD8^+$ ratio under 1.00. Cases with lymphycytosis and lower $CD4^+/CD8^+$ ratio were observed in 50% (4/8) in patients with BOOP and 0% (0/34) in UIP. From these results, the determination of both lymphocyte % and $CD4^+/CD8^+$ ratio are considered as useful tools for differentiating between UIP and BOOP.

Table 3.   BALF cell findings in patients with UIP and BOOP

	IP		BOOP	
	NCS (19)	S (13)	NCS (3)	S (4)
Recovered cells x10^5/ml	1.67±0.88*	2.17±1.61	2.58±1.33	7.17±8.72
L %	7.8±9.7	5.3±5.9	20.9±20.7	29.3±9.9**
N %	7.0±15.4*	2.7±4.1	7.3±3.4*	2.4±2.3
E %	4.2±6.0*	1.4±2.4*	4.2±1.9*	3.2±2.9
$CD4^+/CD8^+$	1.69±1.12*	2.24±2.84	0.67±0.37*	0.53±0.38

*   Significant difference ($p<0.05$) compared to healthy controls (NCS and S)
** Significant difference ($p<0.05$) compared to UIP group

III.   BALF CELL FINDINGS IN PATIENTS WITH IP-CVD (Table 4)

BALF cell findings in patients with IP-CVD were heterogenous but those in PSS were similar to the finding of no lymphocytosis in patients with UIP. The findings in other IP-CVD (RA, SLE, MCTD, DM-PM) were different from those in patients with UIP and PSS, in terms of an increase of lymphocytes and a decrease of $CD4^+/CD8^+$ ratio.

Table 4. BALF cell findings in patients with IP-CVD

	No.	Recovered cells x10^5/ml	L %	N %	E %	CD4$^+$/CD8$^+$
RA	12	1.47±1.41	28.1±6.5*	10.7±6.0*	1.9±1.0*	1.43±0.42*
SLE	5	3.59±0.92*	49.3±9.5*	1.6±0.7*	0.8±0.8	0.54±0.14*
MCTD	4	1.58±0.61*	21.1±8.8	3.0±1.8*	1.5±1.2*	0.70±0.20*
Sjo	5	2.61±0.84*	16.9±8.9	10.7±9.8*	0.8±0.3*	2.93±1.70*
DM/PM	12	1.58±0.41*	24.1±5.6	5.5±2.0*	0.7±0.1	1.20±0.20*
PSS	9	1.08±0.31	4.7±1*	2.8±1.6*	0.8±0.4*	2.45±0.47

 * Significant difference (p<0.05) compared to healthy
   controls (NCS)

IV. DEGREE OF ALVEEOLAR SEPTAL INFLAMMATION AND BALF
     CELL FINDINGS IN PATIENTS WITH UIP AND IP-CVD (Table
     5)
     In patients with UIP (n=34), all cases showed
alveolar septal fibrosis and 67% of them were moderate to
severe. Only 11% showed any alveolar septal inflammation
and 28% showed no inflammation. On the other hand, in
patients with IP-CVD (SLE 1, RA 4, MCTD 1, Sjogren 3, PSS
2, DM-PM 1, total n=12), all showed a finding of alveolar
septal inflammation and 64% of them were moderate to
severe. 36% showed alveolar septal fibrosis but 18%
showed no fibrosis. But there was no relationship between the significant increase of BALF lymphocytes and
the degree of alveolar septal inflammation in our histological specimens.

Table 5. Degrees of alveolar septal inflammation in
          patients with UIP and IP-CVD

	Grade	0	1	2	3
UIP	NCS(21)*	6 (28.6%)	12 (57.1)	1 (4.8)	2 (9.6)
	S(13)	4 (30.8)	8 (61.5)	1 (7.7)	0 (0)
IP-CVD	NCS(11)	0 (0)**	4 (36.4)	3 (27.3)**	4 (36.4)**

 * Number of cases
 ** Significant compared to UIP (NCS)

DISCUSSION

Although the BALF cell findings in healthy individuals were influenced by smoking status and age, the presence of diffuse pulmonary lesions in idiopathic UIP, BOOP and IP-CVD cause a significant change in BALF cell findings compared to healthy controls. From the BALF cell finding, we could find a similarity between idiopathic UIP and PSS with lack of lymphocytosis. BOOP and IP-CVD (except PSS) could be differentiated from idiopathic UIP by evaluating both the significant increase of lymphocyte % and the significant decrease of the $CD4^+/CD8^+$ ratio. BALF lymphocyte % did not always reflect the degree of alveolar septal inflammation in patients with both UIP and IP-CVD. This result was rather different from that of a previous report (3), in which BALF lymphocytosis was found in same patients with IPF and in parallel with alveolar septal inflammation and showed good response to corticosteroid. Though BALF lymphocytosis was found in patients with IP-CVD except PSS, it did not always correlate with the degree of alveolar septal inflammation. Different from granulomatous diseases, the problem of whether BALF lymphocyte % can be substituted for histology in UIP and IP-CVD remains to be reevaluated.

REFERENCES

1. Carrington, C.B., Gaensler, E.A., Coutu, R.E., FitzGerald, M.X., and Gupta, R.G. N. Engl. J. Med. 298: 801-809, 1978.
2. Epler, G.R., Colby, T.V., McLoud, T.C., Carrington, C.B., and Gaensler, E.A. N. Engl. J. Med. 312: 152-158, 1985.
3. Watters, L.C., Schwarz, M.I., Cherniack, R.E., Waldron, J.M., Dunn, T.L., Stanford, R.E., and King, T.E. Am. Rev. Respir. Dis. 135: 696-704, 1987.

Diagnostic Values of Cells, Proteins and Lipids in Bronchoalveolar Lavage Fluid (BALF) in Idiopathic Interstitial Pneumonia (IIP)

Susumu Yasuoka, Kenzi Tani, Kenzi Fuzisawa,
Yoshimi Nakanishi, Fumitaka Ohgushi, and Toshio Ozaki

*Third Department of Internal Medicine, School of Medicine, University of
Tokushima, Tokushima, Japan*

Patients with active IIP could be classified into two types by combining BALF data and the clincal picture. Type I IIP patients showed increases in % lymphocytes and IgG content in BALF,and responded to steroids. Type II IIP patients showed no increase in % lymphocytes and no prominent increase in IgG content, and did not respond to steroids and died within 12 months. The BALF findings of patients with chronic stable IIP (Type III IIP) were variable. Both % PMN (neutrophils + eosinophils) and disaturated phosphatidylcholine(DSPC) content in the BALF were not correlated with the disease activity and prognosis. The % lymphocytes was correlated with the IgG content and inversely correlated with % VC and the % PMN was inversely correlated with the DSPC content. These results indicate that an analysis of BALF is useful in diagnosing the type and activity of IIP.

INTRODUCTION

It has been reported by previous investigators that an analysis of bronchoalveolar lavage fluid (BALF) is useful in clarifying the pathogenesis of various diffuse interstitial diseases. In this report, we examined the diagnostic value of cells, proteins and disaturated phophatidylcholine (DSPC) in the BALF in diagnosing IIP.

SUBJECTS and METHODS

Subjects : 1)Normal male volunteers (NV) aged 20 to 32 years consisted of 32 nonsmokers and smokers. Control patients (CP) aged 40 to 69 years, who had localized lung lesions or complained of hemosputum but had no detectable lung lesions,consisted of 40 nonsmokers (8 males and 32 females) and 60 male smokers. These two groups were used as controls. 2) Patients with IIP consisted of 19 nonsmokers (6 males and 13 females)with a mean age of 60 years (40 to 76 years) and 22 male smokers (including 3 exsmokers) with a mean age of 64 years (50 to 77 years). 3) Patients with sarcoidosis consisted of 38 cases (11 males and 27 females) with a mean ages of 45 years (24 to 50 years),and consisted of 35 nonsmokers and 3 smokers. Patients with summer-type hypersensitivity pneumonitis (HP) consisted of 19 cases (3 males and 16 females) with a mean age of 48 years,and consisted of 17 nonsmokers and 2 smokers.

Methods :1) BAL was performed as described previously[1]. A segment or subsegment of the middle lobe or lingula was lavaged with 50 ml of saline 3 times. The BALF was centrifuged at 250 x g, and the precipitated cells were subjected to a total cell count and differential analysis of cells as described previously[1].The 250 xg supernatant was centrifuged at 27,000 x g for 40 min, and the resultant supernatant was subjected to an assay of protein components and the precipitate (white layer) was used for the disaturated phosphtidylcholine (DSPC) assay. DSPC content was measured as described previously[2]. The contents of protein components and DSPC were expressed as a concentration(μg/ml) or total amount in the BALF.

The significance for difference between the two groups was tested by Student's t-test, and the significance of correlation between the two parameters was assessed by Spermann's rank correlation coefficient.

RESULTS

I. Characteristics of cell profile of BALF from IIP patients

Fig. 1 shows cell profiles of BALF from control (NV and CP) groups and patients with IIP, sarcoidosis and HP. In both NV and CP groups, alveolar macrophages (AM) and lymphocytes constituted 85-90 % and 10 %, respectively, of total cells in nonsmokers, and the total cell number was about twice as large in smokers than in nonsmokers mainly due to an increase in AM. The total cell number of the subjects, especially smokers in the CP group, who were age-matched with IIP patients, was larger than that of the NV group.

The total cell number in BALF from IIP patients was about twice as large the CP group in nonsmokers but not significantly larger than the latter group in smokers. The mean numbers of lymphocytes, neutrophils and eosinophils were increased , but those of the AM were not significantly increased, in both nonsmokers and smokers in the IIP patients, compared with the CP group. The absolute numbers of neutrophils and eosinophils in BALF were about 10-fold larger in IIP patients than in the CP group. Absolute numbers of the lymphocytes were about 3-fold larger in IIP patients than in the CP group.

Total cell numbers in BALF from HP patients were about 5-fold larger than those from nonsmoking CP mainly due to a marked increase in lymphocytes. In this group, lymphocytes constituted about 80 % of the total cells and its absolute numbers were about 30-fold larger in this group than in the CP group. A slight increase in lymphocytes in BALF was characteristic for sarcoidosis patients. Lymphocytes constituted about 30-40 % of the total cells in BALF from patients with sarcoidosis.

Thus, a slight to mild increase of each neutrophils, eosinophils and lymphocytes were characteristic for BALF from IIP patients, in accordance with the reports of previous investigators[3-5] .

II. IgG cocentration in BALF from patients with IIP

In order to clarify characteristic in changes in IgG content in BALF from IIP patients, the mean IgG concentrations in BALF from control and patient groups were measured and are shown Fig. 2.

The IgG level in BALF from IIP patients was slightly but significantly higher than that from the CP group in both nonsmokers(p< 0.001) and smokers(p< 0.001). The increase in IgG level in IIP was almost the same as in sarcoidosis patients, but very slight compared with that in HP.

III. Relatioship between BALF data and type of IIP

The IIP patients were classified into 3 groups according to their BALF data and clinical course (Table I). Patients in an active stage were divided into Type I IIP patients who responded significantly to steroid therapy and lived over 25 months after BAL, and in Type II IIP patients who did not respond or only slightly responded

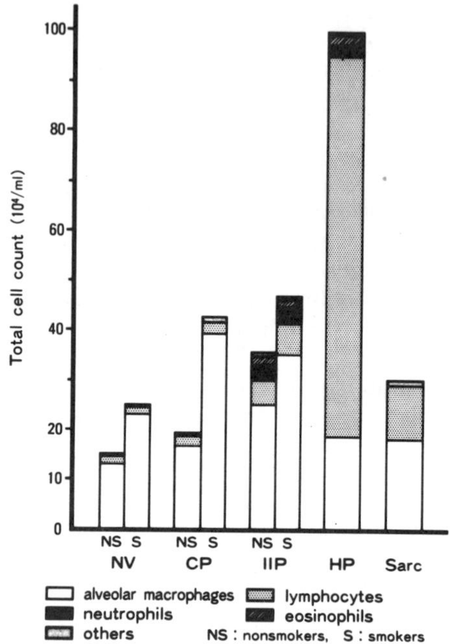

Fig. 1 Cell profile of BALF from patients with IIP

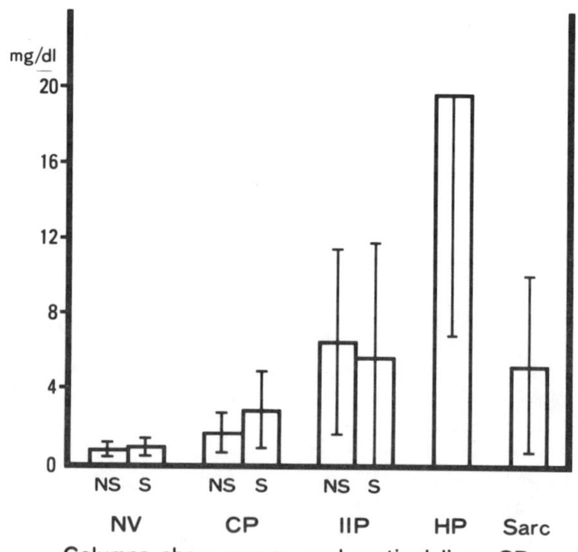

Fig. 2 IgG concentration in BALF from control patients and patients with IIP

to steroid therapy and died within 2 to 12 months after
BAL . All the Type I IIP patients (6 cases) had acute
,diffuse interstitial lesions, with a prominent decrease
in % VC and PaO_2, and the Type II IIP patients consisted
of 2 acute IIP patients and 4 patients in whom acute
exacerbation occurred in the chronic or subacute stage,
with a mild to marked decrease in % VC and PaO_2.
Patients, in whom diffuse interstital lesions were in a
stable stage or in very slow progression, were classified into Type III IIP patients. The BALF data and lung
function data of this group were variable, depending on
the degree of their pulmonary lesions. In about 50 % of
the Type III IIP patients, an interstitial shadow in the
chest X-ray was distributed mainly in the lower lobe,
indicating that the interstitial lesion was localized
mainly in the lower lobe or lower half of the lung.
Therefore, the impairment of lung function was more
slight in Type III IIP patients than in Types I and II
IIP patients (Table I).

The % lymphocytes, % neutrophils and IgG and DSPC
content in BALF from the Types I, II and III IIP
patients are shown in Fig. 3.   The % lymphocytes was
significantly higher in Type I IIP than in Type II IIP ;
it was more than 20 % in all Type I IIP patients while
it was less than 20 % in all Type II IIP patients.   The
IgG content also tended to be larger in Type I IIP than
in Type II IIP. The % neutrophils and % eosinophils,
and DSPC content in BALF from Type I IIP patients were
not significantly different from each other in BALF from
Type II IIP patients.

There was considerable variation (3 to 55 %) in %
lymphocytes in BALF from from Type III IIP patients.
There was no significant difference in % neutrophils and
% eosinophils in BALF among Types I, II and III IIP
patients, although the % eosinophils tended to be lower
in Type II IIP than in Types I and III IIP.

The contents of DSPC, a main component of pulmonary
surfactant, was measured to examine changes in the
pulmonary surfactant in IIP. No Type I IIP patients
showed a DSPC content over 7 µg/ml.   There was no
significant difference in DSPC content in BALF between
Types I and II IIP. On the other hand, as can be seen
in Fig. 3, there was a large variation in DSPC content
in BALF from Type III patients. In Type III IIP
patients, one-third of patients showed a DSPC level over
11 ug/ml, higher than age-matched control patients,

Table I Relationship betwen BALF data and type of IIP

	Active IIP			Stable IIP
	acute I(n=6)	acute or chronic II(n=6)		chronic III(n=26)
BALF				
% Ly	42.3 ±19.9	7.7 ± 5.9	p<0.001	10.4 ±11.3
% Neut	4.7 ± 1.4	7.5 ± 7.8	ns	6.6 ± 8.2
% Eo	8.4 ± 8.4	1.3 ± 1.6	ns	4.5 ± 3.5
albumin	18.2 ±11.1	8.0 ± 4.5	ns	6.2 ± 3.5
IgG	14.7 ± 8.3	6.4 ± 4.0	ns	4.7 ± 2.7
DSPC	3.9 ± 1.6	4.6 ± 3.2	ns	6.4 ± 4.5
Lung function				
% VC	40.4 ± 2.9	67.3 ± 16.2	p<0.005	74.7 ±14.8
A–aDo$_2$	43.2 ±11.0	34.3 ± 4.4	ns	18.4 ± 8.3
Response to steroid	signifi-cant	slight-absent		

Values are means±SD. Ly:lymphocytes, Neut:neutrophils,
Eo:eosinophils , ns:not significant

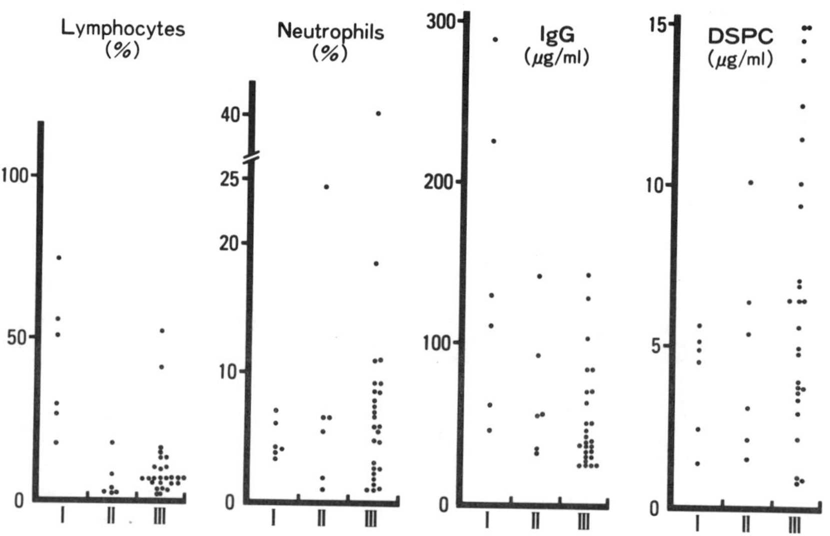

I : acute active, steroid responders

II : acute or chronic active, steroid nonresponders

III : chronic stable

Fig 3 Relationship between BALF data and Type of IIP

one-third showed a DSPC level lower than that of age-matched control patients, and one-third showed a DSPC level similar to that of control patients.

IV. Relationship between BALF data and survival period after BAL in patients with IIP

As shown in Fig .4, patients with IIP were divided into three groups according to their survival period after BAL : Group I died within 12 months, Group II died within 13 to 24 months and Group III lived over 25 months. All the Type I IIP patients belonged to Group III, and all the Type II IIP patients to Group I.

About one-third of the patients in Group III showed over 20 % lymphocytes in BALF while there were no patients who had more than 20 % lymphocytes in Groups I and II. However, there was no significant difference in both % neutrophils, % eosinophils and IgG content in BALF among Groups I, II and III.

As shown in Fig.4, about one-third of Group III patients showed BALF DSPC level over 11 µg/ml, an upper limit in the of nonsmoking CP in age of 40–69 years old. Four patients in Group III showed a very low DSPC level below 2 µg/ml. Half of Group I patients showed a DSPC level from 5 to 10 µg/ml, similar to that of age-matched control patients. These results indicate that a low DSPC level in BALF is not always related to a short survival period or poor prognosis in IIP.

V. Relationship of % lymphocytes and % polymorphonuclear leukocytes (PMN) in BALF to other substances in BALF and lung function data in IIP

As shown in Table 2, % lymphocytes in BALF was significantly correlated with albumin and IgG content in BALF, and not with DSPC content. It was very slightly inversely correlated with % VC but not with DLco and A–aDo$_2$.

The % PMN in BALF was inversely correlated with DSPC content in BALF, but not with albumin and IgG content. There was no significant correlation between % PMN and lung function (% VC ,DLco and A–aDo$_2$).

VI. Relationship between DSPC content in BALF, and other substances in BALF and chest X-ray findings in IIP

DSPC content in BALF was significantly inversely correlated with % PMN (r=−0.430, p< 0.01) and positively correlated with albumin content (r=+0.361, p< 0.05.) in BALF, but not with any lung function data (% VC,DLco and A–aDo$_2$). The DSPC content in BALF was significantly

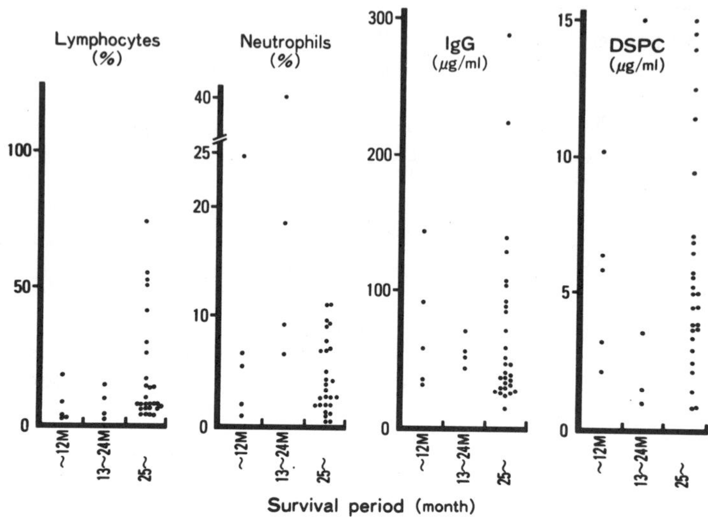

Fig 4 Relationship between BALF data and survival period after BAL in patients with IIP

Table II Relationship of % lymphocytes and PMN in BALF to other substances in BALF and lung function data

	% lymphocytes		% PMN	
	r	p	r	p
BALF				
Albumin µg/ml	−0.128	ns	+0.582	p<0.001
IgG µg/ml	+0.082	ns	+0.628	p<0.001
DSPC µg/ml	−0.430	p<0.01	+0.235	ns
DSPC µg/BALF	−0.469	p<0.01	−0.140	ns
Lung function				
% VC	−0.032	ns	−0.353	p<0.05
DLco	−0.011	ns	−0.224	ns
DLco %	−0.211	ns	−0.200	ns
A−aDo$_2$	+0.248	ns	+0.096	ns

lower in IIP patients who showed a ring shadow with or without a nodular shadow on chest X-ray film (n=22, 8.00 ± 4.10) than in those who showed a predominantly nodular shadow (n=15, 3.04 ± 1.70).

DISCUSSION

A very slight increase in total cell number, and a slight to mild increase in % neutrophils and eosinophils as well as in % lymphocytes in a differential cell count, compared with age-matched control patients, was characteristic for BALF of patients with IIP, and generally agreed with the results of previous investigators [3-5]. It has been reported that the contents of immunoglobulins including IgG in BALF is increased in variuous kinds of diffuse interstitial diseases[3]. The increase in IgG content in BALF was most marked in HP of the diffuse interstitial diseases examined, and similar in IIP and sarcoidosis.

The results of cell profiles and the IgG contents of BALF indicate that a mild inflammation accompanied by an infiltration of PMN and lymphocytes is present in the lungs of patients with IIP. However, similar changes in the cellular and protein components of BALF have been found in other pulmonary diseases, such as collagen-vascular diseases, pneumoconiosis, bronchial asthma and mild airway infection. These results indicate that we can not use an analysis of BALF as a final diagnostic method for IIP.

Combining BALF data with the clinical picture, our patients with IIP were divided into 3 types. Active IIP was divided into steroid responders (Type I) and nonresponders (Type II). A mild increase in % lymphocytes and IgG content in BALF was found in Type I IIP but not in Type II IIP. It is considered from the BALF data that in Type I IIP, acute alveolitis associated with lymphocyte infiltration occurs. Type I IIP patients were associated with prominent impairment of lung function, and responded well to steroid therapy. These results are generally in agreement with the reports of Rudd et al.[5] that patients with acute IIP, who showed an increase in % lymphocytes in BALF and a prominent decrease in % VC, responded to steroids.

Type II IIP patients did not respond or responded only slightly to steroid. The increase in % lymphocytes was not found in this type. We demonstrated previously that a poor response to steroids of this type of IIP patient was partly due to a decrease in the steroid receptors of the immune-inflammatory cells concerned with their pulmonary lesions[6].

Type III IIP coresponds to chronic stable IIP. We did not try steroid therapy for this type of IIP but this type, probably contains both steroid responders and nonresponders.

These results indicate that an analysis of BALF is useful in diagnosing type, activity and responsiveness to drugs of IIP although we cannot use it as a final diagnostic method for IIP.

The present results indicate that % lymphocytes in BALF was related to type, steroid responsiveness and prognosis of IIP to some extent, and correlated with an increase in IgG and albumin in BALF.

Although a slight increases in % neutrophils and % eosinophils in BALF were found in all types of IIP, they were not intimately related to disease activity and prognosis in our patients with IIP. Previously, we reported that the % increase in neutrophils in BALF from patients with IIP was partly due to the fact that the ratio of neutrophils derived from the bronchial region to ones derived from alveolar region was increased in patients with IIP[7].

The DSPC content of BALF was influenced by smoking and aging, as previously reported [8]. The DSPC content in BALF from IIP patients was similar to that from age- and smoking-matched control patients (unpublished data). The DSPC content of BALF was not significantly related to lung function and prognosis, but inversely correlated with % PMN in BALF, in IIP patients. Further study is necessary to clarify the mechanism of the inverse correlation between DSPC content and % PMN in BALF from IIP patients.

1. Nakayama,T, Yasuoka,S, Nakayama,T. et al. Clin. Allergy 13,107-117, 1983.
2. Yasuoka,S.,Manabe,H.,Ozaki,T.and Tsubura,T. J.Geront. 32, 387-391, 1977.
3. Reynolds,h.Y., Fulmer,J.D., Kazmierowski,J.A.et al. J. Clin.Invest 59,165-175, 1977.
4. Haslam,P.L.,Turton,C.W.G., Lukoszek,A. et al. Thorax 35, 328-339, 1980.
5. Rudd,R.,Haslam,P.L.,Turner-Warwick,M. Am.Rev.Repir. .Dis. 124, 1-8, 1981.
6.Ozaki,T.,Nakayama,T., Yasuoka,S. et al.Am.Rev.Respir, .Dis. 126, 968-971, 1982..
7.Yasuoka, S.,Nakayama,T., Kawano,T.et al. Tohoku J Exp Med 146,33-45, 1985.
8. Yasuoka,S.,Tatenuma,Y.,Tani, K. et al. Tokushima J. Exp. Med. 35, 5-12, 1988.

III
PATHOLOGICAL PICTURE

Pathology of Interstitial Lung Disease

B. Corrin

Brompton Hospital, London, UK

From 1980–87 inclusive, 910 biopsies from patients attending the Brompton hospital with pulmonary fibrosis and/or interstitial lung disease were evaluated as follows (failed biopsies and those lacking significant abnormalities being excluded): compatible with sarcoidosis (n=343), compatible with cryptogenic fibrosing alveolitis (n=339), organizing pneumonia (n=123), lymphoproliferative disease (n=32), extrinsic allergic alveolitis (n=25), eosinophilic granuloma (n=12), organizing diffuse alveolar damage (n=6), asbestosis (n=5), lymphangiomyomatosis (n=5), hard metal disease (n=3), compatible with berylliosis (n=2). This paper considers the differential diagnosis of these conditions.

The term chronic interstitial pneumonia refers to any chronic inflammatory process that occurs predominantly in the supporting structures of the lungs rather than within the alveoli. It is often used synonymously with chronic interstitial fibrosis of the lungs because the two frequently co-exist. Many cases are unexplained and may be said to be idiopathic or cryptogenic. Several conditions enter the differential diagnosis.

CHRONIC INTERSTITIAL PNEUMONIA AND FIBROSIS AS A CONSEQUENCE OF CYTOTOXIC INJURY

Some cases of chronic interstitial pneumonia represent the outcome of diffuse alveolar damage (1), a condition that represents acute cytotoxic injury caused by agents that range from fumes to viruses. Thus, interstitial pulmonary fibrosis may be seen after irradiation injury, the ingestion of toxins such as paraquat or anti-cancer drugs, the inhalation of noxious gases, and circulatory collapse caused by sepsis or trauma. Histologically, the early stage is characterised by necrosis of the alveolar lining cells and the formation of hyaline membranes. In the reparative phase, organisation of these membranes and their incorporation into the alveolar wall augments the activity of interstitial fibroblasts so that the alveolar walls become fibrotic. More severe alveolar damage, particularly that seen in paraquat poisoning, floods the alveolar lumen with a fibrin-rich exudate, organisation of which obliterates the air spaces over broad tracts of lung. Within these areas, however, the framework of the alveolar walls can still be appreciated with appropriate stains for elastin or basement membrane. Sometimes it is evident that collapsed alveoli have been incorporated in this obliterative pattern of alveolar fibrosis, a process that is sometimes termed atelectatic or collapse induration (2).

CRYPTOGENIC FIBROSING ALVEOLITIS

The name cryptogenic fibrosing alveolitis is widely used for chronic interstitial pneumonia and fibrosis occurring without any obvious cause (3), but in many countries the terms usual interstitial pneumonia (4) or idiopathic pulmonary fibrosis (5) are preferred. The adjective "usual" was introduced to emphasise differences between this pattern of interstitial pneumonia (UIP) and four others, namely a "desquamative" pattern (DIP), one occurring in association with bronchiolitis obliterans (BIP), one marked by the presence of giant cells (GIP) and one characterised by heavy lymphoid infiltrates (LIP). Some of these are now recognised as quite separate

conditions. For example, LIP is best considered along
with frankly malignant lymphoproliferative conditions
and GIP, many cases of which are now known to be caused
by hard metal alloys (6), with occupational lung
disease. The nature of BIP is obscure but it possibly
represents a further outcome of diffuse alveolar
damage. It is debatable whether UIP and DIP are
separate diseases, or different patterns of one, but
many cases show mixed features (3), and they are
consequently often spoken of as the mural and luminal
(or "desquamative") patterns respectively of one
disease.

Fibrosing alveolitis commences with oedema and
infiltration of the alveolar walls by lymphocytes and
plasma cells, augmented later by fibroblasts and an
increase in the amount of reticulin and collagen.
Often there is also focal hyperplasia of lymphoid
tissue. These interstitial features constitute the
so-called mural changes. The alveoli contain many free
cells, initially thought to be desquamated epithelial
cells (hence DIP) but now known to be largely
macrophages (7). Although appreciable numbers of
neutrophils and eosinophils are present in
bronchoalveolar lavage fluid in fibrosing alveolitis,
very few are evident in tissue sections, suggesting
that macrophages are selectively retained when the
alveoli are lavaged. Rarely, hyaline membranes form,
and these may become converted into fibrous tissue by
organisation, but this feature is largely confined to
the rapidly progressive cases (Hamman-Rich syndrome).
Electron microscopy (8) shows profound damage to the
alveolar epithelium and to a lesser extent the
capillary endothelium.

Advanced cases show replacement of the normal alveolar
structure by dense collagen surrounding cystically
dilated air spaces lined by bronchiolar or cuboidal
alveolar epithelium. Some inflammatory cells persist
in the fibrous tissue, but they are not as prominent as
in the early stages. Reactive smooth muscle
hyperplasia is often very marked, so-called "muscular
cirrhosis of the lung".

The lower lobes are most severely affected and have a

bossellated, finely nodular external appearance.
Pleural fibrosis is uncommon, in contrast to asbestosis
which, apart from the absence of asbestos bodies,
fibrosing alveolitis otherwise resembles. The cut
surface of the lung shows a variable degree of
honeycombing, most marked beneath the pleura, where it
forms a band a few centimetres wide. This rind of
contracted fibrous tissue prevents the lungs from
expanding and is an important contributory factor to
the restrictive respiratory defect.

The pathologist may well find it difficult to offer an
unequivocal diagnosis of fibrosing alveolitis. This is
acceptable as the pathological appearances are not
specific: viral infection, chemical toxins and
radiation damage may all produce similar changes and
the diagnosis is best arrived at after consideration of
the clinical circumstances as well as the histological
appearances. However, after excluding more specific
interstitial diseases, such as asbestosis,
histiocytosis X, extrinsic allergic alveolitis,
sarcoidosis and lymphangioleiomyomatosis, the
histological appearances are sufficiently
characteristic to permit the pathologist to say that
they are fully compatible with a diagnosis of
cryptogenic fibrosing alveolitis.

The pathologist can also offer useful advice on
prognosis. Hyaline collagenisation and loss of
alveolar architecture with honeycombing are obviously
irreversible, but inflammatory changes, both mural and
luminal, are potentially amenable to therapy.

Cryptogenic fibrosing alveolitis is complicated by the
development of lung cancer in up to 13% of fatal
cases (9). When patients are matched for age and
smoking habit, the fibrosing alveolitis is found to
contribute a ten-fold increased risk of lung cancer.
Squamous and adenocarcinoma are the most frequent
histological types. The hyperplasia of alveolar lining
cells found in cryptogenic fibrosing alveolitis is
probably the starting point of both these types of
cancer, for metaplasia and dysplasia are occasionally
observed in the cuboidal alveolar epithelium.

CRYPTOGENIC ORGANIZING PNEUMONITIS (BRONCHIOLITIS OBLITERANS ORGANIZING PNEUMONIA) (10-12)

This condition affects the air spaces much more than the interstitium but mimics interstitial disease clinically and functionally, causing a predominantly restrictive lung defect. Pathologically, it is identical to post-infective organizing pneumonia but taken in conjunction with the clinical features, a distinct clinico-pathological syndrome of unknown cause emerges, recognition of which is important because it responds well to steroids. Men and women are affected about equally and most are in the 40 to 60 year age group. Persistent cough, shortness of breath and malaise are common complaints and the onset is insidious. Chest radiographs show widespread blotchy opacities, which regress in some places whilst progressing in others. Pulmonary function tests generally show a predominantly restrictive ventilatory defect but some patients have a mixed obstructive and restrictive pattern. The erythrocyte sedimentation rate is elevated but no evidence of infection can be detected, either by culture or serologically. On biopsy, the distinguishing feature is the presence of small buds of granulation tissue (bourgeons conjunctifs, Masson bodies) in the air spaces. Chronic inflammation and interstitial fibrosis of the alveolar walls may also be seen but the predominant change is intraluminal. The alveoli are mainly affected but the process also involves the lumen of respiratory bronchioles. Occasionally, residual fibrin is seen in or near the connective tissue buds, which also contain small numbers of lymphocytes, plasma cells and neutrophils in addition to macrophages and fibroblasts. The inflammatory cells tend to cluster in the centres of the connective tissue buds.

SARCOIDOSIS (13)

Sarcoidosis commonly involves the lungs, where numerous small granulomas, or groups of granulomas, develop. As with other granulomatous diseases, the upper lobes are more severely affected than the lower. The lesions often regress but sometimes there is progressive infiltration, leading to widespread pulmonary fibrosis and bronchiectasis.

The sarcoid granulomas closely resemble early tubercles microscopically but differ in that even when large they do not caseate. Epithelioid and multinucleate giant cells, similar to the Langhans' cells of tuberculosis, are found in the centres of the granulomas. The giant cells often contain Schaumann or asteroid bodies but these are not specific for sarcoidosis. Closely associated with the epithelioid cells are lymphocytes of T helper type, whilst suppressor T cells accumulate as a peripheral cuff at the edge of the granulomas.

Sarcoid granulomas are widely disseminated in the lung but are most numerous along the lymphatics. They are therefore particularly well developed near the centriacinar bronchioles and arteries and in the interlobular septa near veins, all of which they may involve. They are very well developed in the main airways, so this is a condition in which fibreoptic biopsies frequently provide sufficient tissue for diagnostic purposes.

Rarely, large masses of sarcoid tissue are formed, the so-called nodular form of sarcoidosis. Necrotising sarcoid granulomatosis is however a separate condition: it displays a similar angiitis but differs from nodular sarcoid in showing large tracts of necrosis.

Sarcoid-like granulomas characterise extrinsic allergic alveolitis but there they are poorly formed, scanty and seen on a background of diffuse chronic interstitial pneumonia, in contrast to sarcoidosis where the granulomas are studded throughout otherwise normal alveolar tissue.

Sarcoid granulomas heal by progressive hyalinisation but even very late lesions are generally recognisable as burnt out granulomas, whereas in extrinsic allergic alveolitis the granulomas resolve without trace within a few months. Active and healed sarcoid granulomas are often seen together.

EXTRINSIC ALLERGIC ALVEOLITIS (HYPERSENSITIVITY PNEUMONITIS) (14)

Farmers' lung is the classic example of this disease
but many different antigens may be responsible, giving
rise to such exotic names as paprika bark strippers'
lung. The pathology is identical in them all. Lung
biopsies taken during the first months show poorly
formed non-necrotising granulomas, which are generally
smaller and less numerous than those seen in
sarcoidosis, and are accompanied by widespread
thickening of the alveolar walls by a diffuse
lymphocytic infiltrate. No fungal elements are found,
but small fragments of foreign material may be present.
The occurrence of giant cells with cytoplasmic clefts
is a useful but non-specific diagnostic aid. In
contrast to sarcoidosis, the hilar lymph nodes are
unaffected. The diffuse background pneumonitis is
another distinguishing feature from sarcoidosis. Also,
the whole inflammatory process tends to show a
peribronchiolar preponderance, these airways being the
portal of entry of the aetiological agents. A further
difference is the presence of knots of granulation
tissue within alveoli and respiratory bronchioles,
evidence of organisation of luminal exudates. Unless
there is further exposure, the granulomas resolve
within about six months, but the inflammation
frequently progresses to an irreversible scarring. In
fatal cases the lungs show honeycombing, with the upper
lobes more affected than the bases, in contrast to
fibrosing alveolitis which is predominantly basal.

PULMONARY HISTIOCYTOSIS X (EOSINOPHILIC GRANULOMA OF THE LUNG) (15)

Three separately described conditions, Hand-Schüller-
Christian disease, Letterer-Siwe disease and
eosinophilic granuloma, have much in common
pathologically, and the term histiocytosis X (HX) was
therefore introduced to encompass all three. The
essential unity of HX is supported by the electron
microscopic identification of a distinctive cytoplasmic
marker organelle in all forms of the disease.
Letterer-Siwe disease, Hand-Schüller-Christian disease
and eosinophilic granuloma may respectively be

considered the acute generalised, the chronic
generalised and the localised forms of HX.

In normal tissues, the marker organelle has only been
described in Langerhans' cells, implying that HX
represents a pathological proliferation of these cells.
The nature of the proliferation remains unclear for
whereas eosinophilic granuloma often heals
spontaneously, and may therefore be presumed to be
reactive, Letterer-Siwe disease typically behaves like
a malignant neoplastic condition. The Langerhans' cell
is a constant feature of the normal epidermis and is
occasionally found in the dermis and lymphoid tissue,
but so far has not been identified in normal lung,
although it has been observed in various pulmonary
diseases, both reactive and neoplastic. Langerhans'
cells carry surface receptors for Fc and C_3 but are
poorly phagocytic and have few lysosomes. They are
believed to be involved in delayed hypersensitivity
reactions.

Langerhans' cells have a moderate amount of
eosinophilic cytoplasm and a single indented nucleus
with a finely dispersed chromatin pattern. Electron
microscopy identifies the marker organelles, the
so-called Birbeck granules. These are small elongated
pentalaminar structures of constant width (40-45 nm)
with a longitudinal periodicity (10 nm) in their
central laminae and a small terminal dilatation. On
biopsy, eosinophilic granuloma of the lung consists of
a focal interstitial infiltration, most marked about
the centriacinar bronchioles and arteries or small
veins in the interlobular septa. The bronchiolar wall
may be infiltrated and weakened so that small cavities
develop. Active lesions consist of nodular collections
of Langerhans' cells that may exhibit mitoses,
intermingled with eosinophils. As the lesions heal,
there develop stellate fibrous scars in which
Langerhans' cells and eosinophils are no longer readily
apparent, having been replaced by pigment-laden
macrophages, lymphocytes and plasma cells. The pigment
in the macrophages is generally Perls' and periodic
acid-Schiff positive and diastase-resistant. At
autopsy, interstitial fibrosis is widespread and there
may be marked "honeycombing". Old and active lesions

are often found together.

Eosinophilic granuloma must be distinguished from eosinophilic pneumonia, reactive eosinophilic pleuritis and fibrosing alveolitis. The interstitial rather than intraluminal location of the eosinophils should indicate eosinophilic granuloma rather than eosinophilic pneumonia, whereas an associated blood eosinophilia would favour the latter. Reactive eosinophilic pleuritis is caused by pneumothorax and is limited to the pleura and subpleural lung tissue. Fibrosing alveolitis is diffuse and lacks the focal distribution of the lesions of eosinophilic granuloma. When HX is completely inactive a definite histological diagnosis may no longer be possible, the lung having reached an end stage of widespread honeycombing common to many diseases.

Immunocytochemistry may be used to demonstrate Langerhans' cells', the plasma membranes of which stain for T6 antigen and the cytoplasm for S100 protein. Positive results are however only of significance in the right pathological setting, for S100 is not a specific marker of Langerhans' cells, and in the lung dendritic reticular cells are a particular source of confusio being increased in a variety of reactive states. Furthermore, true Langerhans' cells are a relatively common reactive cell in many fibrotic and neoplastic diseases. Histological diagnosis is most difficult in the healing phase when Langerhans' cells are poorly represented, in which stage immunocytochemistry is least helpful. Its optimal usage is probably in the examination of small fibreoptic specimens, in which the valuable architectural features evident in an open biopsy cannot be assessed, and in the evaluation of bronchoalveolar lavage cells. Electron microscopy may also be helpful in identifying Langerhans' cells in lavage specimens. However demonstrated, their presence in lavage fluid is very strong evidence of pulmonary HX, more so than in tissue sections.

REFERENCES

1. Liebow AA. In: The Lung. International academy of

pathology monograph No 8.   (Williams and Wilkins eds.),
Baltimore, pp. 332-365, 1967.

2.   Burkhardt A.   Hum Pathol 1986; 17: 971-973.

3.   Scadding JG, Hinson KFW.   Thorax 1967; 22:
291-304.

4.   Liebow AA.   Prog Resp Res 1975; 8:1-33.

5.   Crystal RG, Fulmer JD, Roberts WC, Moss ML, Line
BR, Reynolds HY.   Ann Intern Med 1976; 85: 769-788.

6.   Davison AG, Haslam PL, Corrin B, Coutts II, Dewar
A, Riding WD, Studdy PR, Newman-Taylor AJ.   Thorax
1983; 38: 119-128.

7.   Leroy EP. Virch Archiv 1969; 348: 117-130.   10.

8.   Corrin B, Dewar A, Rodriguez-Roisin R,
Turner-Warwick M.   J Pathol 1985; 147: 107-119.

9.   Kawai T, Yakumaru K, Suzuki M, Kageyama K.   Acta
Pathol Jpn 1987; 37: 11-19.

10. Grinblat J, Mechlis S, Lewitus Z.   Chest, 1981;
80:259-263.

11. Davison AG, Heard BE, McAllister WAC,
Turner-Warwick MEH.   Quart J Med 1983; 207: 382-394.

12. Epler GR, Colby TV, McLoud TC, Carrington CB,
Gaensler EA.   N Engl J Med 1985; 312: 152-158.

13. Rosen Y, Vuletin JC, Pertschuk LP, Silverstein E.
Path Ann 1979; 14 Part 1: 405-439.

14. Coleman A, Colby TV.   Am J Surg Pathol 1988; 12:
514-518.

15. Basset F, Corrin B, Spencer H.   et al.   Amer Rev
Resp Dis 1978; 118: 811-820.

Pulmonary Changes in Connective Tissue Disease

Yasuhiro Hosoda

Department of Pathology, School of Medicine, Keio University, Tokyo, Japan

A clinicopathological study of interstitial pneumonia in 116 autopsy cases with connective tissue disease was carried out. The relationship between the interstitial and vascular changes was also analyzed. Interstitial changes were essentially similar in all connective tissue diseases and nonspecific. In MCTD both interstitial changes and plexogenic arteriopathy were observed in some cases. In PSS, MCTD, SLE and overlap syndrome vascular changes were far-advanced compared with interstitial changes in some cases. Association of carcinoma and bronchiolitis obliterans is rare in this series. In RA no necrobiotic nodules was observed.

Interstitial pneumonia (IP) in connective tissue diseases (CTD) is believed to be associated with some immunological disturbance, although the mechanisms involved are still unknown. Furthermore, the morphological lesions found could be described more or less as non-specific, and to identify a specific change associated with a disease is difficult [1,2].

However, although the IP in CTD are grouped together under a single heading, several characteristics can be pointed out for the IP in each CTD. There have been many reports given by many authors in the field of pathology concerning the IP caused by CTD, and there seems to be a

159

difference among the races regarding the IP, just as
there are ethnic differences with the CTD. We would like
to report our analysis based on observation of autopsy
cases concerning the IP found in CTD, comparing them with
researches which have been made in the Western countries.
    Described here are 116 autopsy cases of CTD, performed
at the pathology department of Keio University and other
affiliated hospitals. We have employed, for progressive
systemic sclerosis (PSS) the '80 ARA criteria [3], for
mixed connective tissue disease (MCTD) the definition set
by Sharp et al. [4], for polymyositis/dermatomyositis
(PM/DM) the criteria of Bohan et al. [5], for rheumatoid
arthritis (RA) the '87 ARA diagnostic criteria [6], for
systemic lupus erythematosus (SLE) the revised ARA criteria [7], and as for the overlap syndrome, we have
designated them as those which fulfill the above-mention-
ed criteria simultaneously, we then reviewed the clinical
picture, especially the respiratory symptoms and salient
laboratory data of the cases, as well as the pulmonary
morphological changes taking special note of the relationship between interstitial changes and the vascular lesion.
In addition, to some cases which had few postmortem
changes, immunohistochemical methods were applied to see
deposition of immunoglobulins and complements. The
interstitial fibrosis (IF) were classed into Grades of
0 to 4, according to their severity [8].

Results

1. PSS: Among the 15 cases, IF were found in 12, 6 of
them Grade 4. They were usually prominent in the pos-
terior aspect of the lower lobes beneath the pleura.
Inflammatory cell infiltration in the thickend interstitium was mild, no hyaline membrane formation was seen in
the alveolar space, and all the lesions belonged to the
so-called "chronic type". In advanced cases, there was
marked destruction of normal pulmonary structure, and
round cell infiltration, consisting mainly of lymphocytes
and plasma cells, was seen in varying degrees. Hypertrophy and hyperplasia of the alveolar epithelium were
generally found in cases with prominent pulmonary change.
In one case with PSS, as an incidental finding, an adenocarcinoma measuring 1 cm in diameter was found. No meta-
stasis was seen. Carcinoma was found in just this one

case, of all the cases with CTD. To analyze changes in
the pulmonary arterial system, histomorphometric methods
were employed. Taking note of the relationship between
the IF and the vascular changes, those areas with IF and
those without, groups with a high grade of IF and those
with a low grade of IF were separated, and the degree of
intimal and mural thickening, as well as mucoid intimal
thickening, considered a characteristic of PSS, was compared among them. In cases with severe IF, the degree of
mural thickening of the muscular type arteries and the
degree of IF matched in many cases, but some with the
degrees widely divergent were found, and in one case,
marked mural thickening was found even in parts with
minimal IF. In cases with a low grade IF, 4 cases with a
fair degree of mural thickening, compared to the degree
of IF here found. Mucoid intimal thickening occurred
frequently in the group with a high grade of IF, and were
found to be scarce in the group with mild IF. Incidence
and severity were greater in areas of pronounced fibrosis,
although it could be found in non-fibrotic areas also
(Fig. 1).

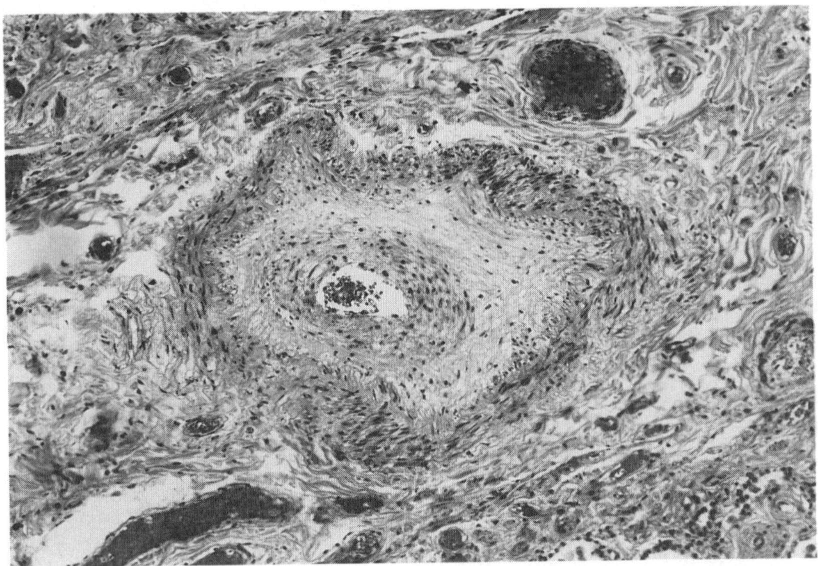

PSS: Mucoid intimal thickening of the pulmonary artery,
     x 100

Fig. 1

The pulmonary vascular changes and interstitial changes
seen in PSS, at least in part, seem to be independent of
each other in their occurrence. No severe hypertensive
pulmonary vascular changes, seen in plexogenic pulmonary
arteriopathy, such as a plexiform lesion , however, was
found. Prominent intimal thickening and cystic medial
necrosis was sometimes found in the elastic type arteries
as well. Generally speaking, no great degree of right
ventricular hypertrophy (RVH) was to be seen, but in one
case with minimal IF there was a distinct RVH. The
degree of IF did not correspond with the duration of the
disease nor with the degree of fibrosis of the skin.

2. MCTD: The pulmonary changes are one of the important
factors determining the prognosis of MCTD [9,10,11].
By studying 15 autopsy cases of MCTD, we have been able
to divide them up into 3 types. The vascular type is one
with mainly hypertensive pulmonary vascular disease
(HPVD), and without changes in the interstitium. The
interstitial type mainly shows IF without HPVD, and the
mixed type has both HPVD and IF at the same time. There
were 8 vascular, 2 interstitial, and 5 mixed types. The
importance of pulmonary hypertension in the cause of
deaths with MCTD was confirmed. Diffuse IF was seen in
7 cases, all of them with varying degrees of lymphocyte-
predominant chronic inflammatory cell infiltration.
Amongst them 3 were complicated by HPVD of Grade 4, two
by HPVD of Grades 3. Plexiform lesions were found in 2
cases. The 5 with HPVD were classified as mixed type.
RVH was apparent in 3 of the 5 cases. Of the 8 cases of
vascular type, there was one with necrotizing angiitis of
the pulmonary artery, and 6 with plexiform lesions.
Thrombus formation was seen in 13 cases regardless of the
respective degrees of pulmonary artery and interstitial
changes. The thrombi were found scattered in small
numbers and no case of recurrent thromboembolism was
observed. Concerning the muscular type pulmonary artery,
using the method of Yazaki and Wagenvoort [12], index of
pulmonary vascular disease (IPVD) was computed. Thirteen
cases of the vascular and mixed types showed IPVD over
2.7, and IPVD both of the 2 cases of interstitial type
showed IPVD under 1.8. In cases with a high IPVD, the
degrees of interstitial and vascular changes did not
match. We examined the muscular type pulmonary arteries
dividing them into proximal and distal segments according

to their outer diameter at the point of 130 μm.
In general, intimal thickening was more prominent in the
distal segments, and medial hypertrophy was more remarkable in the proximal segments. In the vascular type, most
cases showed marked intimal thickening in both the distal
and proximal segments. No correlation existed between
the IPVD and the duration of the disease, but among cases
with clinical courses of 2 years or less, some were noted
for severe intimal thickening. The simultaneous occurrence of IF and plexiform lesions in MCTD makes it distinct from other CTD (Fig. 2).

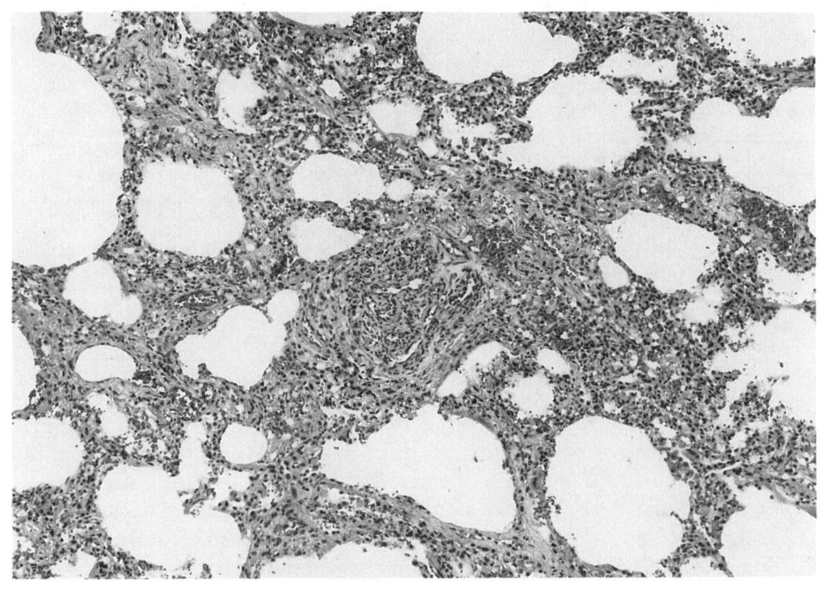

MCTD: Moderate IF and plexiform lesion (center), x 80

Fig. 2

Most of the pulmonary vascular changes in MCTD are identical with plexogenic arteriopathy. In one case, immunohistochemical study revealed deposition of IgG, IgA and
C3 in the walls of the muscular type pulmonary arteries.

3. PM/DM: Among the 21 cases with PM/DM, 12 cases showed
IP. Morphologically, we could classified them into 3
types. The exudative type is characterized by edematous
and cellular thickening of the alveolar septa and hyaline

membrane formation along the alveolar wall and minimal
IF (Fig. 3).

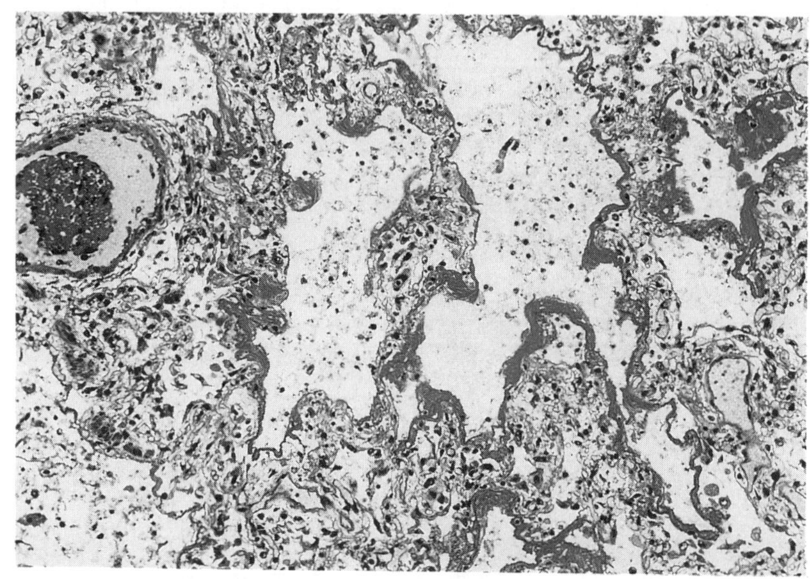

PM: Exudative type of IP, x 100

Fig. 3

The fibrotic type featured by remarkable interstitial
fibrosis involving alveolar septa and disorganization of
the air space. Some are associated with honeycombing,
especially in the basal subpleural regions. Those classified as the intermediate type do not correspond with
either of the 2 types mentioned above. Intra-alveolar
fibrosis, which is thought to be the result of organization of exudates, such as hyaline membrane along the
alveolar wall, and inflammatory cell infiltration in the
alveolar septa are often seen in this type. There were
3 exudative types, 4 fibrotic types, and 3 intermediate
types. All of the three cases of the exudative type died
within 1 month and one case died with diagnosis of
bronchopneumonia within 2 weeks. On the other hand, 3
cases had clinical courses of over 1 year, although 1
case died with aspiration pneumonia in 3 weeks, among
the fibrotic type. Those of the intermediate type died
in 3 months, histologically, they are thought to be the
healing processes of the exudative types. In general

terms, the exudative type could be called an acute type, while the fibrotic type could be called chronic, but even among the fibrotic types are ones with a short clinical course, so that to call them chronic types may not always be adequate. RVH was evident in 2 of the fibrotic types and in one of the intermediate type. The antibody to Jo-1 antigen [13] has analyzed in 7 cases and in 3 fibrotic cases found to be positive. No IP was found in the cases with PM/DM associated with malignancy.

4. RA: Interstitial pneumonia of varying degrees was found in 15 cases of the 21 cases, the 15 consisted of 6 males and 9 females. The rheumatoid factor was markedly positive in 12 cases. Eight cases had systemic vasculitis. No correlation with hypocomplementemia and eosinophilia was found, and the relationship between the diseases and circulating immune complex and smoking habits is obscure. The interstitial change also initiates in the lower subpleural regions in RA. In early stage, as in PSS, the deposition of collagen fibers and minimal to mild inflammatory cell infiltration in the alveolar septa and around the blood vessels and bronchi was observed. Inflammatory cell infiltration, rather, is prominent in advanced cases often around the bronchi. The cells consist mostly of lymphocytes and plasma cells. The presence of lymphoid follicles with germinal centers has been frequently referred, but in our series cases with obvious lymphoid follicles were rare (Fig. 4). Rheumatoid nodules and bronchiolitis obliterans were not found in any case. Dilatation of the air spaces including honeycombing were seen in 8 cases mainly in the lower lobes. In RA, the pulmonary vascular changes coincided with the interstitial changes. In all the cases including the 8 with systemic vasculitis, angiitis of the pulmonary arteries was not seen, and no plexiform lesion was recognized. Right ventricular hypertrophy was found in only 2 cases.

5. SLE: Interstitial changes were found in 6 cases out of a total of 36. Among them 5 were IF, mostly restricted to the lower lobes, with minimal to mild lymphocyte-predominant chronic inflammatory cell infiltrates. One case had an acute course, its main feature was exudative change with the cell infiltrates including neutrophiles and hyaline membrane formation (Fig. 5). In this case there was no renal failure and acute lupus pneumonitis

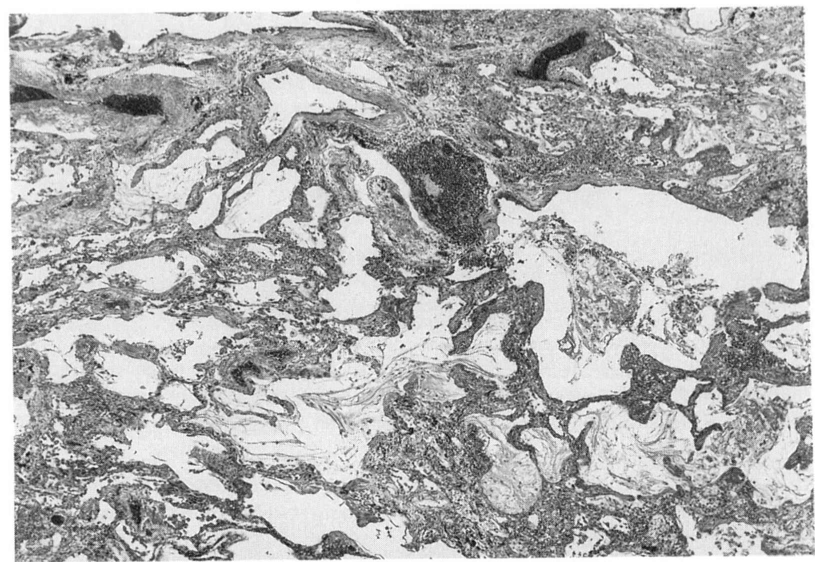

RA: IF with lymphoid cell aggregates, x 40
Fig. 4

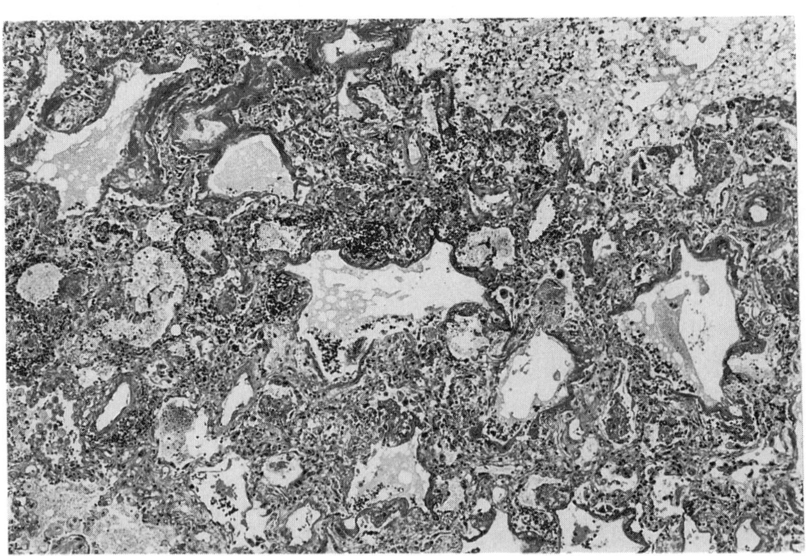

SLE: Hyaline membrane and inflammatory cell infiltrates
in alveolar septa, x 64
Fig. 5

was suspected. Hypertensive pulmonary vascular disease
of Grades 3 - 4 were seen in 6 cases without PF and in
them, 3 showed necrotizing vasculitis of the muscular
type pulmonary arteries. These cases were complicated
by pulmonary hypertension.

6. Overlap Syndrome: In 4 cases out of 9 mild IF was
found, and all 4 had PSS as a clinical and pathological
component. In one case of PSS-SLE overlapping HPVD of
Grade 4 without PF and endarteritis obliterans were found.
Marked RVH complicated this case.

Generally, in this series no immune deposition sufficient for an interpretation was obtained in the interstitium.

To summarize, we have reviewed the pulmonary interstitial and vascular changes in CTD, and found the interstitial changes to be diverse and non-specific. However,
the presence of IF and simultaneous plexiform lesions in
"mixed types" of MCTD can be described as rather specific.

The pulmonary vascular lesions found in PSS, SLE, MCTD
and overlap syndrome were independent of the interstitial
lesions. In contrast, in RA and PM/DM, pulmonary vascular lesions unproportionally pronounced in comparison to
the interstitial change were not found.

The interstitial pneumonia in CTD of Japan has several
features compared with the ones in Europe and the USA.
In general, occurrence of the recently highlighted
bronchiolitis obliterans seemed to be rare, and the association of cancer is also infrequent in Japan. In RA,
development of rheumatoid nodules in the lungs is again
rare.

Acknowledgments
Drs. J.Fukuda and S. Irimajiri, Municipal Kawasaki Hosp.,
kindly permitted reviewing autopsy cases with RA.

References
1. Hunninghake, G.W. and Fauci, A.S. <u>Am. Rev. Resp. Dis.</u>
    119, 471-503, 1979.
2. Stanford, R.E., In: Pulmonary Pathology (D.H. Dail
    et al. eds.) Springer-Verlag, pp.471-482, 1988.
3. Subcommittee for scleroderma criteria of the ARA
    Diagnostic and Therapeutic Criteria Committee.

Arthritis Rheum.23, 581-590, 1980.

4.   Sharp, G.C., Irvin, W.S., Tan, E.M., Gould, R.G. and
      Holman, H.R. Am. J. Med. 52, 148-159, 1972.

5.   Bohan, A., Peter, J.B., Bowman, R.S. et al. Medicine
      56, 255-283, 1977.

6.   Arnett, F.C., Edworthy, S.M., Bloch, D.A., McShane,
      D.J., Fries, J.F., Cooper, N.S., Healey, L.A.,
      Kaplan, S.R., Liang, M.H., Luthra, H.S., Medsger,
      T.A., Mitchell, D.M., Neustadt, D.H., Pinals, R.S,
      Schaller, J.G., Sharp, J.T., Wilder, R.L. and
      Hunder, G.G. Arthritis Rheum. 31, 315-324, 1988.

7.   Tan, E.M., Cohen, A.S., Fries, J.F. et al. Arthritis
      Rheum. 25, 1271-1277, 1982.

8.   Hammar, S.P. In: Pulmonary Pathology (D.H.Dail et
      al. eds.), Springer-Verlag, pp.483-510, 1988.

9.   Hosoda, Y. In: Mixed Connective Tissue Disease and
      Antinuclear Antibodies. (R. Kasukawa et al. eds.),
      Elsevier Sci. Publ., pp.281-290, 1985.

10.   Hosoda, Y., Suzuki, Y., Takano, M., Tojo, T. and
      Homma, M. J. Rheumatol. 14, 826-830, 1987.

11.   Sullivan, W.D., Hurst, D.J., Harmon, C.E., Esther,
      J.H., Agia, G.A., Maltby, T.D., Lillard, S.B., Held,
      C.N., Wolfe, J.F., Sunderrajan, E.V., Maricq, H.R.,
      and Sharp, G.C. Medicine 63, 92-107, 1984.

12.   Yazaki, S. and Wagenvoort, C.A. Br. Heart J. 54,
      428-434, 1985.

13.   Yoshida, S., Akizuki, M., Mimori, T., Yamagata, H.,
      Inada, S. and Homma, M. Arthritis Rheum. 26, 604-
      611, 1983.

Alveolar Tissue Reaction to Lung Injury

Ewald R. Weibel and Marianne Bachofen

Departments of Anatomy and Anaesthesiology, University of Berne, Berne, Switzerland

Alveolar tissue is characterized by a population of extremely delicate cells, the endothelium and the epithelium forming permeability barriers. The reaction of this tissue to injury proceeds in three stages. During the first day leaky cell barriers lead to pulmonary edema. This is followed by organization of exudate with the formation of hyaline membranes and immigration of inflammatory cells. After about one week repair processes ensue with the regeneration of an epithelial lining and of capillaries.

Introduction

The main feature of alveolar tissue is its extraordinarily delicate structure, designed to establish favorable conditions for gas exchange. An extensive capillary network is contained within alveolar walls which form a very large internal surface — nearly the size of a tennis court. This is supported by a thin sheet of tissue — merely 1/50 the thickness of a sheet of airmail stationery — which forms the barrier between air and blood; it is thin to allow easy diffusion of gases. But it must also serve mechanical and metabolic support functions, and for this it is organized into three layers: a capillary endothelium forms the wall of the capillary network, an alveolar epithelium lines the alveolar spaces, and an interstitial space with fibers and cells binds the two cell linings together. All three layers are exceedingly thin, but they extend over large areas as they form continua throughout the labyrinth of alveolar walls.

When considering the reaction of this tissue system to lung injury we must first note that any injurious agent that reaches the alveoli by either the airways or the blood vessels meets a large surface on which to act: the chances of an injurious event are therefore high. But then the injured tissue elements, particularly the cells, are very sparse and delicate, so that their potential to fend off the injury must be limited. And since the delicacy of tissue design is a prerequisite for efficient lung function, i.e. for gas exchange, successful injury must needs result in some degree of acute pulmonary failure. To understand the typical sequence of events that follow lung injury we must first discuss the nature and peculiarity of the alveolar cell population [1], and then examine the ways by which this cell population changes as the injury develops and eventually is repaired [2].

Cellular structure of the blood-air barrier

The structures of the alveolar wall are built on a three-dimensional system of connective tissue fibers as a backbone, which are interlaced with the capillary network [3, 4]. The capillaries are thus directly suspended on the fibrous skeleton of the lung, specifically on the fine septal fibers which are anchored on two major connective tissue tracts to form a fiber continuum: (1) the peripheral fiber system that emanates from the pleura and penetrates deep into the lung parenchyma as interlobular septa; and (2) the axial fiber system that consists of the tissue sheaths of airways and extends into the acini as the network of fibers surrounding the alveolar ducts where it appears as the lattice of alveolar entrance rings on which alveolar walls are fastened.

The capillaries are bounded without interruption by a layer of endothelial cells (Fig.1) that are continuous with the lining of the pulmonary arteries and veins. Capillary endothelial cells form thin cytoplasmic sheets which are poor in organelles but contain pinocytotic vesicles [5].

The alveolar septa are lined, on both sides, by the alveolar epithelium which forms a continuous, uninter-

rupted cell barrier consisting of two cell types. _Type I_
cells (Fig.1) are, to some extent, similar to endothelial cells, forming very broad cytoplasmic sheets poor in
organelles. These sheets are much more extended than
those of the endothelium and may even branch and cross
over to the other side of the septum [6]. _Type II cells_
(Fig.2) are cuboidal and rich in organelles; they are
metabolically highly active as the producers of pulmonary surfactant [7]. In terms of cell number the type II
cells are somewhat more frequent than type I cells, but
the latter coat about 97% of the alveolar surface [8].
The alveolar _surface lining layer_, composed of an
aqueous hypophase topped by a surfactant film of lipoprotein, is the active product of epithelial cells, particularly of type II cells. It contains its own cell
population, the alveolar _macrophages_ which are derived
from monocytes.

The structure of the _interstitium_ is determined by the
relationship between fibers and capillaries (Fig.1);
both form networks that are interlaced in such a fashion
that fibers appear only on one side of the capillary
[3]. Endothelium and epithelium are each provided with a
basement membrane; these become fused where no fibers
are interposed thus forming the thin barrier part which
does not have an interstitial space and therefore cannot
take up fluid. An actual interstitial space forms around
the fibers, that is on one side of the capillary and in
what is sometimes called the "posts" in the capillary
meshes. This is where one finds interstitial cells which
comprise mainly _fibroblasts_ (Fig.1),as well as very few
free cells, such as mast cells and an occasional leuco-
cyte or plasma cell. The fibroblasts have a peculiar
disposition. They are branched and contain contractile
fibrils which connect to the basement membranes of endothelium and epithelium and may thus regulate the compliance of the interstitial space for fluid accumulation
[10].

It is also noteworthy that the _septal interstitial space_
is continuous within the plane of the septum and extends
towards the peripheral connective tissue; it can hence
function as a waterway for water and solutes that perme-
ate the alveolar wall [10]. Excess fluid can thus be
transported to the interstitial fluid sumps associated
with the connective tissue sheaths around blood vessels
and conducting airways, and be drained into lymphatics.

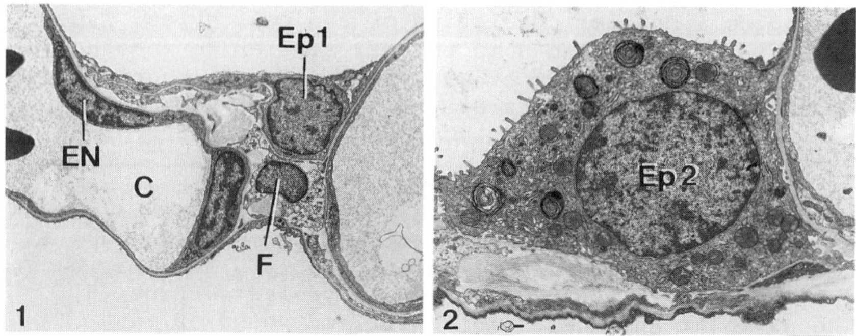

<u>Figs 1 and 2:</u> Normal human lung. Fig. 1: Capillaries (C) with endothelial cells (EN), type I epithelial cell (Ep 1) and fibroblast (F). Fig. 2: Type II epithelial cell with lamellar bodies.

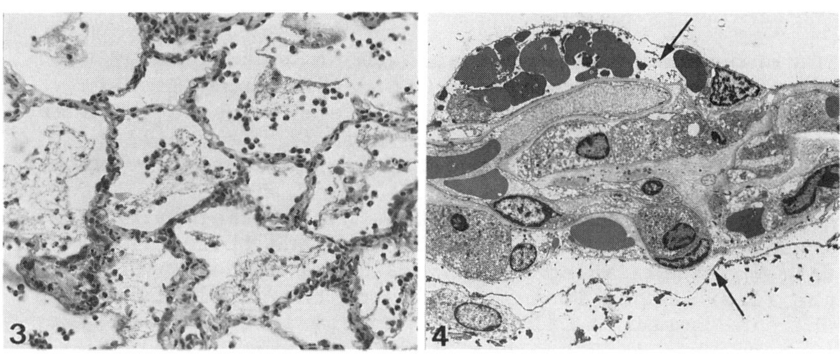

<u>Figs 3 and 4:</u> Acute ARDS. Pulmonary edema with cell and protein rich exudate seen in light (3) and electron microscope (4). Note destruction of epithelium (arrows).

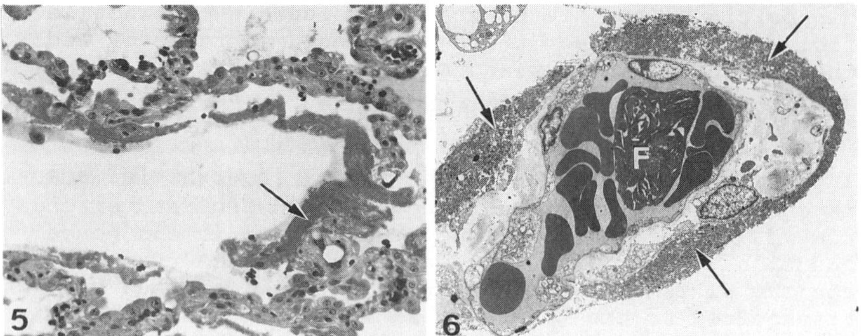

<u>Figs 5 and 6:</u> Formation of hyaline membranes (arrows) in ARDS lasting several days seen in light (5) and electron microscope (6). Note fibrin clot in capillary (F).

<u>Sequential changes in acute lung injury</u>

The mechanisms that initiate acute lung injury and eventually lead to the adult respiratory distress syndrome (ARDS) are manifold, but they all result in rather typical and uniform structural alterations [2, 11]. Invariably, a leaky blood-gas barrier, featuring interstitial and alveolar edema, is the predominant feature in the acute stage; inflammatory and then proliferative tissue reactions mark the subsequent stages of the disease. In general, this process can be subdivided into three stages.

During the <u>first day</u> following injury profuse <u>exudation</u> of blood plasma and of some blood cells into the interstitium and into alveolar spaces occurs (Fig.3), clear evidence that the integrity of the cell layers of the alveolar septa has been disturbed. The architecture of lung parenchyma is largely preserved, but electron microscopy reveals focal destructions of endothelial and epithelial cells (Fig.4), although the majority of the cells still appear intact. Particularly when the injury is due to septicemia the exudate contains many granulocytes, and one finds signs of activation of the clotting system since fine fibrin strands appear in the exudate as well as in capillaries.

The following days of the <u>first week</u> are marked by further destruction of lining cells, by organization of the exudate, and by an intensified appearance of inflammatory cells (Figs.5 and 6). Hyalin membranes — a mixture of fibrin and cell debris — form at the alveolar surface, particularly where the epithelial basement membrane has been denuded by detachment and destruction of type I cells, the most delicate and vulnerable of the alveolar cells (Fig.6). Capillaries are destroyed: microthrombi form as endothelial cells desintegrate. The architecture of alveolar septa now is severely altered, and one finds an immigration of inflammatory cells, mostly granulocytes, into the widened tissue spaces as well as into alveolar exudate.

Towards the end of and <u>beyond the first week</u> the reaction of the lung tissue proper becomes increasingly apparent. The first and most conspicuous reaction is the <u>repair of epithelial defects</u> by proliferating cuboidal cells (Figs. 7 and 8). Within two weeks most of the alveolar surface, still submerged under edema fluid, may become lined with a cuboidal epithelium. This characteristic cuboidal "transformation" of the epithelial layer

is a non-specific, or rather "tissue-specific", reaction
to epithelial cell damage which has affected mostly the
delicate type I cells. One reason for this proliferation
of type II cells is their role as progenitor cells for
the entire epithelial lining: the squamous type I cells
are unable to undergo mitotic division; they must be replaced by cuboidal type II cells which can replicate and
undergo subsequent transformation into squamous type I
cells. This process takes several weeks to be completed
and is associated with a gradual resorption of alveolar
exudate.

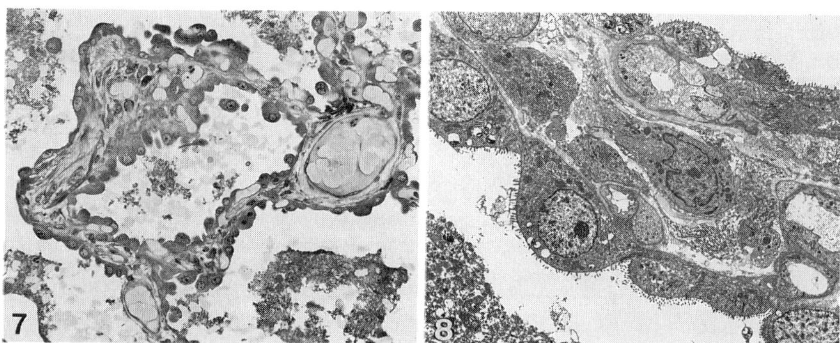

Figs 7 and 8: Type II cells proliferate in ARDS lasting
three weeks forming cuboidal alveolar epithelium.

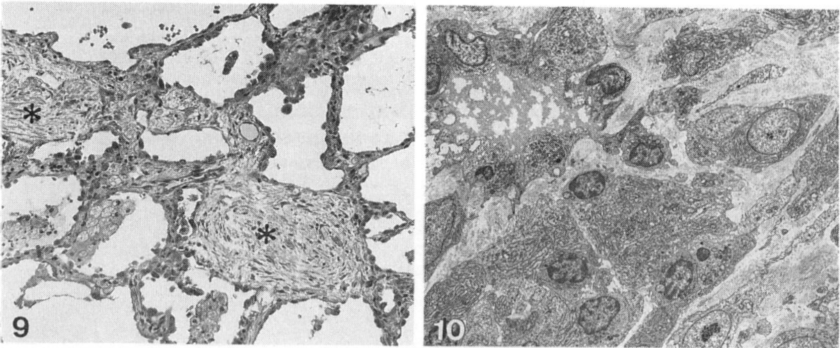

Figs 9 and 10: Interstitial changes are heterogeneous in
ARDS lasting several weeks. Coarse fiber masses (*) are
seen next to slender septa in light micrograph (9).
Interstitium is rich in plasma cells (10).

This repair process is accompanied by changes in the
septal tissue. Myofibroblasts proliferate and may contribute to the contraction of damaged septa, and the
deposition of connective tissue fibers initiates the
formation of scars which eventually lead to <u>fibrosis</u>
(Fig.9). New capillaries are formed, and the inflammatory cell population becomes transformed into one rich
in plasma cells and lymphocytes (Fig.10). The resulting
alveolar septa are coarse. The architecture of lung parenchyma can be grossly distorted, as some of these new
"septa" may originate from groups of folded up alveolar
walls, partly destroyed and glued together by organized
exudate. Lung parenchyma now exhibits a quite heterogeneous structure with large fibrotic masses interspersed
in more delicate nearly normal looking septa whose capillaries are provided with a thin air-blood barrier,
once the proliferated epithelium has been transformed
into type I cells again.

<u>Relations between structure and function</u>

The acute and severe failure of respiratory function in
the early stage cannot be explained by the destruction
of tissue structure alone. Profuse alveolar exudates
eliminate much of the functional gas exchange surface.
But further problems arise in the microcirculation, as
the capillaries have a much lower hematocrit than in
venous blood and leucocytes occupy a large part of capillaries. These changes persist through all subsequent
stages and are associated with a considerable thickening
of the tissue barrier [2].

A morphometric study reveals that the parameters which
determine pulmonary diffusing capacity for oxygen, DL_{O2},
are grossly altered in cases with severe gas exchange
impairment in the third phase of the disease: the alveolar and capillary surface areas, the capillary blood
volume, and the hematocrit are reduced to half the normal value, and the harmonic mean barrier thickness is
increased fivefold, with the result that DL_{O2} is reduced
to less than 10% of normal. But it is likely that this
diffusing capacity cannot be fully exploited: additional
impairment of gas exchange by ventilation-perfusion ine-
qualities and the formation of right-to-left shunts are
apt to lead to very severe reduction in arterial oxygen-
ation of blood.

Mechanisms of tissue damage

Although the basic pattern of tissue injury appears
rather uniform, clear differences are observed in different lungs with regard to number and types of intra-
and extravascular cells, or in the amount of fibrin deposition and microthrombi. To understand the mechanisms
one would like to find similarities with well defined
experimental models. Three possible pathways leading to
tissue damage have received particular attention:
(a) injuries mediated by accumulation and activation of
granulocytes in the pulmonary microvasculature [12];
(b) damage of endothelial cells by platelets or coagulation products [13, 14]; (c) primary direct barrier lesions elicited by endotoxin and humoral mediators [15],
or by other toxic agents.

Two findings are worth noting in that respect: (1) already in the very acute stage a conspicuous accumulation
of leucocytes, mainly granulocytes and monocytes, is a
consistent finding in ARDS lungs of quite different origin, although it is most pronounced in cases associated
with septicemia; (2) signs of activation of coagulation
are also a common finding in ARDS, irrespective of etiology, but fibrin deposits in capillaries or alveolar
exudate are rarely found earlier than 24-48 hours after
the onset of the disease, so that they appear to be sequelae of endothelial damage rather than cause.

Some principles of lung tissue reaction to injury

It appears that, during the initial phases, lung tissue
cannot react adequately to injury. Its most prominent
cells, the endothelial and type I epithelial cells, are
damaged, and apparently lack the capacity to swiftly repair the leaks — or then the extent of injury overwhelms
whatever repair capacity these cells have, a repair capacity which must needs be limited considering the paucity of cellular organelles, such as endoplasmic reticu-
lum and ribosomes, in relation to the vast expanse of
their membranes.

The next phase is marked by the reaction pattern of im-
migrant cells, particularly leucocytes and thrombocytes,
which contribute to accentuate the damage and then initiate the organization of exudate and the proliferation
of fibroblasts. The interaction of platelets, neutrophils, and (damaged) endothelial cells releases a multi-
tude of mediators that govern these events [14].

The cell population of lung tissue proper reacts only in
a second or third phase and is directed towards repair-
ing the damages incurred. This reaction appears to depend on proliferation of cells, and it takes a few days
to trigger mitotic cell division in a cell population
with a normally slow turnover rate. Particular problems
occur with damage to alveolar epithelium as it affects
primarily the type I cells which normally cover 97% of
the alveolar surface, whereas type II cells appear to be
more resilient to damage. Regeneration of an epithelial
lining depends entirely on proliferation of type II
cells which serve as stem cell population for the alveolar epithelium [16], since type I cells are terminally
differentiated cells incapable of mitotic division. This
may explain why damage to alveolar epithelium is so
severe and takes so long to repair. In comparison, the
repair of capillaries appears to be swifter, but even
here many if not most of the capillaries found in the
repair phase have been newly formed by angiogenesis. It
is still unclear how and to what extent these events are
governed by growth factors of various kinds, such as
mitogens released by blood platelets in a wound healing
effort, or by local tissue-specific factors related, for
example, to mesenchymal-epithelial interaction. It is
interesting, however, that some patterns of the tissue
reaction and transformation resemble processes of mor-
phogenesis observed during lung development.

Acknowledgment: This work was supported by grant
3.036.84 from the Swiss National Science Foundation.

References

1. Weibel, E.R. Lung Cell Biology. In: Handbook of
   Physiology, Vol.4, Am.Physiol.Soc., Bethesda, MD,
   pp.47-91, 1985.
2. Bachofen, M., Weibel, E.R. Sequential morphological
   changes in the adult respiratory distress syndrome.
   In: Pulmonary Diseases and Disorders (A.P. Fishman,
   ed.), MacGraw-Hill, New York, pp.2215-2222, 1987
3. Weibel, E.R The Pathway for Oxygen. Harvard
   University Press, Cambridge, MA, 1984.
4. Weibel, E.R Functional Morphology of Lung
   Parenchyma. In: Handbook of Physiology, Vol. 3/1,
   Am.Phys.Soc., Bethesda, MD, pp.89-111, 1986.
5. Milici, A.J., Watrous, N.E., Stukenbrok, H., Palade,
   G.E. J.Cell Biol. 105, 2603-2612, 1987.

6. Weibel, E.R Acta Anat. 78:425-443, 1971.
7. Wright, J.R., Clements, J.A. Am.Rev.Respir.Dis. 136, 426-444, 1987.
8. Crapo, J.D., Barry, B.E., Gehr, P., Bachofen, M., Weibel, E.R. Am.Rev.Respir.Dis. 125, 332-337, 1982.
9. Schneeberger, E.E., Karnovsky, M.J. Circ.Res. 38, 404-411, 1976.
10. Weibel, E.R., Bachofen, H. Structural design of the alveolar septum and fluid exchange. In: Pulmonary edema, (A.P. Fishman and E.M. Renkin, eds.). Am.Physiol.Soc., Bethesda, MD, pp.1-20, 1979.
11. Bachofen, M., Weibel, E.R. Clinics in Chest Med. 3, 35-56, 1982.
12. Till, G.O., Johnson, K.J., Kunkel, R., Ward, P.A. J.Clin.Invest. 69, 1126-1135, 1982.
13. Malik, A.B., Johnson, A., Tahomont, M.V. Ann.NY.Acad.Sc. 384, 213-234, 1982.
14. Heffner, J.E., Sahn, S.A., Repine, J.E. Am.Rev.Respir.Dis. 135, 482-492 1987.
15. Brigham, K.L , Meyrick, B. Am.Rev.Respir.Dis. 133, 913-927, 1986.
16. Evans, M.J., Cabral, L.J., Stephens, R.J., Freeman, G. Am.J.Pathol. 70, 175-198, 1973.

Pathological Study of Idiopathic Interstitial Pneumonia

Shigeki Saiki

St. Luke's International Hospital, Tokyo, Japan

Since 1974, idiopathic interstitial pneumonia has been as a reserach project and a course of national survey was conducted throughout Japan. In 1980, the project team published surmmary of the pathological findings of autopsy and biopsy cases as well as clinical information obtained.

I would like to present pathological criteria of idiopathic interstitial pneumonia based on the above data and explain the mechanism of remodeling of the pulmonary structure in terms of honey combing in idiopathic interstitial pneumonia.

The gross characteristics of idiopathic interstitial pneumonia are the lack of pleural adhesion anywhere and pleural effusion. Both lungs are involved equally and the lower lobes exhibit more advanced lesion, usually these are markedly contracted exhibiting corrugated pleural surface.

In other words, the pleural surface shows rather uniform cystic projections lined by anthracotic marking.

The cut surface shows multiple cysts along the pleura replacing the normal parenchyma, a picture is often referred to a honey combing of the lung parenchyma. The size of the cysts are 2 - 3 mm in diamater with largest reaching 8mm.

Some cysts appear connected with each other and directly drain to ectatic bronchi. This is a remarkable difference from the cysts seen in emphysema.

The honey combing of the lung parenchyma apparently

starts its conformation just beneath the pleura and
and progresses inwardly and the most cases of idiopathic
interstitial pneumonia at autopsy shows peripheral honey
combs and spared central· area around the thick bronchi
   The microscopically, the lung parenchyma adjacent to
the honey combed area shows alveolar septa and sparce
round cell infiltration. Alveolar type II pneumocytes
appear swollen and a few macrophages are seen in the
alveolar spaces. There's no polymorphonuclear infiltration. One prominent feature is the development of
proteinous exudate in a form of hyaline membrane. With
elastic fiber staining organization of hyaline membranes
around the alveolar ducts or sacs are common findings.
The low power view shows microcystic spaces with
thickened walls in which fine bundles of collapsed
elastic fibers are present. These elastic fibers are
derived from the alveolar septa. In other words, the
walls of microcysts consist of collapsed alveoli and
occationally of alveolar ducts.
   The normal lung schematically shown exhibits the
architecture expanding from the terminal bronchiole to
alveolar ducts and sacs beneath the pleura, with the
lobuli separated by interlobular connective tissue.
   In idiopathic interstitial pneumonia, this basic
structure of the lung becomes modified through couses of
alveolar collapse with the end result of honey comb lung.
   Initially several groups of alveolar spaces become
collapsed and alveolar ducts are widened.
   In a more advanced lesion, crescent-like materials,
hyaline membranes, in a process of organization, are
noticed covering the surface of alveolar ducts or
occationally are laid over the alveolar septa. The
alveolar ducts are markedly distended showing cystic
changes. The original alveolar septa contains a few
round cells and in the alveolar spaces are a small
amount of macrophages. The linig epithelium of the
alveoli is swollen and appears denuded.
   Schematically shown, the alveoli become small with
overlaying hyaline membranes, and widened alveolar ducts.
The alveolar septa is edematous with a small amount of
round cells and type II pneumocytes are more conspicuous.
   The dilated alveolar ducts are partially coverd by
tall columnar cells as is often called as glandular
metaplasia. In the stroma of the cyst wall are fine
elastic fibers of the alveolar septa and thickend fibers
probably derived from the ring fibers of alveolar ducts.

In other words, multiple alveoli are folded into the texture of the cyst wall stroma. There are glandular and squamous metaplasia over the surface of cyst walls, and alveoli are obliterated and collagen fibers in the cyst wall stroma. Hyaline membranes are no longer seen.

The lesions of an established honey comb lung show no normal pulmonary architecture with all the area replaced by cysts. One important finding is the state of interlobular spaces. In the idiopathic interstitial pneumonia, the interlobular septa is characteristically spared from the fibrotic process. The cyst wall contains reddish stained collagen fibers and in some areas focally thickened bundles of smooth muscles.

I would like to that honey combing process in idiopathic interstitial pneumonia is a lobular event taking places in the lobulus as a unit. Thus the size of the cysts in idiopathic interstitial pneumonia becomes fairly uniform in contrast to the end stage of eosinophilic granuloma or asbestosis in which irregularity of the size of the cyst is more conspicuous reflecting the irregularity of parenchymal destruction.

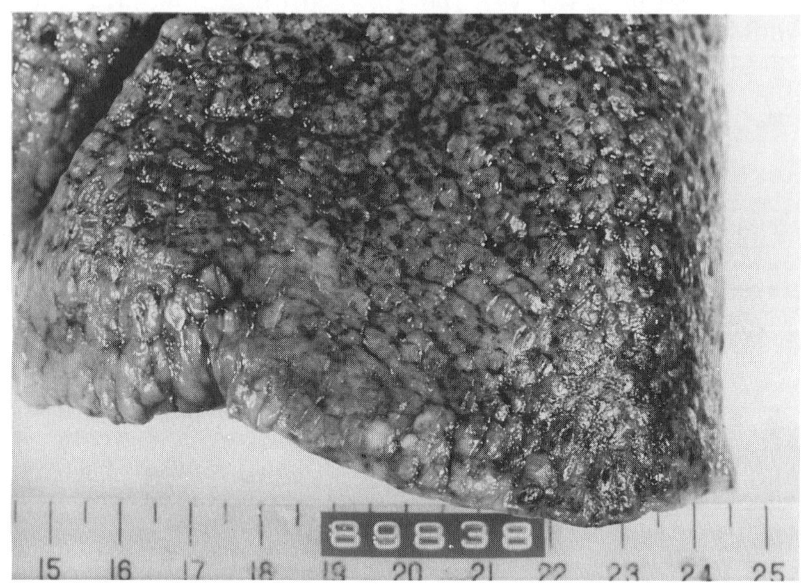

Fig. 1.
Corrugated pleural surface of the lower lobe of a case of idiopathic interstitial pneumonia. Each lobe corresponds to bronchioloectatic cysts.

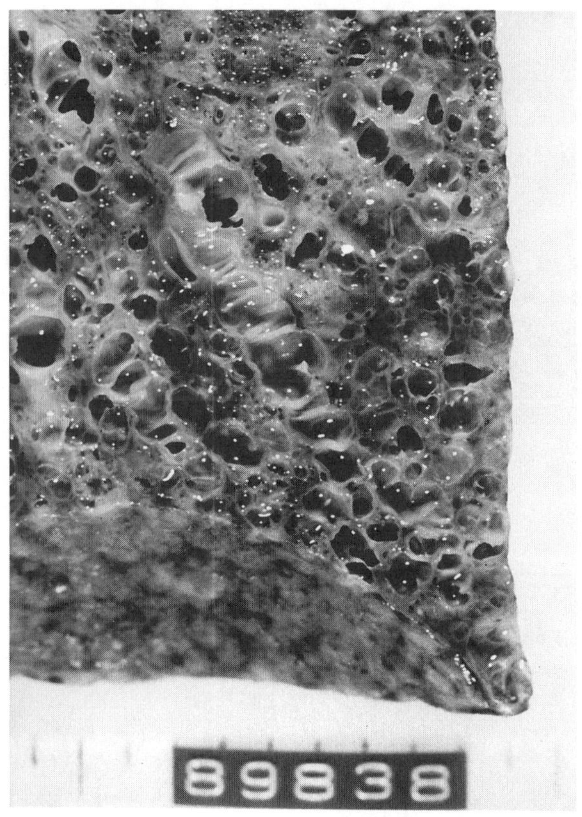

Fig. 2.
  Cut surface of a case of idiapathic
interstitial pneumonia showing a
typical picture of honey comb lung.
Bronchioloectatic cysts relatively
uniform in size are located subpleurally.

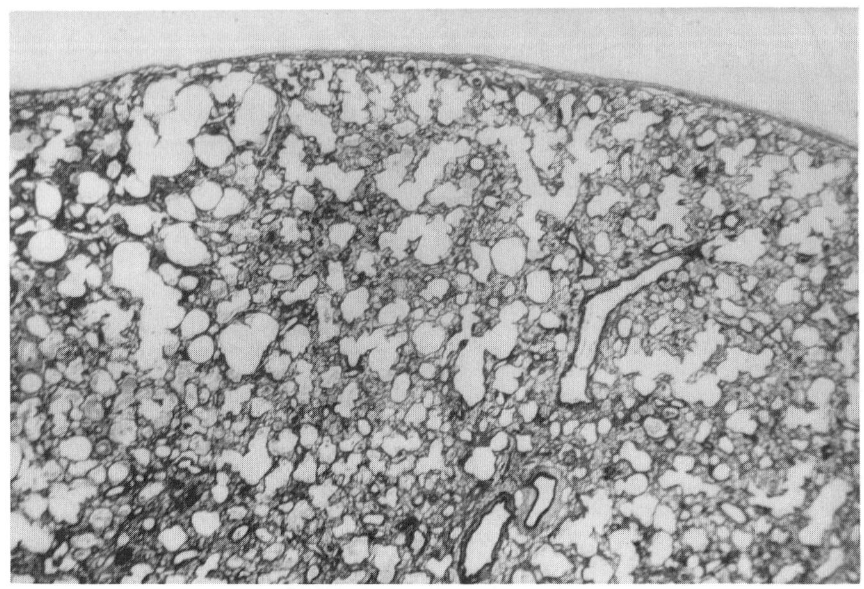

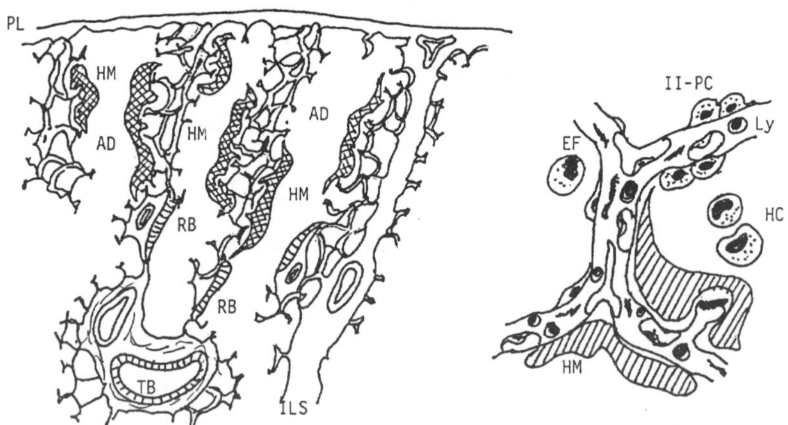

Fig. 3.
    Initial phase of idiopathic interstitial
pneumonia. Groups of alveolar septa became
atelectatic with dilatation of alveolar duct.
    The structural derangement is more easily
understood in the schema.

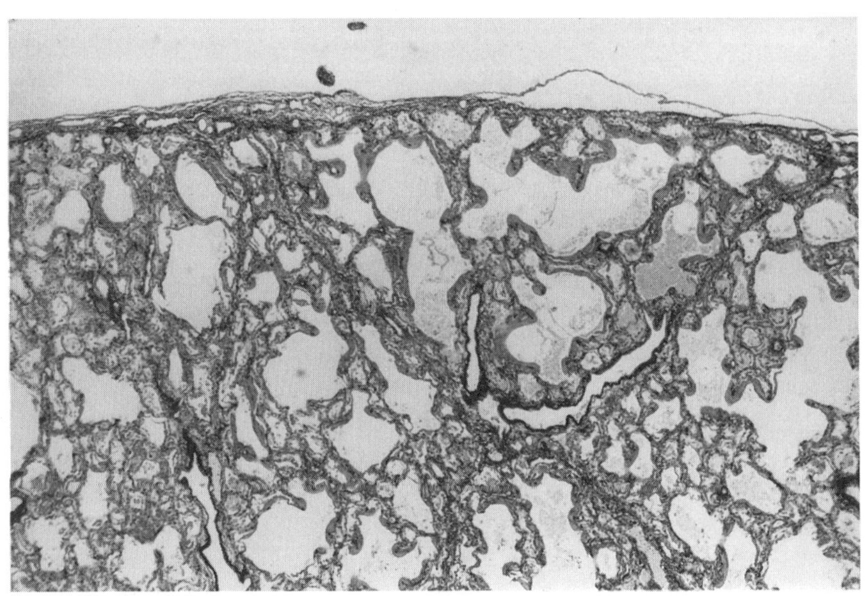

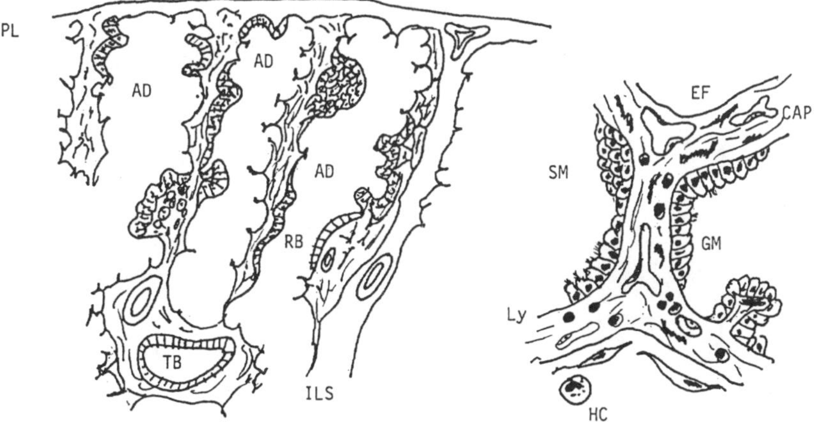

Fig. 4.
    In the more advanced stage, the alveolar ducts
become more widened with collapsed areas of
alveoli getting compressed, where a process of
organization taken place. The epithelium
covering the organized collapsed alveoli
frequently shows glandular metaplasia and
squamous metaplasia.

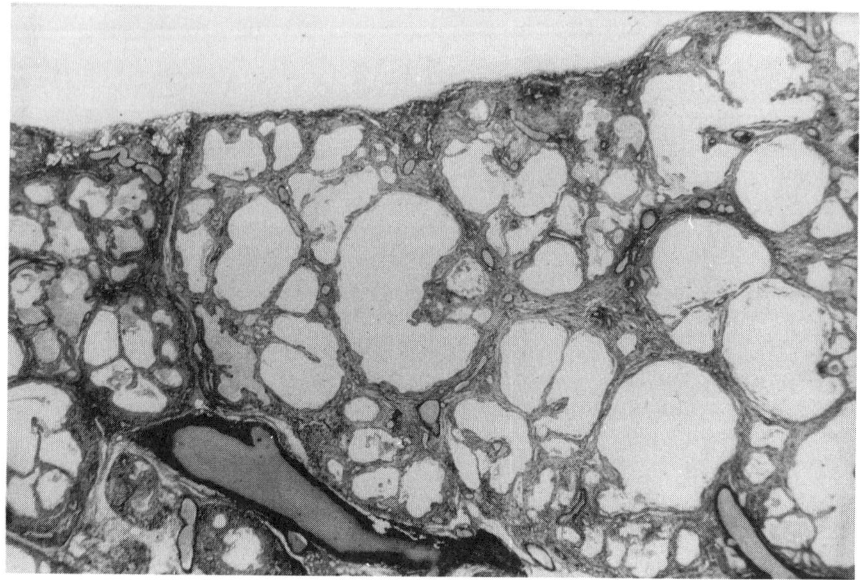

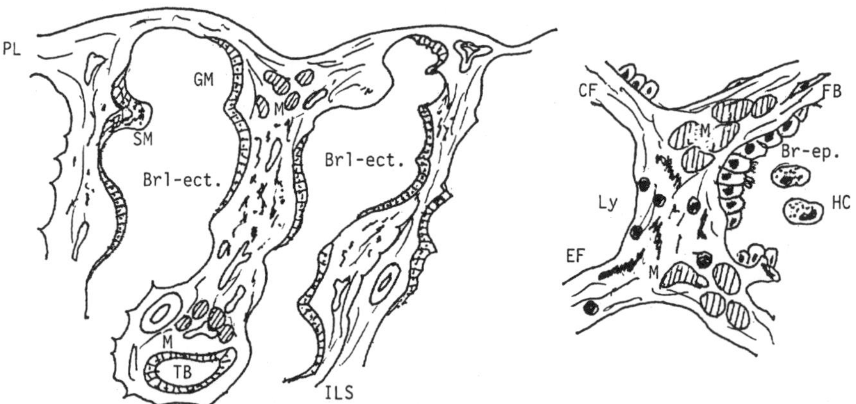

Fig. 5.
   Honey comb lung consists of cystically
dilated alveolar ducts and respiratory
bronchioles and the septating connective
tissue which are originally collapsed groups
of alveoli and alveolar ducts.
   The schema exhibits so-called bronchioloectatic spaces representing the cysts in
honey comb lung.

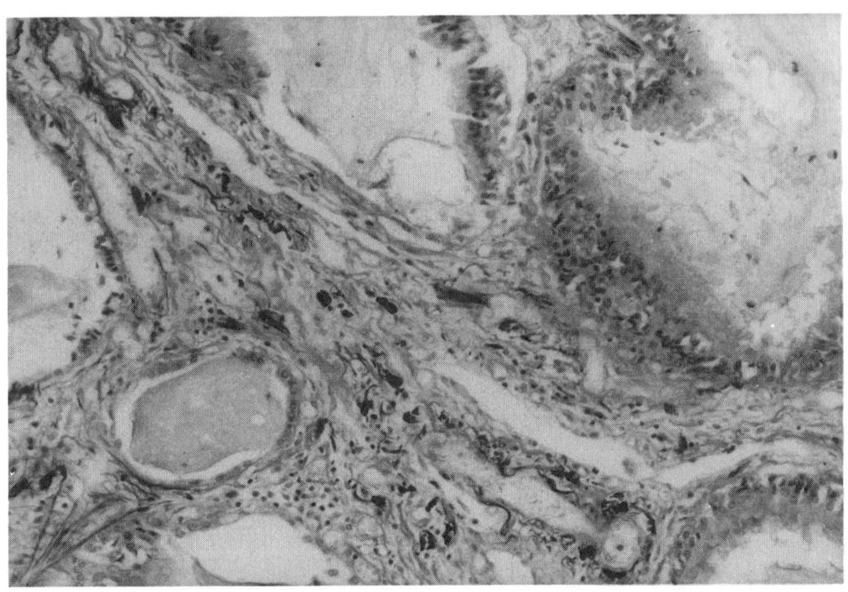

Fig. 6.
   Elastic fiber staining of the fibrosed lung
tissue exhibits crumpled elastic fibers, of
the alveolar septae; an evidence of collapse
of alveoli.

Alveolar Septal Inflammation: A Comparative Pathological Study of IPF and BOOP

Masanori Kitaichi

Chest Disease Research Institute, Kyoto University, Kyoto, Japan

Among 377 Japanese cases who showed bilateral pulmonary disorders and underwent open lung biopsy, the author recognized 62 cases of interstitial pneumonia of unknown etiology: 38 cases of usual interstitial pneumonia(UIP), two cases of desquamative interstitial pneumonia(DIP), 20 cases of bronchiolitis obliterans organizing pneumonia(BOOP) and one case each of lymphocytic interstitial pneumonia(LIP) and diffuse alveolar damage(DAD). Comparing UIP and BOOP, honeycoming was observed significantly more often in UIP, while alveolar septal inflammation and alveolar septal fibrosis were observed significantly more diffusely in BOOP. Spontaneous regression of pulmonary disorder was observed in only 4 cases of BOOP.

INTRODUCTION

Interstitial pneumonia is an intra-lobular inflammatory disorder of the lungs predominantly involving alveolar walls. Classification of interstitial pneumonia has been discussed in the past two decades[1]. Diagnostic criteria of usual interstitial pneumonia(UIP) and desquamative interstitial pneumonia(DIP) has been defined by the study of open lung biopsy cases done by Carrington et al.[2], although DIP was originally described by

Liebow et al. in 1965.   Idiopathic pulmonary fibrosis (IPF) is defined as a chronic, usually progressive pulmonary disorder showing UIP or DIP in the pulmonary histology and the diagnosis of IPF requires an open lung biopsy[3].   Meanwhile, lymphocytosis in bronchoalveolar lavage fluid and the extent of alveolar septal inflammation are reported favorable indices for observing the response from steroid therapy in patients with IPF[4]. Bronchiolitis obliterans organizing pneumonia (BOOP) was reported as a type of interstitial pneumonia with bronchiolitis obliterans having better prognosis than IPF or UIP[5].

To recognize and classify cases of interstitial pneumonia of unknown etiology and to compare histological findings, the author studied Japanese patients who showed bilateral diffuse pulmonary disorders and subsequently underwent an open lung biopsy.

MATERIALS AND METHODS

SOURCE OF THE CASES AND MODE OF LUNG BIOPSY: 377 Japanese cases who showed diffuse pulmonary disorders and underwent an open lung biopsy were studied clinico-pathologically, which included 150 cases in the author's hospital between 1966 and 1988.   Usually two sites from two different lobes of a lung were biopsied.

CLASSIFICATION OF INTERSTITIAL PNEUMONIA: The diagnostic criteria of UIP and DIP were based upon the report by Carrington et al.[2] and those of BOOP were based upon the report by Epler et al.[5].   The criteria of LIP were based upon the description by Colby et al.[6] while those of diffuse alveolar damage(DAD) were based upon the description by Katzenstein et al.[7].

ASSESSMENT OF ALVEOLAR SEPTAL INFLAMMATION, ALVEOLAR SEPTAL FIBROSIS AND HONEYCOMBING: The three kinds of histological findings were divided into four grades according to the extent of involvement: absent (score 0), mild (score 1), moderate (score 2) and severe (score 3). If honeycombing (dilated terminal air spaces surrounded with fibrous changes mainly at the level of respiratory bronchioles) was observed in less than a third of the most involved biopsy sample, the grade of honeycombing (HNCB) was assessed as mild.   If HNCB was observed in more than two thirds of the biopsy sample, the grade of HNCB was assessed as severe.   The grade of HNCB in between was assessed as moderate.   If alveolar septal inflammation(ASI) or alveolar septal fibrosis(ASF) was observed in less than a third of the alveolar area which was not involved in HNCB their grade was assessed as mild.   If ASI or ASF was observed in more than two thirds of the alveolar area uninvolved in HNCB their grade was assessed as severe.   The grade of ASI or ASF in between was assessed as moderate.   When ASF was associated with significant septal cell infiltration, ASI was also assessed as present.

RESULTS

1. RECOGNITION AND CLASSIFICATION OF INTERSTITIAL PNEUMONIA OF UNKNOWN ETIOLOGY

62 cases of interstitial pneumonia of unknown etiology were recognized and could be classified into UIP, DIP, BOOP, LIP and DAD.   Etiological factors of infection, inhalation of exogenous agents and associated collagen vascular diseases were excluded by pre- and post-biopsy clinical information including serological examinations for organisms and bacteriological examinations of patients' secretions and biopsy tissues.

UIP: For the recognition of UIP, the finding of highly variegated structure, including the entire spectrum from normal alveolar walls to fibrotic, end-stage lesions in the same tissue sample [2], was considered as most important.   38 cases were recognized as idiopathic UIP.   ASI was absent in 11 cases (29%), mild in 24 cases (63%), moderate in 2 cases (5%) and severe in one case (3%).   ASF was mild in 13 cases (34%), moderate in 19 cases (50%), and severe in 6 cases (16%).   HNCB was absent in one case (3%), mild in 12 cases (32%), moderate in 7 cases (18%), and severe in 18 cases (47%) (Fig. 1-3).

DIP: Two male cases with ages of 54 and 49 years were recognized as idiopathic DIP.   ASI was mild in one case and severe in another case.   ASF was severe in both cases. HNCB was absent in one case and moderate in another (Fig. 4, 5).   The two cases died from progressive respiratory insufficiency 48 and 68 months after the lung biopsy respectively in spite of steroid hormone treatment.

These 38 cases of UIP and two cases of DIP were recoqnized among the author's hospital series.   Only a

TABLE 1. DIFFERENTIAL DIAGNOSIS OF BOOP

Finding negative for BOOP	Suspected Pulmonary Disorders
- necrosis or infarction	infection pulmonary infarction lymphoproliferative disorder Wegener's granulomatosis(WG)
- marked cellular infiltration in pleura or interlobular septa	lymphoproliferative disorder eosinophilic pneumonia
- solid nodular proliferation of lymphocytic cells	lymphoproliferative disorder
- marked eosinophilic exudates	diffuse alveolar damage (DAD) including infectious etiology eosinophilic pneumonia lymphoproliferative disorder
- hyaline membranes	DAD
- granulomatous lesions	infection hypersensitivity pneumonitis lymphoproliferative disorder eosinophilic pneumonia, WG
- marked infiltration of eosinophils more than observed in UIP	eosinophilic pneumonia
- marked reparative metaplastic changes of bronchiolar epithelial cells	infection(Mycoplasma, viruses)
- marked infiltration of PMN neutrophils	infection multiple bronchiolopneumonia
- vasculitis	infection, WG, lymphoproliferative disorder

case of DIP had pre-biopsy steroid hormone treatment.

BOOP: Although BOOP is a type of pulmonary lesion-- showing (1) bronchiolitis obliterans with granulation tissues or organized exudates in the lumen of membranous and/or respiratory bronchioles, (2) organizing pneumonia with granulation tissues in alveolar ducts and alveoli and (3) interstitial pneumonia with infiltration mainly of mononuclear cells in the alveolar walls associtaed with mild to moderate fibrous thickening--in order to recognize BOOP, in addition to the negative results for organisms using Ziehl-Neelsen and Grocott's methenamine silver stains it was necessary to confirm that the findings listed in TABLE 1 were absent in the biopsy specimens.

20 cases were recognized as idiopathic BOOP. 14 cases had no steroid hormone treatment before lung biopsy while 6 cases had steroid hormone treatment before the biopsy. ASI was absent in one case (5%), mild in 4 cases (20%), moderate in 6 cases (30%), and severe in 9 cases (45%). ASF was mild in 4 cases (20%), moderate in 5 cases (25%) and severe in 11 cases (55%). HNCB was absent in all cases (Fig. 6, 7).

LIP: A 33 year-old female with a 14-month duration of dry cough, exertional dyspnea and bilateral pulmonary infiltrates was recognized as idiopathic LIP. Biopsy specimens showed severe ASI, mild ASF and mild HNCB (Fig. 8).

DAD: A 61-year-old female with a two-month duration of fever of unknown origin, exertional dyspnea and bilateral pulmonary infiltrates was recognized as idio-pathic DAD. Lung biopsy samples were negative for viruses and bacilli in cultures. The case died 35 days after the biopsy from progressive respiratory insuffi-ciency in spite of large doses of steroid hormone treatment before and after the biopsy. Biopsy specimens showed severe ASI and severe ASF with focal hyaline membranes and lacked HNCB (Fig. 9).

2. COMPARISON OF IDIOPATHIC UIP AND IDIOPATHIC BOOP

Comparing idiopathic cases of UIP and BOOP, cases of BOOP showed higher grades of ASI and ASF and lesser grades of HNCB in the pulmonary histology. Spontaneous regression of pulmonary disorders was recognized in only 4 cases of BOOP (TABLE 2).

TABLE 2.   COMPARISON OF IDIOPATHIC UIP AND IDIOPATHIC
            BOOP

	UIP (n = 38)	BOOP (N=20)
Sex (Males/Females)	28/10	12/8
Age at the Biopsy(years old):	23-70	40-69
Mean ± SD (years old)	57.4 ± 9.1	58.1 ± 7.3
Clinical History or		
Observation Period before	1-240 M	0.5-60M
the Biopsy: Mean(months)	45.8 ± 54.9	6.4 ± 14.0 (1)
Findings of Biopsy Samples:		
- ASI: (score: mean ± SD)	0.83 ± 0.64	2.15 ± 0.93(2)
- ASF: (score: mean ± SD)	1.82 ± 0.69	2.35 ± 0.81(3)
- HNCB:(score: mean ± SD)	2.11 ± 0.95	0 (4)
Follow-UP Period after the	0.5-84 M	1-48 M
Biopsy: Mean (months)	20.7 ± 17.9	10.3 ± 12.1(5)
Spontaneous Regression	0/38(0%)	4/20(20%) (6)
after the Biopsy		

(1), (2) and (4): $p<0.01$.   (3), (5) and (6): $p<0.05$.

DISCUSSION

Through the present study, it may be recognized that the concept and criteria of UIP described by Carrington et al. [2] holds the landmark position for the recognition and classification of interstitial pneumonia of unknown etiology. According to the previous report from Denver [4], moderate-to-severe ASI was observed in 39% of 26 cases of IPF. In the present study, however, moderate-to-severe ASI was observed in only 10% of 40 cases of IPF and in only 8% of 38 cases of idiopathic UIP while moderate-to-severe ASI was observed in 75% of 20 cases of idiopathic BOOP. Spontaneous regression of pulmonary disorder was observed in only 4 cases of BOOP. An international study on IPF may be required.

REFERENCES

1. Liebow A.A. Prog Resp Res 8, 1-33, 1975.
2. Carrington, C.B., Gaensler, E.A., Coutu, R.E., FitzGerald, M.X., and Gupta, R.G. N Eng J Med 298, 801-809, 1978.
3. Crystal, R.G. In: Harrison's Principles of Internal Medicine (E. Braunwald et al. eds.), McGraw-Hill Book Company, pp. 1099-1100, 1987.
4. Watters, L.C., Schwarz, M.I., Cherniack, R.E., Waldron, J.M. Dunn, T.L., Stanford, R.E., and King, T.E. Am Rev Resp Dis 135, 696-704, 1987.
5. Epler, G.R., Colby, T.V., McLoud, T.C., Carrington, C.B., and Gaensler, E.A. N Eng J Med 312, 152-158, 1985.
6. Colby, T.V., and Carrington, C.B. Pathol Annual 18, 27-70, 1983.
7. Katzenstein, A.A., and Askin, F.B. In: Surgical Pathology of Non-Neoplastic Lung Disease, W.B. Saunders Company, pp. 9-42, 1982.

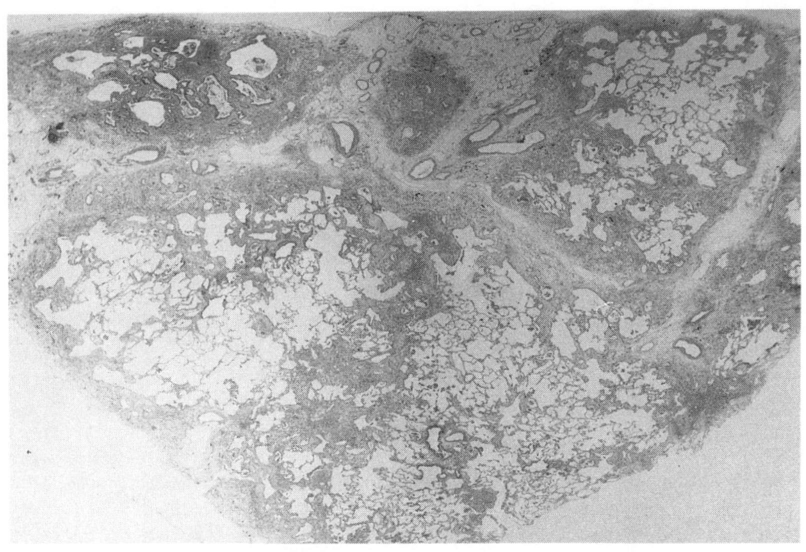

Fig. 1. UIP. The lung specimen shows honeycombing (left upper) and fibrotic lesions predominantly in the peripheral zones of lobules. A lobule (lower half) shows patchy distribution of fibrosing processes intermingled with normal alveolar walls (H & E, 1x5).

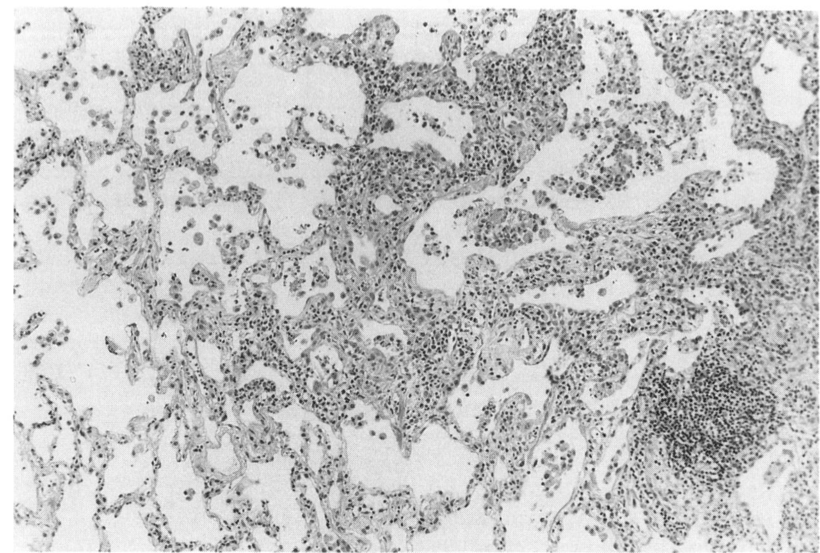

Fig. 2. Alveolar septal inflammation in a case of UIP.
Alveolar walls show thickening with infiltration of
lymphocytes and plasma cells (H & E, 10x5).

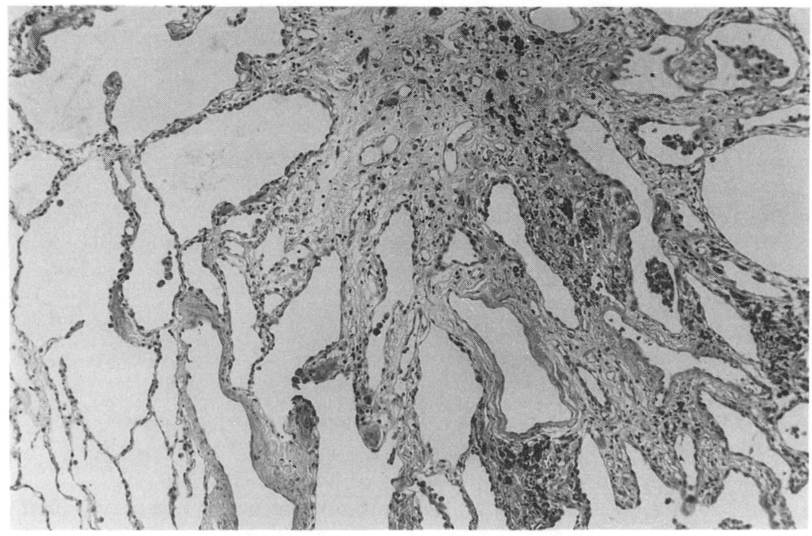

Fig. 3. Alveolar septal fibrosis in another case of UIP.
Alveolar walls show fibrous thickening with normal ones
in the adjacent area (H & E, 10x5).

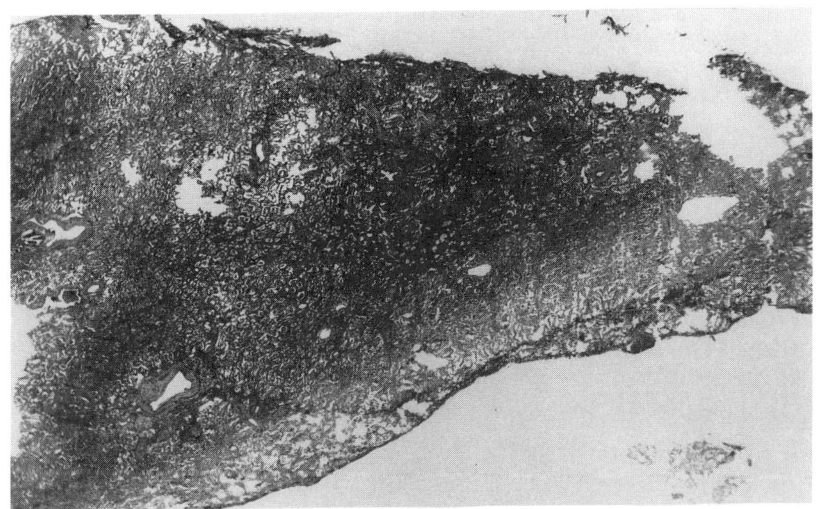

Fig. 4. DIP. The lung specimen shows relatively uniform involvement with abundant large mononuclear cells filling air spaces of alveoli, alveolar ducts and bronchioles (H & E, 1x5).

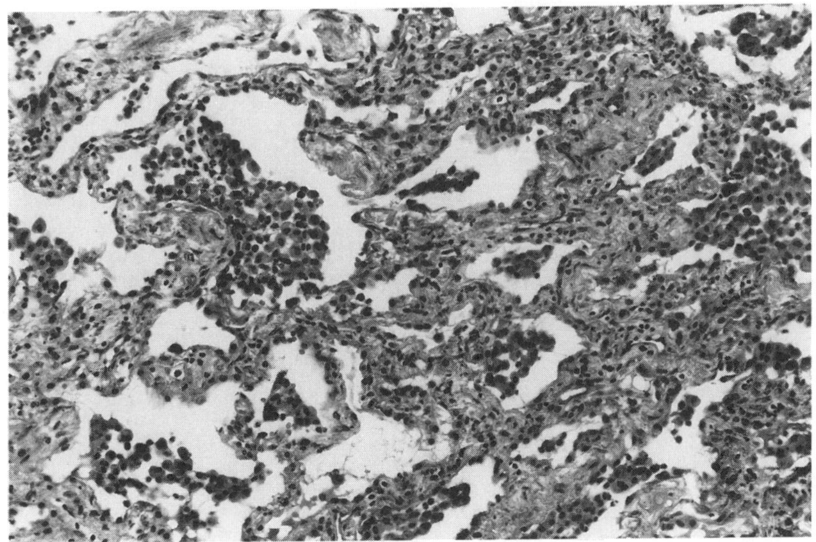

Fig. 5. DIP. Higher magnification of Fig. 4 showing alveolar septal inflammation and fibrosis (ASI and ASF). Alveolar walls show fibrous thickening and infiltration of lymphocytes, plasma cells and eosinophils (H&E, 20x5).

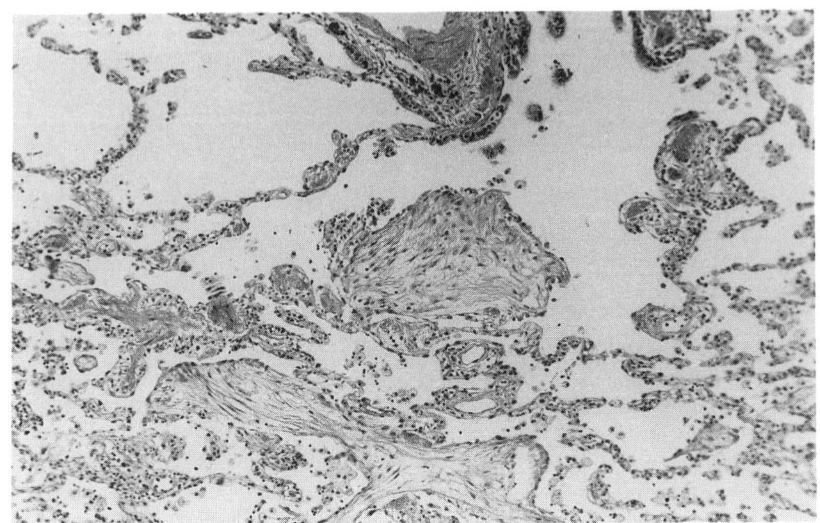

Fig. 6.   Alveolar septal inflammation in a case of BOOP.
A respiratory bronchiole and alveolar ducts show granulation tissues.   Alveolar   walls   show   infiltration   of
lymphocytes and plasma cells (H & E, 10x5).

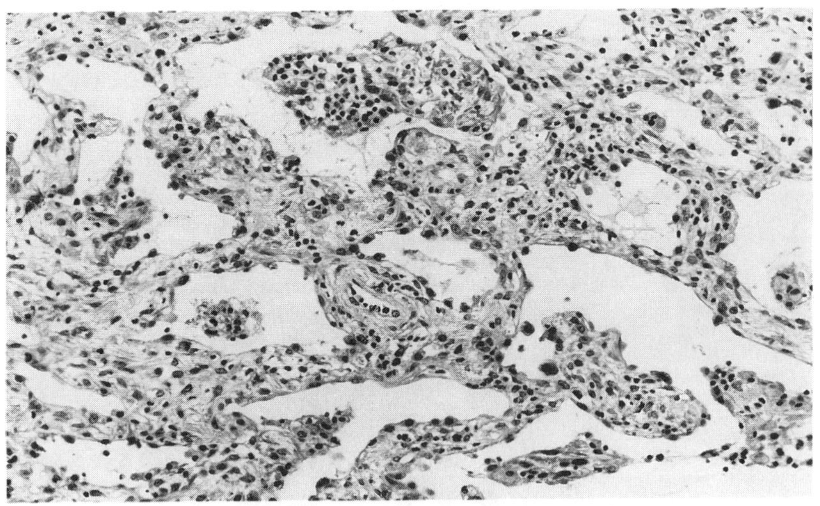

Fig. 7.   Alveolar septal inflammation and fibrosis (ASI
and ASF) in another case of BOOP.   Alveolar walls show
fibrous   thickening   and   infiltration   of   lymphocytes,
plasma cells and several eosinophils (H & E, 20x5).

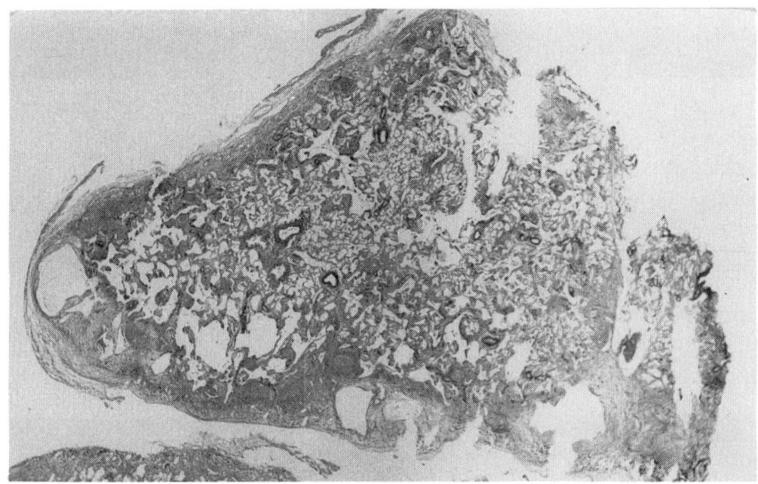

Fig. 8. LIP. The lung specimen show subpleural honeycombing and diffuse infiltration of lymphocytes, plasma
cells, histiocytes and eosinophils in alveolar walls with
mild fibrous thickening (H & E, 1x5).

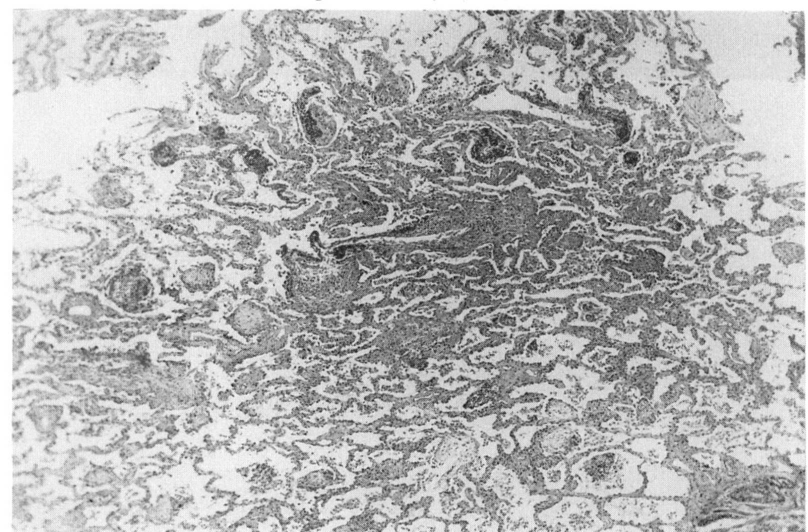

Fig. 9. DAD. The lung specimen shows diffuse fibrous
thickening of alveolar walls with infiltration of lymphocytes, plasma cells and eosinophils associated with
organizing exudates and a few hyaline membranes in
alveoli and alveolar ducts (H & E, 4x5).

IV
PATHOGENESIS

Epidemiological Approaches to Idiopathic Pulmonary Fibrosis

Kazuro Iwai* and Yutaka Hosoda**

* *Research Institute of Tuberculosis, Japan Anti-Tuberculosis Association, Tokyo, Japan*
** *Radiation Effect Research Institute, Hiroshima, Japan*

Prevalence studies on idiopathic pulmonary fibrosis (IPF) in each district of Japan, by using mass survey films and autopsy records, revealed a significantly higher rate of IPF in rural than in urban areas. Correlation between annual consumption of agricultural chemicals and death rate due to IPF in each district showed a significant relationship in 2 of 35 chemicals. A case-controlled study on 86 sets of 1 IPF case, 1 hospital and 2 healthy controls was made over 200 questionnaires. No definite and specific factors were found, but smoking, agricultural and some industrial exposure seemed to relate to development of IPF.

Interstitial pulmonary fibrosis (IPF) is a disease of unknown etiology with severe prognosis, for which we have no effective or radical therapy at present. Some immunological process may contribute to the pathological feature of the disease, but we don't know what triggers the pathological process. In order to approach the pathogenesis of the disease, we have carried out three studies from an epidemiological standpoint, those are prevalence rate in each district of Japan, correlation between the prevalence rate and consumption of agricultural chemicals and a case-controlled study on environmental and constitutional factors.

1. <u>Prevalence rate of IPF by districts in Japan.</u>

An introductory study was made using annual mass survey films from 7 prefectures in Japan. Miniature chest X-ray films of inhabitants of over 15 years of age were carefully read and the cases which show diffuse fibrotic shadows were selected. After anamnesis, X-ray examination and lung function test by spirometer, cases suggestive for COPD, occupational dust disease or collagen lung disease were excluded.

The prevalence rate of IPF in the 7 prefecture differed markedly from prefecture to prefecture. The prevalence was low in Hokkaido, Miyagi and Osaka, and high in Okayama and Ehime prefectures. The subjects were further classified according to residential area, and the prevalence was calculated by these areas. In contrast to our initial assumption, the prevalence rate of IPF was higher among the inhabitants of rural areas than those in urban areas with a significant p-level.

The next study was carried out by using the data book of autopsy records in Japan. The Japanese Society of Pathology published this annual data book, which included around 90% of all the autopsies in this country since 1959. Data since 1974 was entered into a computer for analysis. The average autopsy rate to total death in Japan is around 5%. All of the cases which were diagnosed pathologically to be "interstitial fibrosis and pneumonia", were sorted by computer. Japanese pathologists like to use the term "interstitial pneumonia" even when fibrosis is prominent, as they think fibrosis is a sequela of pneumonia. So, both interstitial pneumonia and fibrosis were selected. Then the cases suggestive for non-idiopathic interstitial pneumonia or lung fibrosis were excluded.

During the 12 years from 1974 to 1985 a total of 2,315 cases of IIP/IPF were selected. Total number of registered autopsies of people over 15 years of age in the same period was 342,279. Thus, the rate of IIP/IPF cases in the autopsy population was calculated to be 0.68%. Applying this rate to the total number of deaths in Japan yields around 4,500 deaths per year due to IIP/IPF. From the population size of Japan of people over 15 years of age, the annual death rate of IIP/IPF was presumed to be approximately $5/10^5$ population.

Age distribution curve of the disease reveals a high peak in 60 to 70 year-olds; and males were affected in greater frequency. These may be explained both by the accumulation of environmental factors and impaired immunoregulation system in older people.

Table I Rate of IIP/IPF Autopsy to Total Autopsy
and to Population

District	Rate of IIP/IPF to total autopsy(%)	Presumed death rate of IIP/IPF (per 10^5 pop.)
Hokkaido	0.84	6.02
Tohoku	0.68	5.76
Kanto [1] except Tokyo	0.72	4.62
Tokyo	0.59	3.54
Hokuriku	0.90	7.96
Chubu [2]	0.72	5.46
Kinki [3]	0.63	4.67
Chugoku	0.75	6.88
Shikoku	0.84	8.23
Kyushu [4]	0.57	5.16
Whole Japan	0.68	5.16

cf: 1) to 4) indicate the districts where large cities locate; 1) Yokohama, Kawasaki 2) Nagoya 3) Osaka, Kyoto, Kobe 4) Fukuoka, Kitakyushu

Presumed death rate of IIP/IPF in each district of Japan
varied from district to district similar to the previous
mass survey data, after adjustment by autopsy rate in
each districts. Shikoku, Hokuriku, Chugoku districts,
which are primarily agricultural, showed higher rates
than that of other districts. (Table I) Rate of differences between urban and rural areas were noted again and
large cities with population of over a million demonstrated significantly lower death rates as compared to
rural areas.

Studies on the relationship between death rate of IIP/IPF
and population density in each districts in Japan, revealed a negative correlation. The correlation coefficient was calculated to be −0.687 which shows significance in the 1% p−level.

2. Correlation between the death rate of IIP/IPF and consumption of agricultural chemicals.

From the above mentioned data, a question arises as to
whether some of the widely used agricultural chemicals
relate to the development of the disease. The relationship between consumption level of these agricultural
chemicals in each district in Japan and the rate of death
by IIP/IPF was studied. We obtained a data book published
by the Ministry of Agriculture and Forestry, of agricultural chemicals used in this country which lists annual
consumption levels of each drug by prefecture.

35 agricultural chemicals which are consumed at levels of
over 1000 tons per year over all of Japan were chosen.
Of the 35 chemicals, 4 are poisonous, 24 are powerful,
and the remaining 8 are ordinary drugs. We compared the
amount of the chemicals consumed per cultured area to the
death rate of IIP/IPF calculated from autopsy records.
Among the 35 chemicals tested, organic arsenic powder and
NAC (1−naphrhyl−N−methyl−carbamate) showed a significant
correlation to the death rate of IIP/IPF with correlation
coefficients of over 0.7 (Fig. 1), though the slope is by
no means steep. Paraquot, which is known to provoke
severe interstitial lung damage when it is ingested, did
not show any correlation.

3. Case-controlled study

Finally, we performed a case-controlled study on clinically diagnosed IPF cases with matched paired controls. The cases of IPF which were diagnosed clinically by using the criteria made by the Research Committee of Interstitial Pneumonia in Japan, were collected. One hospital control which has the same sex and age as the case, was selected from the same hospital, regardless of disease (mostly lung disease) and whether the case was treated on out- or in-patient basis. Two healthy controls of the same sex and age as the case were selected at random from inhabitants living in the same residential area. All of these subjects were interviewed at home by trained interviewers and were questioned on approximately 200 items in the same way. The collected cases accounted to be 101 in total, 88 in the hospital control, and 178 in the healthy control. However, after reviewing these subjects and matching them, the number of cases dropped to 86. Therefore, the hospital control was also 86, and healthy control became 172. Analysis was made mainly on these matched cases and controls but, at the same time, a comparison was also made of these three groups as a whole. As for the matched pair, relative risk was estimated on each questioned item, and the differences were examined statistically.

19 questions were asked on predilection for food, 15 on beverages, wine and tobacco, 3 on hobbies, 17 on general health condition until the disease, 39 on previous disease history, 18 on long term medicine intake, 10 on family disease history (including intermarriage), 10 on the use of cosmetics for women, 32 on any chemicals used in home, 33 on occupational exposure, 12 on residential area, and 2 on the home heating system.

Regarding food preference, there was a negative correlation to eating fish, both in the healthy and hospital controls, indicating that eating fish might reduce the development of IPF. Comsumption of meat, black tea and coffee also showed a negative correlation to the healthy control, but not to the hospital control. This shows that diseased people tend to consume less western-style beverages and drink more green tea.

Table II   Questionary Items Which Showed Significant
Relative Risk to Healthy and/or Hospital Controls

	Relative Risk	
	To Healthy Control	To Hosp. Control
Food		
Fish	0.48 *	0.35
Meat	0.57 *	NS
Beverage		
Green tea	2.60 **	NS
Black tea	0.25 **	NS
Coffee	0.45 *	NS
Wine	0.43 **	NS
Tobacco	2.93 **	NS
Previous Illness		
Rubeola	NS	10.99 *
Herpes zoster	3.22 *	NS
Pneumonia	3.12 **	NS
Long-term drug intake		
Antibiotics	3.44 **	NS
Hypertension	0.44 *	NS
Home chemicals		
Anti-corrosive	1.78 **	NS
Cosmetics		
Make up	0.13 *	NS
Rouge	0.06 **	
Agricultural exposure		
Rice field	4.85 *	NS
Chance of Inhalation of Agricult. Chem.	3.22 *	NS
Industrial Exposure		
Metal	1.34 *	1.36 **

* $p < 0.05$ ** $p < 0.01$

As for smoking, high positive relative risk was noted to healthy control with a significance of 1% p-level, and to the hospital control the relative risk was 1.49, though it is not significant. Group analysis of smoking habits also indicated a higher smoking rate in the case group (50.0%) than in the hospital(30.5%) and healthy controls (35.3%).

Regarding previous illness, the case group had a high significant relative risk to herpes and pneumonia, and they were often treated by anti-biotics in the past. This may reflect events after the subclinical onset of the disease. No significant relation to intermarriage was seen to the healthy and hospital controls but group analysis showed a slightly higher rate of intermarriage among the case group (9.0%) than the hospital (5.7%) or the healthy control (3.5%) groups.

As for chemicals used in home, anti-corrosive drugs showed a significant relative risk, but the actual risk is not so high. The relative risk in healthy control pairs is lower than 1.0 for cosmetics. This could result from an inaccurate recollection of cosmetic use before and after the onset of the disease.

Regarding occupational exposure, rice field work and probable inhalation of agricultural chemicals showed a significantly higher relative risk to the healthy control pairs but not to the hospital controls. These may be factors for the development of pulmonary diseases but they are not specific for that of IPF in a significant level. Among various kinds of industrial exposure, only exposure to metal dust showed significant relative risks to both the healthy and hospital controls, but for this exposure the relative risk is not so high.

Discussion

In epidemiological approaches to idopathic pulmonary fibrosis, a principal concern is accuracy of the diagnosis for the collected cases. In a mass survey, when screening is done by examining miniature X-ray films, a primary source of error is failure of include the secondary fibrosis following the other lung diseases.

These non-idiopathic pulmonary fibrosis were excluded
using anamnesis and lung function tests. In the
autopsy-record study, individuals who has lung fibrosis
accompanying collagen diseases, infectious/allergic lung
diseases due to known microbiological agents, pneumoconiosis, therapeutic radiation or anti-cancer drug
administration were excluded from the subjects under
study by reading the brief summary diagnosis in the
autopsy records. Secondly, adjustment for different sex-
and age-distribution is necessary in a mass survey study
for prevalence rate comparison among the subject-groups
in each prefecture, and adjustment of the autopsy rate to
the total death in each district is required in an
autopsy record study.

Japanese pathologists often use the term of diffuse
interstitial "pneumonia" instead of "fibrosis", as they
regard fibrosis as a sequela of pneumonia. The majority
of cases which were diagnosed to be idiopathic interstitial pneumonia (IIP) were presumed to be idiopathic
pulmonary fibrosis (IPF), as the distribution of IPF
and that of IIP in the present autopsy series in each
district of Japan showed the same pattern (data was not
shown). Therefore, both IIP and IPF were summed into a
single disease group. (IIP/IPF)

In the autopsy record study, negative correlation was
noted between the prevalence rate of the disease and the
population density in each district. The disease was
found more in primarily agricultural districts with no
large city having a population over one million people.

In Japan in recent years, consumption levels of agricultural chemicals is high and toxic action of these chemicals has been a concern for the farmers who spray them,
as well as for consumers of agricultural products. Not a
few of the agricultural chemicals in use are poisonous or
powerful drugs, causing irritation to surface mucosa and
skin as well as toxic effects on some organs of humans
who spray and inhale them. Asthma-like symptoms or lung
edema or even pneumonitis may develop in some instances.
Among 35 agricultural chemicals tested, two showed
significant correlation to the death rate of IIP/IPF.
However, the slope of relative risk is not steep, and the
disease was also found in considerable numbers in highly

populated areas. Therefore, these two chemicals seemed
not to have a specific, highly significant causative
relationship to IIP/IPF, but to be one of the factors
or cooperative one leading to the development of the
disease.

The case-controlled study revealed many positive and
negative factors for the health controls, but except for
a negative correlation for "eating fish" and a positive
correlation for "metal dust exposure" there were no
factors common to both healthy and hospital controls.
The data showing that IPF is seen less frequently among
people who eat fish frequently may indicate some unknown
nutritional effect of fish or, on the other hand, it may
reflect the fact that many IPF patients live inland in
agricultural areas where less fish is consumed. Concerning the relationship of metal dust depostion and IPF,
previous study(1) showed that the amount of Ni deposited
in the hilar/mediastinal lymph nodes was significantly
larger in IPF patients than in control patients. In
addition, Inoue(2) demonstrated large depositions of Si
in the lung tissue of IPF patients, and this may relate
to the fact that the disease is seen more in rural areas.

In summary, it is likely that no single but multiple
exogenous factors may correlate to the onset of the
disease, and the disease are thought to develop under
an autoimmune process which has been triggered by lung
tissue damage due to various kinds of noxious agents.
Viral and hereditary studies are requested to conduct
further.

References

(1) IWAI, K., Hashimoto, N., Sato, T. et al.: Elemental
    analysis of heavy metals deposited in the hilar/
    mediastinal lymph nodes of IPF patients. Annual
    Report of "Epidemiology of Intractable Disease"
    Research Committee, Ministry of Health and Welfare,
    1985. (in Japanese)
(2) INOUE, M.: Qualitative and quantitative analysis on
    intrapulmonary inorganic dusts in idiopathic inter-
    stitial pneumonia. Hokkaido Igaku Zasshi 61, 745-
    754, 1986. (in Japanese)

Immunological Approach to IPF: Emphasis Upon Viral and Collagen-Specific Antibodies

Nobuyuki Kobayashi and Terumasa Miyamoto

*Department of Medicine and Physical Therapy, Faculty of Medicine,
University of Tokyo, Tokyo, Japan*

The implications of viral infection and
humoral autoimmunity to collagen in the
pathogenesis of idiopathic pulmonary fibrosis (IPF) were investigated. No specific antiviral antibody indicating a
possible correlation between IPF and viral
infection was found. Types I, III and V
collagen-specific antibodies were detected
in 33%, 22% and 13%, respectively, of 98
sera of patients with IPF. The levels of
antibodies to the three types of collagens
in immune complex (IC)- positive sera were
significantly higher than those in IC-
negative sera. Autoimmunity to collagens,
particularly that directed to type I collagen, may participate in the development
of pulmonary fibrosis.

Introduction

In recent years, extensive studies of the lower
respiratory tract, including the analysis of bronchoalveolar lavage fluid [1,2], have helped identify mechanisms leading to the development of pulmonary fibrosis.
Many etiologic agents, including viruses, inorganic or
organic dusts and a variety of self-antigens in the lung
[3-5], have been proposed as causes of idiopathic pulmonary fibrosis (IPF), but the cause of the disease is

still unknown. Immune complexes (IC), frequently detected in serum and bronchoalveolar lavage fluid of patients with IPF and in fibrotic lung specimens [6,7], have been generally believed to trigger lung injury and to play a pathogenic role in subsequently developing fibrosis of the lung, although the antigen has not yet been identified.

Table I. Viruses to which the antibodies were examined

Chicken pox (HZ)	Rubella (Rbl)
Influenza A (I-A)	Parainfluenza 1 (PI1)
Influenza B (I-B)	Parainfluenza 2 (PI2)
Measles (Msls)	Parainfluenza 3 (PI3)
RS virus (RS)	Parainfluenza 4 (PI4)
Mycoplasma (Myc)	EBV-VCA IgG (VG)
Herpes simplex (HSV)	EBV-VCA IgM (VM)
Cytomegalovirus (CMV)	EBV-EA DR-IgG (EAG)
Chlamydia (Chlm)	EBNA (NA)
Echo 4 (E4)	EBV-VCA IgA (VA)
Echo 9 (E9)	EBV-EA DR-IgA (EAA)
Coxsackie A4 (CA4)	Adenovirus 1 (Ad1)
Coxsackie A7 (CA7)	Adenovirus 2 (Ad2)
Coxsackie A9 (CA9)	Adenovirus 3 (Ad3)
Coxsackie B1 (CB1)	Adenovirus 4 (Ad4)
Coxsackie B2 (CB2)	Adenovirus 7 (Ad7)
Coxsackie B3 (CB3)	Adenovirus 8 (Ad8)
Coxsackie B4 (CB4)	Adenovirus 11 (Ad11)
Coxsackie B5 (CB5)	
Coxsackie B6 (CB6)	Adult T-cell Leukemia (HTLV-1)

Table II. Frequencies of anti-viral antibodies

	IPF whole	IPF patho (+)	Normals
HSV	76/98 (78.6)*	27/31 (87.1)	33/45 (73.3)
CMV	96/98 (98.0)	31/31 (100)	43/45 (95.6)
Rbl	98/98 (100)	31/31 (100)	43/45 (95.6)
PI-3	95/98 (96.9)	30/31 (96.8)	45/45 (100)
EB-VCA IgG	95/96 (99.0)	30/30 (100)	43/45 (95.6)
Ad-1	90/98 (91.8)	28/31 (90.3)	41/45 (91.1)

* % values are shown in the parenthesis

A relationship of viral infection to the pathogenesis of IPF has been suggested since viral-like intranuclear inclusion bodies were demonstrated in the lining and free alveolar cells in patients with desquamative interstitial pneumonia (DIP) [8]. However, it is now postulated that these inclusion bodies are not specific to DIP and do not represent viral particles [9,10]. In addition, attempts to isolate a viral agent from biopsied lung materials have proved unsuccessful. However, these findings might not negate the possibility that a certain unknown virus could participate in the pathogenesis of the disease.

In fibrotic lung disorders, because a variety of collagen types are deranged and altered in amount, immunologically competent cells may recognize collagen as "foreign" and collagen may act as an antigen provoking or perpetuating a fibrotic process of the lung [4,11, 12]. Since the cellular sensitivity to type I collagen was demonstrated in IPF patients by Kravis et al. [4], type I collagen has been thought to be an antigen to IPF. To reassess the contribution of viral infection and collagen autoimmunity to the development of IPF, we investigated the presence of antibodies to a variety of viruses and collagens in IPF patient sera.

Viral antibodies

The viruses to which the antibodies were examined are listed in Table 1. Ninety-eight serum samples of IPF patients and 45 serum samples of normal controls were analyzed for viral antibodies. IPF serum samples were obtained from the members of the Research Committee of Interstitial Lung Disease supported by the Japanese Ministry of Health and Welfare. Thirty-one of the 98 patients were pathologically diagnosed as IPF.

Antibodies to six viruses were frequently detected in sera of whole IPF patients and of pathologically defined IPF patients (Table 2). These viruses were herpes simplex virus, cytomegalovirus, rubella virus, parainfluenza 3 virus, Epstein-Barr virus (IgG to viral-capsid antigen) and adeno 1 virus. However, all of these antibodies were detected in normal control sera as frequently as in IPF sera. Vergnon reported that IgG and IgA antibodies to viral-capsid antigen (VCA) of EB virus were frequently present in IPF sera [13]. However, we detected IgA to VCA of EB virus in only 10 of the 53 IPF patients.

Of all the viruses examined, the IgG antibody level to VCA of EB virus was significantly elevated only in the pathologically diagnosed IPF sera when compared to normal subjects. We subsequently measured the circulating immune complexes using C_{1q} solid-phase radioimmunoassay [14] and by murine monoclonal rheumatoid factor assay [15]. The EBV-VCA IgG antibody level did not correlate with the level of circulating

IC measured by two different methods (Fig.1). These
results suggest that the viral antigen in IPF might not

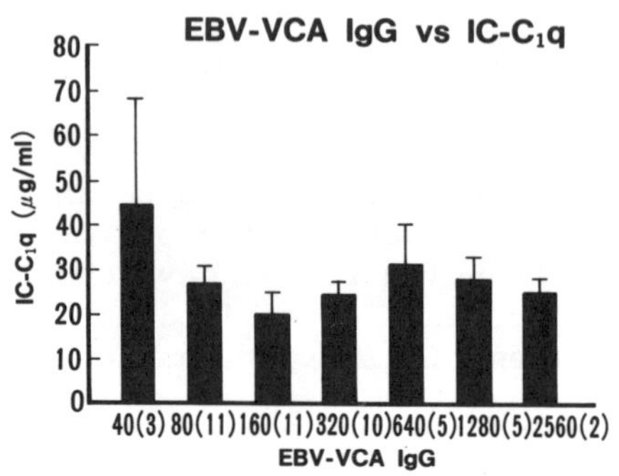

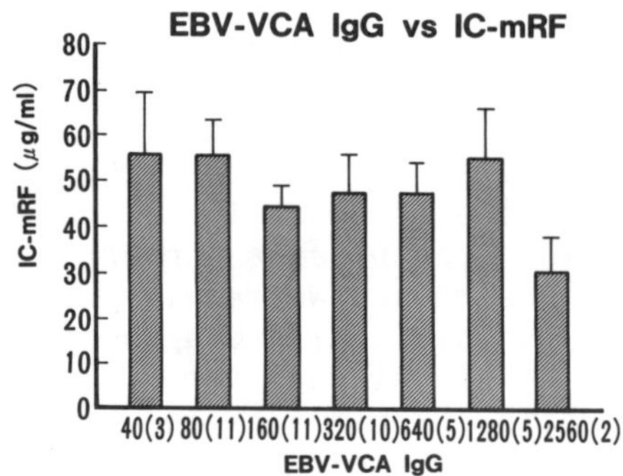

Fig. 1.   Relationship between EB virus-VCA IgG and
immune complexes (IC) in sera of IPF patients.
IC was measured by C_{1q} solid-phase radioimmunoassay and by murine monoclonal rheumatoid
factor assey.

consist of pathogenic IC. However, this does not rule
out the possibility that a certain virus could alter a
self antigen or modulate the immune system in such a
way that would promote the fibrotic process of the lung.

Collagen-specific antibodies

Collagen is the most abundant connective tissue

macromolecule in the normal lung, accounting for 20% of lung dry weight. So far, at least, five collagen types have been isolated from the normal lung, and their distribution and their origin have been determined [16]. In the normal lung, the most abundant collagen species is type I collagen, which represents approximately 60% of the total content of lung collagen. The next one is type III collagen, about 30%, and the third one is type V collagen, accounting for a little less than 10%. The content of type IV collagen is small, but it is a major component of the basement membrane. In the fibrotic lung, the ratio of type I to type III collagen changes. There is an increase of type I collagen content and a decrease of type III collagen content [17,18], although in the early phases of the fibrotic process a predominance of type III collagen content is suggested [19,20]. An elevated level of type III procollagen peptide in BAL fluid is a reflection of increased synthesis of type III collagen in the early stages of lung fibrosis [21]. We found an increase in type V, and a decrease in type IV collagen content [22], in addition to an increased ratio of type I to type III collagen content, in fibrotic human lungs compared with normal human lungs. The decreased content of type IV collagen may reflect damage to the basement membrane during the inflammatory and fibrotic process of the lung. These alterations in the relative content of specific collagen types might be important in the development of pulmonary fibrosis, but further analysis of the production and degradation of each type of collagen is necessary.

In the present study, we examined the presence of autoantibodies to types I, III and V collagens in sera of patients with IPF. Serum samples were obtained from 98 patients with IPF (63 males and 35 females), between 32 and 82 years old, with a mean disease duration of 3.9 years. Control serum samples were obtained from 39 normal subjects, between 38 and 65 years old. Of all patients with IPF, seven had acute onset or acute exacerbation of the disease and the other individuals had chronic diseases with slowly progressive interstitial pulmonary fibrosis. Types I and III collagens used as antigens were isolated from bovine skin and type V collagen was isolated from human placenta. Their purity was assayed by amino acid analysis and SDS-polyacrylamide gel electrophoresis.

Antibody to collagen was detected using enzyme-linked immunosorbent assay (ELISA). The assay was performed in polystyrene microtiter plates coated with collagen as described by Rennard et al. [23]. The antigens were plated at a concentration of 1 μg/100 μl in each well. One-hundred μl of diluted serum was transferred to the collagen-coated well and incubated for 1 hour at 37°C. After being washed, 100 μl of peroxidase-conjugated goat anti-human IgG antibody was added and the plate was incubated for 1 hour at 37°C. After additional washing, the substrate was added and the absorbance was read at 490 nm in an automated microtiter plate reader.

Rabbits were immunized with type I collagen and their antisera were collected. Rabbit antisera to type I collagen were raised, and were analyzed by ELISA to determine optimal conditions and reproducibility. Serial dilutions of immune and normal rabbit sera were tested on type I, III and V collagen-coated wells. Rabbit antiserum to type I collagen displayed significant reactivity when assayed on the type I collagen-coated well, but not on the type III or V collagen-coated wells. Minimal absorbance was exhibited by normal rabbit serum. An inhibition study was subsequently performed using rabbit antisera. Aliquots of antisera were preincubated with type I, III, or V collagens and then tested by ELISA. Antiserum was strongly inhibited by type I collagen, but not by type III or V collagens, indicating that type I collagen was essentially free of types III and V collagens.

Sera obtained from IPF patients and normal controls were tested for antibodies to types I, III and V collagens. The mean levels of types I, III and V collagen-specific antibodies in IPF patients were significantly higher than those in normal subjects (p<0.01) (Fig. 2). An absorbance value higher than two standard deviations above the control sera mean was considered positive. By this criterion, type I, III and V collagen-specific antibodies were detected in 33%, 22% and 13%, respectively, of IPF patient sera. In particular, type I collagen-specific antibody was frequently detected in IPF sera.

Circulating immune complexes (IC) were detected in 26 out of 74 patients with IPF (35%) using C_{1q} solid phase radioimmunoassay. The levels of antibodies to

three types of collagens in IC-positive sera were significantly higher than those in IC-negative sera (p<0.01
or p<0.05) (Fig. 3). Between the acute onset or acute
exacerbation group and chronic stable group of IPF, no
difference was observed in anti-collagen antibody titers

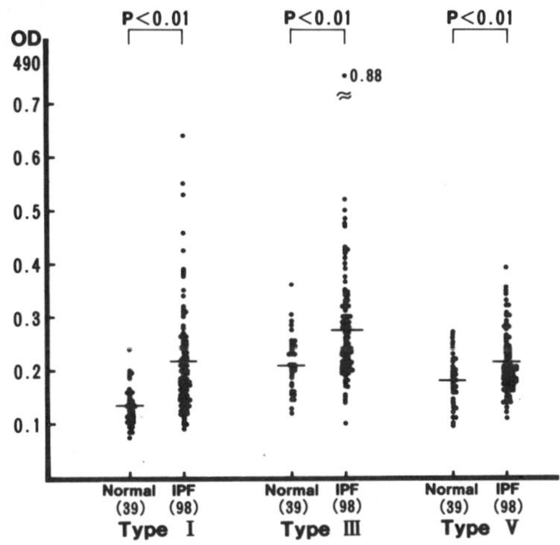

Fig. 2.   Type I, III and V collagen-specific antibody
         titers in sera of patients with IPF and normal
         subjects.

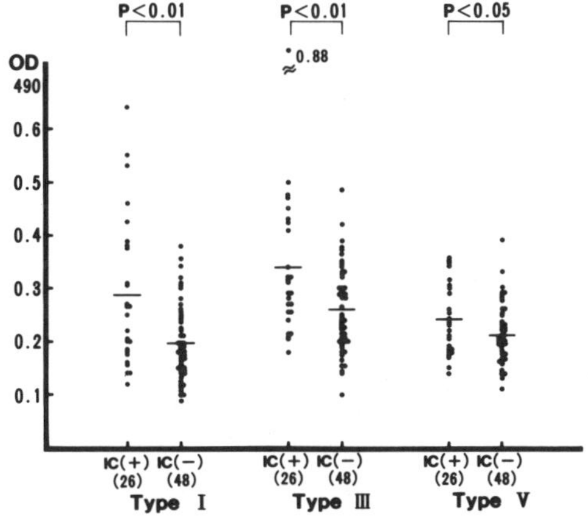

Fig. 3.   Relationship between collagen-specific antibody
         titers and circulating immune complexes (IC) in
         sera of patients with IPF and normal subjects.

(Fig. 4).   However, two out of seven patients in the
acute group exhibited markedly elevated levels of types
I and III collagen-specific antibodies. One patient had
acute onset of IPF and the serum sample was obtained
before steroid therapy. Another patient had a rapidly
progressing disease and his sample was obtained after
steroid therapy. The other 5 samples of the acute group
were obtained after steroid therapy. There were statis-

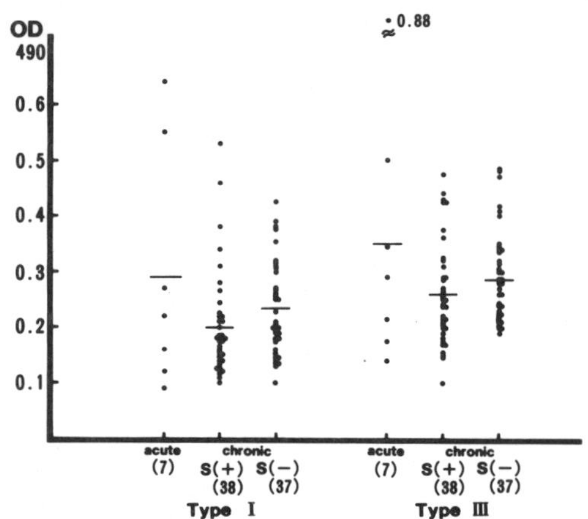

Fig. 4.   Type I and III collagen-specific antibody
           titers in acute and chronic stages of IPF.
           S (+): with steroid therapy
           S (-): without steroid therapy

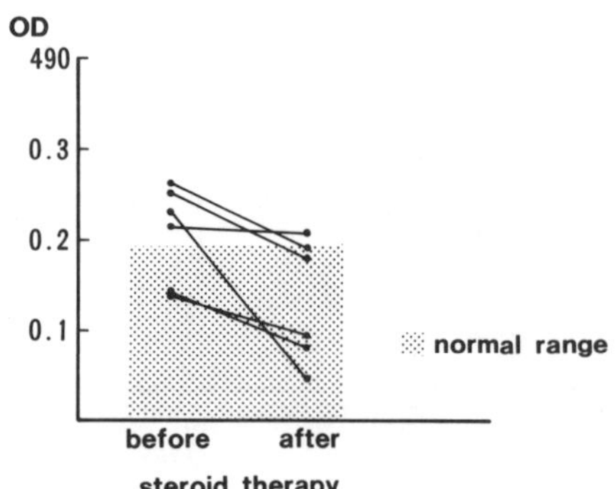

Fig. 5.   Effect of steroid therapy on type I collagen-
           specific antibody.

tically significant correlations (p<0.01) among the levels of types I, III and V collagen-specific antibodies. An inhibition study was performed in two IPF sera showing high levels of anti-collagen antibody. Preincubation with type I collagen decreased the absorbance values dose-dependently, whereas no inhibition of the absorbance value was observed in normal sera.

We evaluated the effect of steroid therapy on anti-collagen antibody. Six paired sera of IPF obtained before and after steroid therapy were analyzed. Type I collagen-specific antibody was detected in 4 of 6 samples before steroid administration. In three cases, the antibody titer decreased to the normal range after therapy (Fig. 5), suggesting that steroids might reduce the humoral immunity of collagen in these patients.

Since Kravis [4] reported that peripheral blood lymphocytes in IPF patients released lymphokines on exposure to type I collagen, the antigenicity of alveolar wall components, especially type I collagen, has been postulated to play a role in the pathogenesis of IPF [1, 11]. Our observation that type I collagen-specific autoantibody was relatively frequently detected in IPF sera may support the hypothesis; type I collagen is the antigen of IPF. However, anti-collagen antibodies were found in at most 30% of the patients with IPF and they have been detected in other disorders [12, 24-26]. Moreover, it is not clear whether type I collagen would be an antigen component of IC that is frequently detected in IPF sera. Although there is no convincing evidence at present that type I collagen is the etiologic antigen of IPF, humoral and cellular autoimmunity to collagen might be involved in the development of pulmonary fibrosis, presumably under a modified immune system in the lung. Anti-collagen antibodies seemed to be detected in the active phase of IPF and the steroid might suppress humoral sensitivity to collagen. In bleomycin-induced pulmonary fibrosis in rats, a transient cellular sensitivity to homologous type I collagen was demonstrated during the period of increased collagen synthesis [27]. This indicates that autoimmunity to type I collagen is caused by exposure to bleomycin and subsequent injury in the lung. Therefore, it is also thought that the production of autoantibody to collagen is a result of the destruction of lung connective tissue. Even so, humoral immunity might be implicated in further expansion of lung injury and subsequently occurring lung fibrosis.

Conclusions

We found no specific anti-viral antibody indicating a possible correlation between IPF and some viral infection. The mean levels of types I, III and V collagen-specific antibodies in sera of IPF patients were significantly higher than those in normal subjects. The levels of antibodies to three types of collagens in IC-positive sera were significantly higher than those in IC-negative sera. Autoimmunity to collagens, especially those directed to type I collagen, might participate in the pathogenesis of pulmonary fibrosis or might reflect the destruction of lung connective tissue.

References

1) Crystal, R.G., Bitterman, P.B., Rennard, S.I., Hance, A.J. and Keogh, B.A.: Interstitial lung diseases of unknown cause. Disorders characterized by chronic inflammation of the lower respiratory tract. New Engl. J. Med., 310: 154-166, 1984.
2) Schraufnagel, D.E., Claypool, W.C., Fahey, P.J., Jacobs, E.R., Rubin, D.B. and Snider, G.L.: Markfield symposium. Interstitial pulmonary fibrosis. Am. Rev. Respir. Dis., 136: 1281-1284, 1987.
3) Haslam, P., Turner-Warwick, M. and Lukoszek, A.: Antinuclear antibody and lymphocyte responses to unclear antigens in patients with lung disease. Clin. Exp. Immunol., 20: 379-395, 1975.
4) Kravis, T.C., Ahmed, A., Brown, T.E., Fulmer, J.D. and Crystal, R.G.: Pathogenic mechanisms in pulmonary fibrosis. Collagen-induced migration inhibition factor production and cytotoxicity mediated by lymphocytes. J. Clin. Invest., 58: 1223-1232, 1976.
5) Crystal, R.G., Fulmer, J.D., Roberts, W.C., Moss, M.L., Line, B.R. and Reynolds, H.Y.: Idiopathic pulmonary fibrosis: clinical, histologic, radiographic, physiologic, sintigraphic, cytologic, and biochemical aspects. Ann. Intern. Med., 85: 769-788, 1976.

6) Dreisin, R.B., Schwarz, M.I., Theofilopoulos, A.N.
    and Stanford, R.E.:   Circulating immune complexes
    in the idiopathic interstitial pneumonias.   New
    Engl. J. Med., 298: 353-357, 1978.

7) Hunninghake, G.W., Keogh, B.A., Gadek, J.E.,
    Bitterman, P.B., Rennard, S.I. and Crystal, R.G.:
    Inflammatory and immune characteristics of idiopa-
    thic pulmonary fibrosis.   In: Clinical immunology
    update (E.C. Franklin, ed.), Elsevier Biomedical,
    New York, pp. 217-233, 1983.

8) Liebow, A.A., Steer, A. and Billingsley, J.G.:
    Desquamative interstitial pneumonia. Am. J. Med.,
    39: 369-404, 1965.

9) Patchefsky, A.S., Banner, M. and Freundlich, I.M.:
    Desquamative interstitial pneumonia.   Singnificance
    of intranuclear viral-like inclusion bodies.   Ann.
    Intern. Med., 74: 322-327, 1971.

10) Kawanami, O., Ferrans, V.J., Fulmer, J.D. and
     Crystal, R.G.:   Nuclear Inclusions in alveolar
     epithelium of patients with fibrotic lung
     disorders.   Am. J. Pathol., 94: 301-322, 1979.

11) Morgan, J.E., Barkman, H.W. and Waring, N.P.:
     Idiopathic Pulmonary fibrosis.   Sem. Respir. Med.,
     5: 255-262, 1984.

12) Meckel, A.M., Delustro, F., Harper, F.E. and LeRoy,
     E.C.:   Antibodies to collagen in scleroderma.
     Arthritis Rheum., 25: 522-531, 1982.

13) Vergnon, J.M., Vincent, M., Dethé, G., Mornex, J.F.,
     Weynants, P. and Brune, J.:   Cryptogenic Fibrosing
     alveolitis and epstein-barr virus: An association ?
     Lancet ii: 768-771, 1984.

14) Yoshinoya, S. and Pope, R.M.:   Detection of immune
     complexes in acute rheumatic fever and their rela-
     tionship to HLA-B5. J. Clin. Invest., 65: 136-145,
     1980.

15) Takahashi, K., Yoshinoya, S., Miyamoto, T., Sugi,
     M., Ichige, M. and Hamaoki, M.:   Murine monoclonal
     rheumatoid factor as a staff for detection of cir-
     culating immune complexes.   Jpn. J. Allergol., 36:
     313-321, 1987.

16) Clark, J.G.:   The molecular pathology of pulmonary
     fibrosis.   In: Connective tissue Disease (J. Vitto
     et al. eds.), Vol 12 in The Biochemistry of Dis-
     ease.   Marcel Dekker, New York-Basel, pp.321-343,
     1987.

17) Seyer, J.M., Hutcheson, E.T. and Kang, A.H.: Collagen polymorphism in idiopathic chronic pulmonary fibrosis. J. Clin. Invest., 57: 1498-1507, 1976.

18) Last, J.A.: Changes in the collagen pathway in fibrosis. Fundam. appl. Toxicol., 5: 210-218, 1985.

19) Raghu, G., Striker, L.J., Hudson, L.D. and Stricker, G.E.: Extracellular matrix in normal and fibrotic lungs. Am. Rev. Respir. Dis., 131: 281-289, 1985.

20) Selman, M., Montano, M., Ramos, C., Chapela, R., González, G. and Vadillo, F.: Lung collagen metabolism and the clinical course of hypersensitivity pneumonitis. Chest, 94: 347-353, 1988.

21) Kirk, J.M.E., Bateman, E.D., Haslam, P.L., Lanrent, G.J. and Turner-Warwick, M.: Serum type III procollagen peptide concentration in cryptogenic fibrosing alveolitis and its clinical relevance. Thorax, 39: 726-732, 1984.

22) Kobayashi, N., Murata, K., Takizawa, H., Horiuchi, T. and Miyamoto, T.: Collagen types in human and rat lungs and their changes with fibrotic process. Jpn. J. Thorac. Dis., 26: 55-62, 1988.

23) Rennard, S.I., Berg, R., Martin, G.R., Foidart, J.M. and Robey, P.G.: Enzyme-linked immunoassay (ELISA) for connective tissue components. Anal. Biochem., 104: 205-214, 1980.

24) Stuart, J.M., Huffstutter, E.H. and Townes, A.S.: Incidence and specificity of antibodies to types I, II, III, IV, and V collagen in rheumatoid arthritis and other rheumatic diseases as measured by ^{125}I-radioimmunoassay. Arthritis Rheum., 26: 832-840, 1983.

25) Michaeli, D. and Fudenberg, H.H.: Antibodies to collagen in patients with emphysema. Clin. Immunol. Immunopathol., 3: 187-192, 1974.

26) Suou, T. and Hirayama, C.: Antibodies to denatured bovine collagens in sera of patients with liver disease. Clin. Exp. Immunol., 39: 119-124, 1980.

27) Schrier, D.J., Phan, S.H. and Ward, P.A.: Cellular sensitivity to collagen in bleomycin-treated rats. J. Immunol., 129: 2156-2159, 1982.

Idiopathic Pulmonary Fibrosis: Pathogenesis

Nobuaki Shigematsu*, Shinichiro Hayashi*,
Nobuhiro Kamikawaji**, Hideo Ogino*, Katsuro Yagawa*,
and Takehiko Sasazuki**

* *Research Institute for Diseases of the Chest, Faculty of Medicine, Kyushu University, Fukuoka, Japan*
** *Medical Institute of Bioregulation, Kyushu University, Fukuoka, Japan*

The pathogenesis of idiopathic pulmonary fibrosis(IPF) still remains unknown, however, several lines of evidence indicating that immune complexes in lung may play as a trigger for the serial inflammatory process is accumulated. We measured circulating immune complexes in patients with IPF, using 4 different methods, in which PEG-CC seemed to be the most sensitive method in case of IPF.

Furthermore, we investigated immunological factors which might be associated with pathogenesis of the disease. Antibodies against some viruses were examined, resulting in relatively high titer in the patient group. HLA typing was also done. B51 and Bw62 antigens were significantly more frequent in patients with IPF. Moreover, patients with acute progression found to belong only to B51 group. These findings as well as a case, whose alveolitis seemed to be affected by administration of ofloxacin, suggest that such factors that modulate immunological responses may play an important role in the pathogenesis of IPF.

Introduction

Idiopathic pulmonary fibrosis(IPF) is a clinical syndrome affecting predominantly the alveoli, associated with a strong tendency toward relentless progressive fibrosis. There have been accumulated several pieces of immunologial evidence indicating the role of immune complexes(IC) as a trigger for the serial inflammatory process [1,2,3], while there still remains unknown which method for detection of IC is appropriate and which antigen is associated with this immune complexes. Vergnon et al. [4] suggested a possible role of Epstein -Barr as a causative agent of IPF. To verify their findings, we examined antibodies against EB virus, herpes zoster virus and herpes simplex virus. For the susceptibility, genes of major histocompatibility antigens are known to be closely related to immunological responses. Furthermore, some drugs such as new quinolone agents are reported to enhance those responses [5]. we investigated if these factors affecting on immunological responses might be associated with pathogenesis or clinical course of patients with IPF.

Material and Methods
Patients: Circulating immune complexes(CIC) were examined in sera from patients with interstitial lung diseases who referred to the Department of Respiratory Diseases, Kyushu University Hospital. They included 14 patients with IPF, 8 with rheumatoid lung disease and 9 cases of interstitial pneumonia associated with other collagen diseases. 20 healthy volunteers were included to normal control.

HLA typing and measurement of antiviral antibodies were made with 27 cases of IPF patients. 16 cases of patients with other interstitial lung diseases and 20 cases of normal controls. Their mean age was 63.5, 53.4 and 32.7, respectively.

Measurement of CIC: Measurement of CIC was achieved using polyethylene glycol precipitate complement consumption test(PEG-CC), Clq solid phase ELISA, Raji cell RIA and Macrophage Fc receptor RIA.

Measurement of antiviral antibody: Antibodies against EB virus, Herpes simplex virus and Herpes zoster virus were measured. Indirect immunofluorecent assay was used for anti-EB virus antibodies, while antibodies gainst Herpes viruses were measured by complement fixation test.

Modulation of lymphocyte response by drugs: To study modulation of lymphocyte response by ofloxacin, we

cultured human peripheral lymphocytes with phytohemaggulutinin and various amount of the drug for 48 hr.
Ciplofloxacin was also used as stimulant. 16 hr before
the end of the culture, ^{3}H-thymidine was added. Then
incorporation of thymidine was measured.

Results
    Results of measurement of CIC are shown in Figure 1.
By PEG-CC, patients with IPF and with rheumatoid lung are
found to have significantly increased CIC than those of
normal control. On the contrary, CIC could not detected
well in both two groups by C1q ELISA, while CIC are
significantly increased in patients with other collagen
disease. Data by Raji cell RIA shows significantly
elevated amount of CIC in all three disease groups.
Immune complexes capable of binding to Fc receptors on
macrophages were increased in some cases of any groups.
Those difference between each assay suggest that CIC may
be different in component among these three diseases.

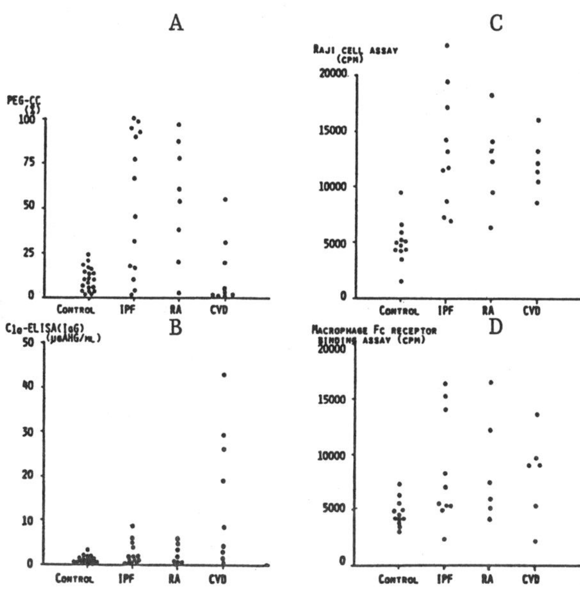

Figure 1. CIC was measured by using A:
PEG-CC, B: C1q ELISA, C: Raji cell RIA,
D: Macrophage Fc receptor-RIA.

Serial analysis of CIC was made in a patient with IPF (Figure 2). CIC level was measured by using PEG-CC, Raji cell assay, C1q ELISA and anti-C3 ELISA. Each method showed elevated level of CIC at first period of admission. This patient was administered 60mg daily of oral prednisolone and 150mg of azathioprine and was well controlled. As the dose of prednisolone was reduced, however, her alveolitis became active again. As shown Figure 2, CIC measured by PEG-CC were seemed to vary in parallel with the activity of alveolitis, although C1q ELISA, Raji cell RIA and anti-C3 antibody ELISA could show elevated immune complexes only in earlier period. Therefore PEG-CC was thought to be most sensitive method for assessing activity of IPF.

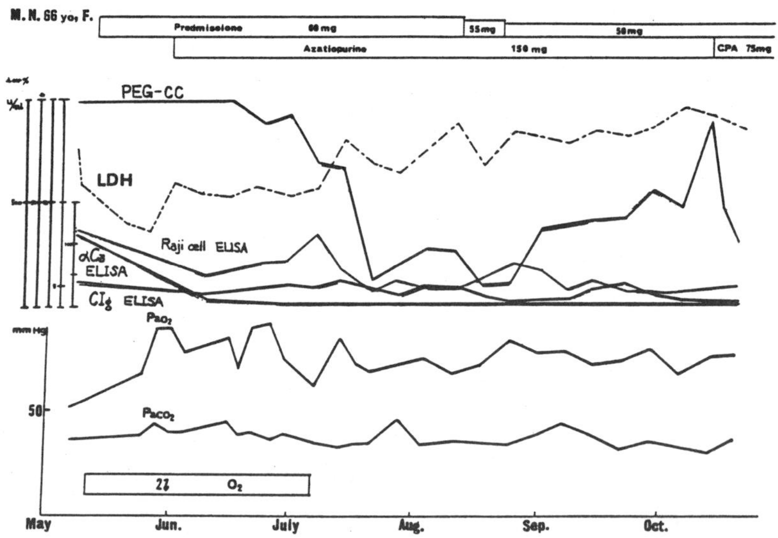

Figure 2. Serial measurement of CIC in a case of IPF.

Herpes zoster virus serological profile was within the normal range in all three groups, however, 26 out of 27 patients with IPF had the antibody against herpes simplex virus (Figure 3). On the contrary, 16 out of 20 healthy controls had no antibody against herpes simplex virus. Serological profile of control patients against herpes simplex virus was between two other groups. Because antibody positive rate against herpes simplex virus in Japanese was known to increase with age, the positive rate rises with age. Because mean age of IPF

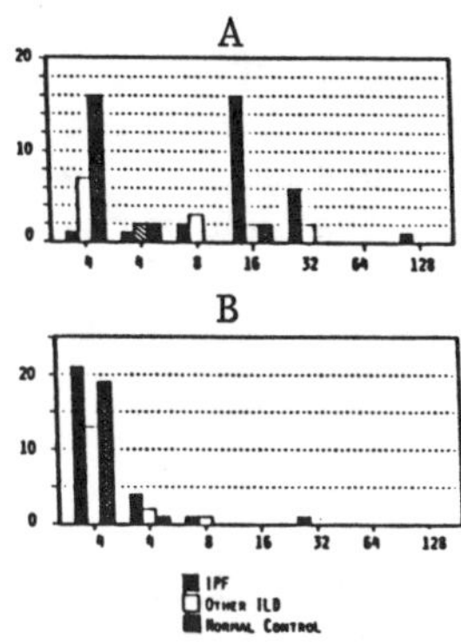

Figure 3. Antibody titer against Herpes simplex(A) and Herpes zoster virus(B).

group is considerably higher than other groups, our data may simply represent the virus exposure history of the three groups.

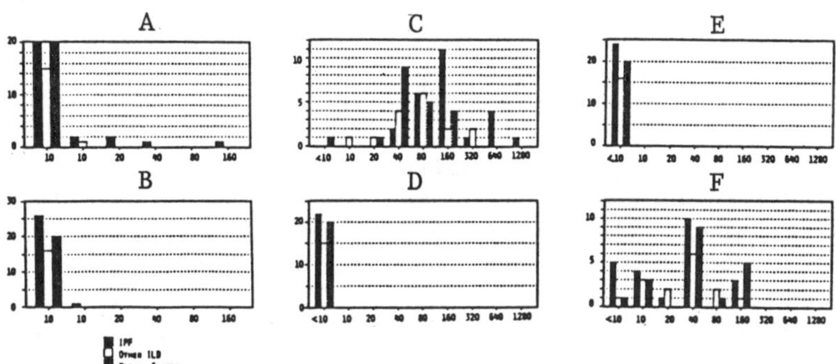

Figure 4. Antibody titer against EBV. A: anti-early antigen(EA) IgG, B: anti-EA IgA, C: anti-viral capsid antigen(VCA) IgG, D: anti-VCA IgM, E: anti-VCA IgA, F: anti-EBNA IgG.

As shown in Figure 4, anti-EB virus viral capsid antigen(VCA) IgG profile showed similar pattern as was noted in herpes simplex virus profile. Median titer was 160 in patients with IPF, whereas 40 in healthy controls. When titer more than 160 was assumed to be significant, because no healthy control had titer more than 160, 6 out of 25 had high IgG titer against EB virus VCA. There was no detectable IgM antibody against VCA. IgA antibody against VCA could not be detected. EBNA antibody was detected in all three groups, however, there was no significant differences within these groups. Some IPF

patients had IgG antibody against early antigen. No IgA
response against EA was detected. Serological data about
EB virus may suggest the possible etiological role of
this virus in development of IPF. But, because we failed
to find difference in antibody titer against EB virus
between IPF and patient control in BAL fluid (Table 1),
it is suggested that high titer may be a simple result of
modulated immune systems in IPF.

EBV ANTIBODIES IN BALF

	N	VCA IgG <10x	VCA IgG 10x	VCA IgG 20x	VCA IgG 40x	VCA IgA <10	EBNA <10
IPF	4	1	2	0	1	4	4
OTHER ILD	4	2	0	1	1	4	4

N: NUMBER OF SUBJECTS TESTED

Table 1.

The frequency of HLA antigens is shown in Table 2.
Frequencies of B51 and Bw62 was significantly high in
patient group, while there is no significant difference
in the frequency of class II antigens between two groups.
Clinical course of patients with IPF is somewhat various.
To clarify if prognosis is related to genetic background,
these patients are classified into four groups by speed
of progression. Group 1 contains patients progressed
most acutely, while patients with slowest progression are
separated into group 4. As shown in Table 3, patients
with acute progression belong only to B51 group.

A

HLA	Control (n=120) n	Control (n=120) Af	IPF (n=29) n	IPF (n=29) Af	RR	x^2	p
A26	23	0.23	7	0.24	1.1	0.01	ns
A31	16	0.13	3	0.10	0.8	0.33	ns
B 51	15	0.13	8	0.28	2.7	4.07	<0.05
B 15	17	0.14	9	0.31	2.7	4.61	<0.05
Bw62	16	0.13	9	0.31	2.9	5.24	<0.05
Bw61	33	0.28	6	0.21	0.7	0.56	ns
Cw3	52	0.43	14	0.48	1.2	0.25	ns

B

HLA	Control (n=120) n	Control (n=120) Af	IPF (n=26) n	IPF (n=26) Af	RR	x^2	p
DR1	23	0.19	2	0.08	0.4	1.26	ns
DR2	51	0.43	9	0.35	0.7	0.55	ns
DR4	44	0.37	11	0.42	1.3	0.29	ns
DR5	16	0.13	7	0.27	2.4	2.97	ns
DRw6	28	0.23	7	0.27	1.2	0.15	ns
DRw8	26	0.22	6	0.23	1.1	0.02	ns
DRw9	30	0.25	4	0.15	0.5	0.63	ns
DRw52	64	0.53	15	0.58	1.2	0.16	ns
DRw53	71	0.59	15	0.58	0.9	0.0	ns
DQw1	94	0.78	17	0.65	0.5	1.97	ns
DQw3	65	0.54	14	0.54	1.0	0.0	ns
DQw4	27	0.23	7	0.27	1.3	0.23	ns

Table 2. Frequency of major histocompartibility antigen,
A: class I, B: class II, in patients with IPF.

<u>CLINICAL COURSE & HLA</u>

| HLA | ACUTE ⟵ ⟶ CHRONIC | | | | TOTAL |
	I	II	III	IV	
B51	4 (50%)	1 (13%)	2 (25%)	1 (13%)	8
Bw62	0 (0%)	2 (25%)	4 (50%)	2 (25%)	8
Others	0 (0%)	2 (17%)	5 (42%)	5 (42%)	12
TOTAL	4 (15%)	5 (19%)	11 (41%)	7 (26%)	27

Table 3. Relationship between HLA class I type and clinical course of IPF.

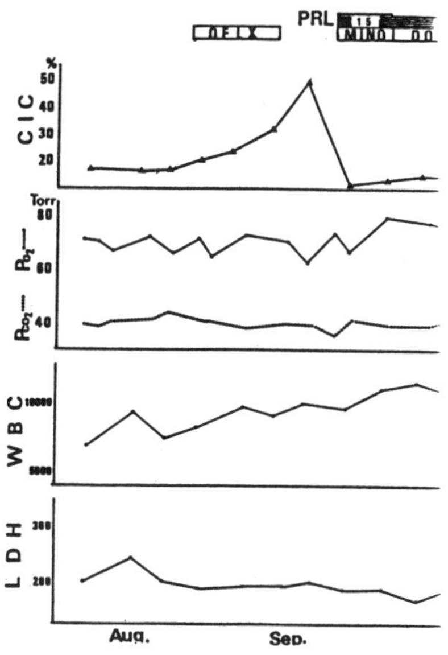

Figure 5. A case of patients with IPF, whose alveolitis was seemed to be excerbated by administration of ofloxacin.

Some drugs were known to modulate immune reaction. We observed a case of IPF exacerbated probably due to administration of ofloxacin (Figure 5). A patient complaining exertional dyspnea admitted to our hospital on July, 1986 and was diagnosed as IPF by findings of

chest X ray and TBLB specimen. Because her illness was
thought to be stable, she had been followed without
medication for 5 weeks. However, at the end of July she
got having fever probably due to Pseudomonas aeruginosa
detected in sputa specimen. Administration of ofloxacin
was started on August, 8th. and fever and Pseudomonas in
sputa seemed to get well-contrelled. However, her dyspnea took a turn to worse at that time. In addition,
circulating immune complexes measured by polyethylene
glycol precipitate complement consumption test increased.
Another TBLB specimen was examined to suggest acute
exacerbation of the disease. Those events suggest that
ofloxacin may play as a trigger for worsening of her
illness.

To study modulation of lymphocyte response by
ofloxacin, we cultured human peripheral lymphocytes with
phytohemaggulutinin and various amount of the drug.
Ciplofloxacin was also used as stimulant. As shown in
Figure 6,ofloxacin and ciplofloxacin enhanced 3H-thymi-
dine uptake of lymphocytes stimulated by PHA to around
120% both in IPF patients and normal controls.

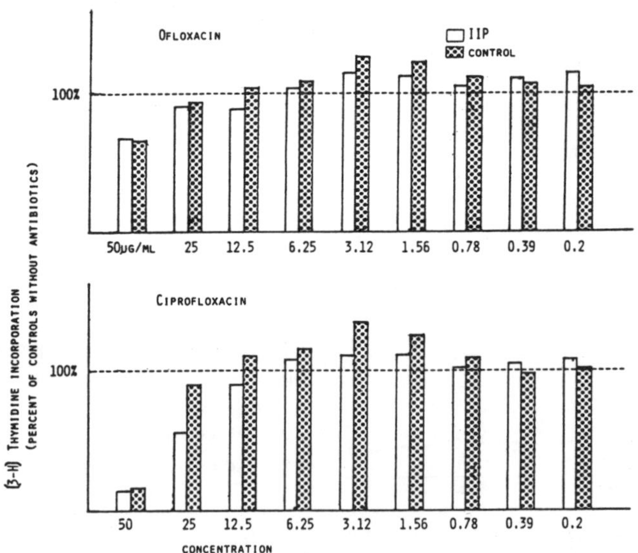

Figure 6. Effect of ofloxacin and cipro-
floxacin on human lymphocyte blastogenesis
by PHA.

Discussion

Pathogenesis of IPF still remains unknown, however, there have been accumulated several pieces of immunological evidence indicating the role of immune complexes as a trigger for the serial inflammatory process [1,2,3]. We measured CIC in sera from patients with IPF, using 4 different methods. CIC in the active patients was found to be increased in all assay other than Clq ELISA. There was difference between the results from each assay, which may be due to the difference of immune complexes in component, such as immunoglobulin or complement. Serial analysis of CIC in a patient shuwed that PEG-CC well reflect the activity of alveolitis. Those findings reemphasized the inportance of immune complexes on pathogenesis of IPF.

Vergnon et al. [4] reported the possibility that EB virus might be the causative agent of IPF. To verify their finding, we examined antibodies against EB virus, herpes zoster virus and herpes simplex virus. Antibody titer against herpes simplex virus and against EB virus viral capsid antigen was elevated in patient group. However, our data about herpes simplex virus are thought to represent simply the virus exposure history. Serological data about EB virus may suggest the possible etiological role of this virus in development of IPF. However, because we failed to find difference in antibody titer against EB virus between IPF and patient control in BAL fluid, it is suggested that high titer may be a simple result of modulated immune systems in IPF.

It is known that genes of major histocompatibility antigens are closely related to immunological responses. Frequency of B51 and Bw62 was significantly high in patients with IPF, while there was no significant difference in appearance of class II antigens between patients with IPF and normal populations. Furthermore, patients with acute progression belong only to B51 group. These findings suggest that genes located near class I locus may relate at least in part to the pathogenesis of this disorder.

Some therapeutical agents, such as new quinolone drugs, were reported to enhance the response of human peripheral lymphocyte to lectins [5]. We confirmed that ofloxacin and ciplofloxacin also enhanced ^{3}H-thymidine uptake of lymphocytes stimulated by PHA in patients with IPF. Together with our observation of a case exacerbated

probably due to administration of ofloxacin, this finding
suggest that drugs capable of modulating lymphocyte
reactions may affect activity of the disease.

References
1.   Dreisin, R.B., Schwarz, M.I., Theofilopoulos, A.N.,
      and Stanford, R.E. New Engl. J. Med. 298, 353–357,
      1978.
2.   Eisenberg, H., Simmons, D.H., and Barnett, E.V.
      Chest 75 suppl, 262–263, 1979.
3.   Gadek, J., Hunninghake, G., Zimmerman, R., Kelman,
      J., Fulmer, J., and Crystal, R.G. Chest 75 suppl,
      264–265, 1979.
4.   Vergnon, J.M., Vincent, M., DeThe, G., Mornex, J.F.,
      Weynants, P., and Brune, J. Lancet 2, 768–771, 1984
5.   Forsgren, A., Bergh, A., Brandt, M., and Hansson, G.
      Antimicrob. Agents Chemother. 29, 506–508, 1986

Role of Alveolar Macrophage in the Development of Pulmonary Fibrosis

M. Yamakido, S. Ishioka, and Y. Awaya

Second Department of Internal Medicine, Hiroshima University School of Medicine, Hiroshima, Japan

For the purpose of analyzing a role of alveolar macrophage in the development of pulmonary fibrosis, with the use of pulmonary fibrosis model mice induced by bleomycin, a study was made on bronchial alveolar lavage fluid (BALF) findings and on the temporal changes in pulmonary alveolar macrophage (PAM) function.

In conclusion, in BLM-induced pulmonary fibrosis model was observed functional changes in PAM accompanying the overproduction of pulmonary surfactant and PAM was activated. It was suggested that these changes might induce interstitial fibrosis.

Introduction

Animal models have been extensively employed in the study of bleomycin-induced pulmonary fibrosis, because the morphological changes observed closely resemble pulmonary fibrosis in humans [1]. Bleomycin directly injures the endothelial cells of the pulmonary capillaries and the alveolar epithelium [2]. As a result, alveolar macrophages are exposed to a drastic environmental change in the lung.

In order to elucidate the role of alveolar macrophages in pulmonary fibrosis, bleomycin was used to induce pulmonary fibrosis in mice. This report presents results obtained in an analysis of pulmonary lavage fluid and the function of alveolar macrophages.

Material and Methods
    Bleomycin was administered intraperitoneally at
a dose of 7.5 mg/kg/day to 12-week-old male mice for
10 consecutive days. The same dose of saline was
administered in a similar manner to a control group
of mice.
    Animals of both groups were sacrificed and pulmo-
nary lavage was performed on the last day of the bleomycin injection, and at the end of the second week,
and also at the end of the fourth week. Following
centrifugation of lavage fluid, the supernatant was
used for measurement of lysosomal enzyme activity, total
protein, phospholipids, and fibronectin. In addition,
macrophage suspensions was used for measurement of
superoxide and interleukin 1 production in vitro.

Results
1. Pathological examination
    A hematoxylin-eosin (H.E.) stained specimen
obtained two weeks after the end of bleomycin injections
showed that swelling of type II alveolar epithelium,
appearance of foamy macrophages, and infiltration of
mononuclear cells in the interstitium in subpleural
region.
    The H.E. specimen from the mice of fourth week
reveals destruction of alveolar structure and thickening of the interstitium and when it was stained with
Azan-Mallory stain, it is evident that there is a
thickening of the interstitium which is attributable
to accumulation of collagen fibers.
    By using Luxol fast blue stain which is specific
to phospholipids and is stained deep blue, we found at
the end of the second week the cytoplasm of alveolar
macrophages was stained deeply blue. This suggests
that phospholipids as pulmonary surfactants were
phagocytized by alveolar macrophages two week after
the end of bleomycin injections.
2. Changes of BALF after the injection of Bleomycin
    Fig. 1 shows the total cell count and differential
count of the cellular components of the pulmonary lavage
fluid. A significant increase in cell count is observed
in the bleomycin-exposed group at all stages of observation (0, 2, and 4 weeks). In particular, the difference
observed in the second week was remarkable. In the

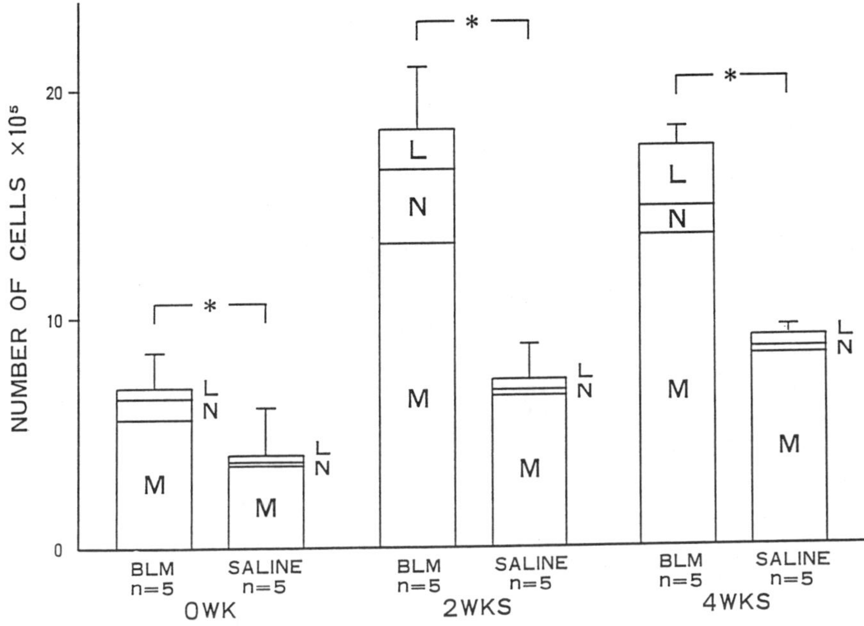

Fig. 1 Total and differential cell counts in pulmonary lavage fluid

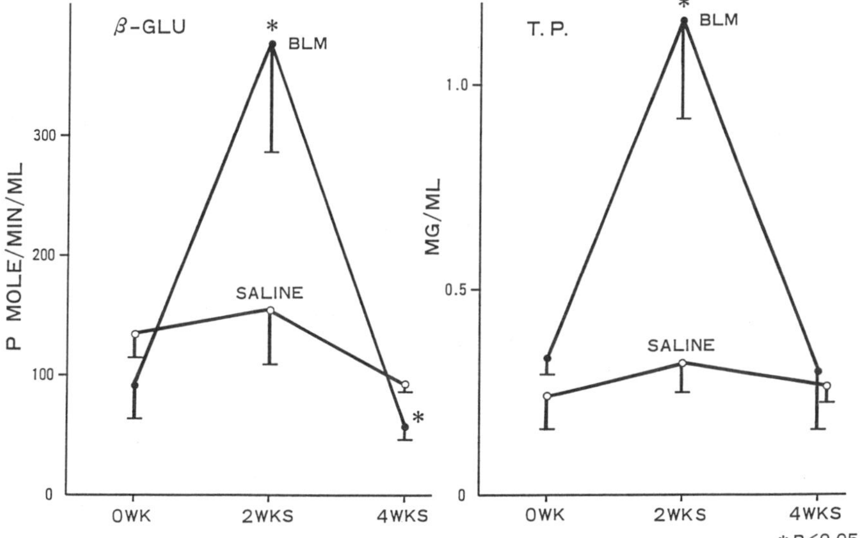

Fig. 2 -Glucuronidase activity and total protein in pulmonary lavage fluid

differential count, a slight neutrophilia was observed in the second week, and in the fourth week a slight increase in lymphocytes could be seen.

Fig. 2 shows the activity of -glucuronidase, one of the lysosomal enzymes, and total protein volume in the pulmonary lavage fluid. In the second week, both are increased significantly in the bleomycin group, but they are decreased in the fourth week. Though not shown in the slide, a similar tendency was observed in acid phosphatase and N-acethyl -glucosaminidase.

In the bleomycin group, phospholipids were apparently increased in the initial analysis and in week 2, but fibronectin gradually increased over the period of observation. Fibronectin in the bleomycin group showed a significant increase compared to those of the controls (Fig. 3).

In addition, superoxide production in the bleomycin group was significantly increased in week 2 compared to controls, but was reduced in week 4. IL-1 release by alveolar macrophages stimulated with lipopolysaccharide in the bleomycin group was also increased in week 2, but was reduced in week 4. Furthermore, alveolar macrophages of the bleomycin group spontaneously release IL-1 even when not stimulated by LPS (Fig. 4).

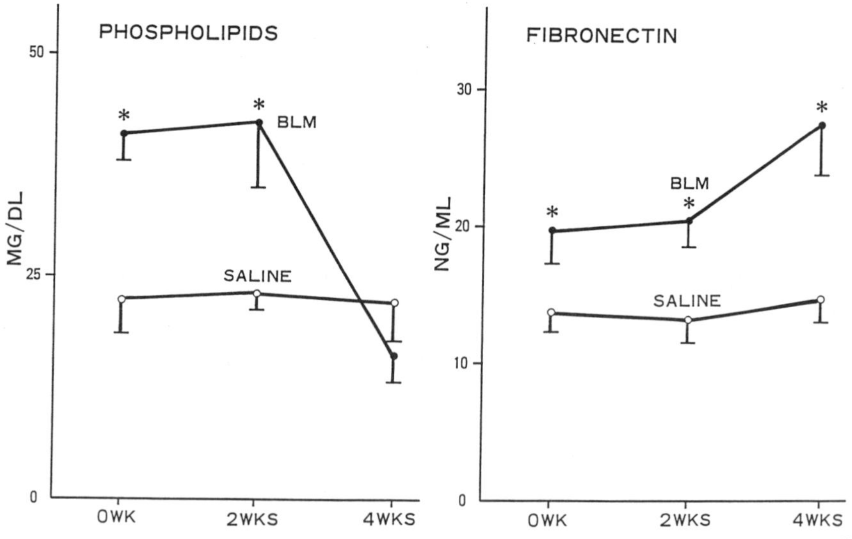

Fig. 3 Phospholipids and fibronectin in pulmonary lavage fluid

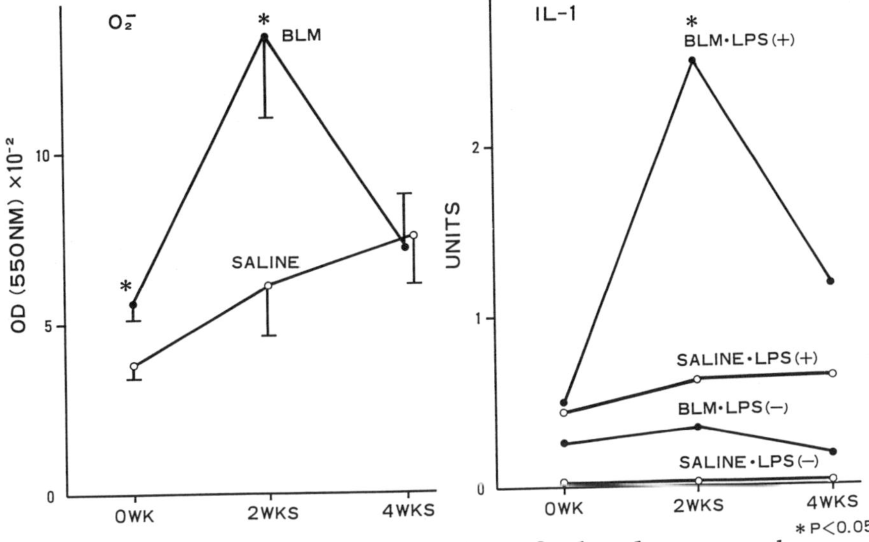

Fig. 4 02⁻ and IL-1 production of alveolar macrophage

3. The effect of pulmonary surfactants on isolated
alveolar macrophage function
     This experiment is based on the observation of that
an increase of surfactant in lavage fluid observed
during the early process of fibrosis and on the histological findings of the ingestion of surfactant by
macrophage.
     Crude pulmonary lavage fluid, a surfactant fraction
(obtained following centrifugation for 20 minutes at
27,000G), bovine artificial pulmonary surfactant, and
dipalmitoyl-phosphatidylcholine or (DPPC) were added,
with or without adding of LPS, to cultures of normal
alveolar macrophages, and released IL-1 was measured.
The surfactant fraction and bovine surfactant stimulated
the release of IL-1, while, DPPC inhibited the release
of IL-1.

Discussion
     The changes in the heretofore described indices of
the bleomycin group are shown by week relative to the
values observed in the control group. An early increase
in phospholipids, considered to have originated from
type II alveolar cells, was observed, while the increase
in total protein, which reflects the hyperpermeability
of small vessels, was marked in the second week. Super-

oxide and lysosomal enzyme levels, which are tissue injury factors derived from macrophages, were highest in the second week, but decreased sharply in the fourth week. IL-1 levels, the fibroblast proliferation factor, were increased in the second week. Although the level was lower in the fourth week, it was higher relative to the controls. Fibronectin gradually increased from week 0 to week 4.

The pulmonary surfactant fraction and bovine surfactant stimulated the release of IL-1, while DPPC inhibited the release of IL-1.

This suggests that ingestion of surfactant by macrophage and the accompanying functional changes of macrophage will not take place with the presence of phospholipid alone but require the intact surfactant which contains apoprotein. This would seem to be a logical finding in view of the fact that macrophage posseses apoprotein receptors [3,4]. Therefore, the intact surfactant is probably the factor to stimulate the release of IL-1.

Finally, we propose a hypothesis on the mechanism involved in bleomycin-induced development of pulmonary fibrosis. Bleomycin directly injures the alveolar epithelium and vascular endothelium to increase the exudation of blood components, proliferation of type II alveolar cells, and overproduction of surfactant. Due to these environmental changes, it is considered that a functional change and activation of alveolar macrophages occurs which leads to the production of tissue-injury factors, such as lysosomal enzyme and superoxide and fibroblast proliferation factors, such as IL-1 and FN. If it is assumed that fibrosis is the process whereby the host responds to tissue injury, we speculate that an increase in IL-1 and fibronectin, following the inflammatory process of the interstitium, is appropriate. There are many points which need to be verified in support of this inference, but it is proposed as a hypothesis based on the experimental evidence obtained to date.

References
1. Ekimoto, H., Takahashi, K., Matsuda, A., and Umezawa, H. Jpn. J. Cancer Chemother. 10, 2550–2557, 1983. (in Japanese)
2. Fasske, E., and Morgenroth, K. Chest 91, 428–435, 1987.
3. Faggiotto, A., Ross, R., and Harker, L. Arteriosclerosis 4, 323–356, 1984.
4. Gerrity, R. Am. J. Pathol. 103, 181–190, 1981.

Biochemical Significance of Glycoconjugates in Fibrogenesis of the Lung

Masakichi Motomiya*, Hideo Arai*, Hiromi Nagai*,
Tatsuya Abe*, Shigeru Shimoda*, Toshio Sato*,
Kimihiko Takusagawa*, and Hiroshi Munakata**

* *Research Institute for Tuberculosis and Cancer, Tohoku University
School of Medicine, Miyagi, Japan*
** *Department of Biochemistry, Tohoku University School of Medicine,
Miyagi, Japan*

Glycosaminoglycans (GAG's) and fibronectin
(FN) from the lung of humans and experimental animals were partially characterized.
It was suggested that dermatan sulfate
increases in association with fibrotic
changes of the lung. Presumably total
amounts of GAG's regulate the rate of maturation of collagen fibers. The presence of
GAG's in bronchoalveolar lavage fluid reflects injuries of the lung and suggests
that fibrotic changes occur thereafter.
Also it was found in the experimental bleomycin lung that FN increases prior to fibrogenesis. A glycoprotein of mucin type was
isolated from a case with pulmonary alveolar
proteinosis. These data suggest a close
association between glycoconjugates and
fibrogenesis of the lung.

The glycosaminoglycans (GAG's) of the lung forms a fine
network through the interstitium and are very closely
related to the structural elements. Hence the GAG's
together with collagen and elastic fibers contribute to
the maintenance of the integrity of the structure and
function of the lung. Fibronectin (FB), a high molecular
glycoprotein with adhesive properties, is found on cell
surface and intercellular matrix of the lung. FB exhibits a variety of biological and biochemical functions

including interactions with gelatin, heparin and hyaluronic acid. The present paper deals with isolation and characterization of GAG's and FB from the diseased human and animal lungs and from bronchoalveolar lavage fluid (BALF) from cases with sarcoidosis, pulmonary alveolar proteinosis or interstitial pneumonitis. Also an attempt was made to characterize a glycoprotein of mucin type in BALF from a case with pulmonary alveolar proteinosis.

Materials and Method

The peripheral lung tissue was minced and extracted with ethanol to remove lipids and formalin and was air-dried completely. The dried tissue was digested with pronase and deproteinized. The supernatant was dialyzed against water and mixed with ethanol saturated with NaCl. The resulting precipitate was taken up in NaCl and mixed with a slight excess of cetyl pyridinium chloride. The resulting precipitate was taken up in NaCl and the fraction of crude GAG's was recovered by an addition of ethanol (1). The amount of GAG's was expressed in terms of uronic acid (2). The fraction of crude GAG's thus obtained was loaded on a column of Dowex-1. Elution was effected with increasing concentrations of NaCl in a stepwise manner. The ratio of individual GAG species was determined by using the difference in substrate specificity of specific GAG-degrading enzymes (hyaluronidase from streptomyces hyalurolyticus, chondroitinase AC & chondroitinase ABC) as described previously (1).

Animal Experiments

Experiment 1: Guinea pigs received five consecutive intramuscular injections of Freund's complete adjuvant. The morphological and biochemical studies were made of the lung 20 weeks after the final injection. The GAG-species were identified and quantitated as described above (1).

Experiment 2: Sprague-Dawley rats received 8 intra-peritoneal injections of paraquat at intervals of 4 days. The animals were sacrificed 8 days after the final injection of paraquat. The lung was removed.

Microscopic specimens of the lung were prepared. At the same time collagen (3) and GAG's were quantitated.

Experiment 3: Sprague-Dawley rats received an intra-tracheal instillation of bleomycin. The animals were sacrificed on days 0, 7, 16, 28 and 56. FN from the lung was extracted with urea and was quantified by means of ELISA (4). The anti-FN antiserum used in the present experiment did not react with collagen 1, 111, IV or V (5). Lung FN was indistinguishable from human plasma FN when tested with this anti-FN antiserum.

Lavage fluid

Bronchoalveolar lavage was done as described by Hunninghake et al (6). The number of cells were counted in a hemocytometer. The cytocentrifuged specimen was May-Giemsa-Grünwald stained for differential count. The BALF was filtered through two layers of gauze freed from mucus and cell components, centrifuged, concentrated, lyophilized and used for biochemistry. Diagnosis of pul-monary alveolar proteinosis was established by histologi-cal examination of a specimen obtained by transbronchial lung biopsy (TBLB). Diagnosis of sarcoidosis was based on ophthalmological findings, histology of a specimen obtained by TBLB, or on biopsy findings of a lymph node.

Characterization of a glycoprotein of mucin type from a case with pulmonary alveolar proteinosis

The clear supernatant after centrifugation of BALF was chromatographed on a column of Sepharose CL-4B. The fraction eluted at the void volume of the first chromato-graphy was rechromatographed using the same column. The homogeneous fraction thus obtained was subjected to β-elimination (7). Total hexose, hexosamine and sulfate were determined by the color reaction. Polyacrylamide gel electrophoresis was carried out in the presence of sodium dodecyl sulfate.

Electron microscopic examination

Human lungs derived from autopsy and operation were used. Specimens were cut into 50–100 μm thick slices, fixed in

0.1 M cacodylate buffered 2.5 % glutaraldehyde containing
500 ppm of Ruthenium Red for 1 h, rinsed twice at 5 min
intervals with 0.1 M cacodylate buffer (pH 7.4) and post-
fixed in 0.1 M cacodylate-buffered 2 % OsO_4 containing
500 ppm Ruthenium Red for 1 h. The tissue was then
dehydrated in a series of graded ethanols and embedded in
Epon 812 (8).

Results

GAG's in the lung: The GAG fraction in the lung comprised hyaluronic acid (HA), chondroitin sulfate, (CHs)
dermatan sulfate (DS), heparan sulfate (HS). Heparin was
absent. The absence of keratan sulfate was one of the
criteria of homogeneity of the lung GAG fraction.
It was found in a sample from the human fibrotic lung
that the relative ratio of dermatan sulfate was increased
as in Table I (9).

Table I

Relative Percentage of Individual GAG Species
in Fibrotic and Control Lungs

GAG species	Fibrotic lung	Control lung
HA	27 %	30 %
CHsA(C)	32 %	40 %
DS	16 %	5 %
HS	24 %	25 %

In animal experiment 1, fibrotic changes were observed
around granulomas in the guinea pig lung in the 20th
week. The relative percentage of dermatan sulfate was
higher in the fibrotic than in control lung (Table II)
(10).

Table II

Quantification of Individual GAG species

GAG Species	Fibrotic Lung	Control Lung
HA	5.3 %	24.7 %
ChsA(C)	54.7 %	33.0 %
DS	15.8 %	5.4 %
HS	24.2 %	37.6 %

In the experimental paraquat lung (experiment 2), an increase of the total amount of GAG's in association with an increase of hydroxyproline was confirmed (Table III).

Table III

Quantification of GAG's and Hydroxyproline
in Experimental Paraquat Lung of Rats

	Paraquat lung	Control Lung
GAG's	1.53mg/100mg	1.22mg/100mg
hydroxyproline	174.8 ± 11.5*	154.2 ± 8.1*

* μg/10 mg

In sarcoidosis cases whose BALF contained detectable amounts of GAG's, interstitial shadows persisted on chest x-ray film despite treatment with steroids (Table IV).

Table IV

Quantification of GAG's in Cases with Sarcoidosis

Case No.	GAG's in BALF	Interstitial shadow
Case 1	–	disappeared
Case 2	–	disappeared
Case 3	–	disappeared
Case 4	+	persisted
Case 5	–	disappeared
Case 6	–	disappeared
Case 7	+	persisted

+ presence of detectable amounts of GAG's
– below the level of detection

Fibronectin in BALF:

The levels of FN/albumin ratio in BALF from patients with sarcoidosis who had gallium uptake in the lung field were higher than those in BALF of sarcoidosis cases without gallium uptake in the lung field.

Pulmonary alveolar proteinosis: In three patients with
pulmonary alveolar proteinosis, alveolar and/or interstitial shadows recurred or persisted despite repeated
bronchoalveolar lavages. In one patient whose BALF had
no detectable amounts GAG's, only one lavage brought about
complete recovery.

FN from experimental bleomycin lung

The level of FN from the bleomycin lung was highest on
the 7th day after instillation of bleomycin and returned
to a normal level on the 56 th day, when fibrosis was
evident histologically. (Fig. 1)

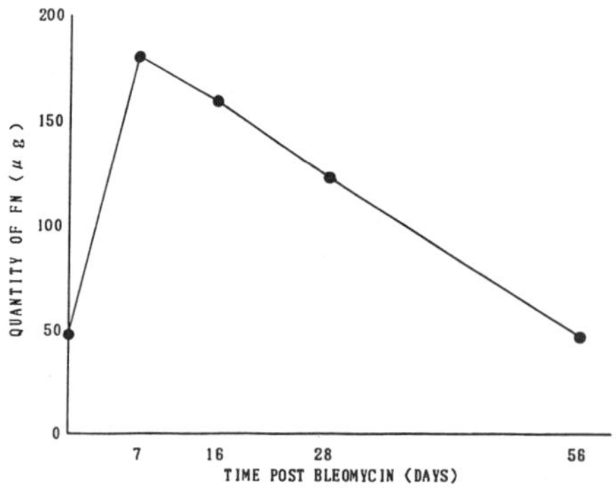

Fig. 1.   Level of FN with time in experimental bleomycin
          lung

Characterization of glycoprotein of mucin type in BALF
from a case with pulmonary alveolar proteinosis:

A high molecular weight glycoprotein was isolated from
the lavage fluid by gel chromatography with Sepharose
Cl-4B. The glycoprotein migrated as a homogenous band
on electrophoretogram. The chemical analysis and the
results of β-elimination reaction showed the presence of
0-linked carbohydrate chains characteristic for a mucin
type glycoprotein. (Chemical composition as shown in
Table V).

Table V
Chemical Composition of Glycoprotein

Galactose	8.2*
Mannose	0.8*
Fucose	3.3*
N-Acetylglucosamine	10.9*
N-Acetylgalactosamine	8.5*
Sialic acid	8.7*

*   g/100g dry sample

Electron microscopy

When collagen fibrils were stained with Ruthenium Red
and post-stained with uranyl acetate and lead acetate,

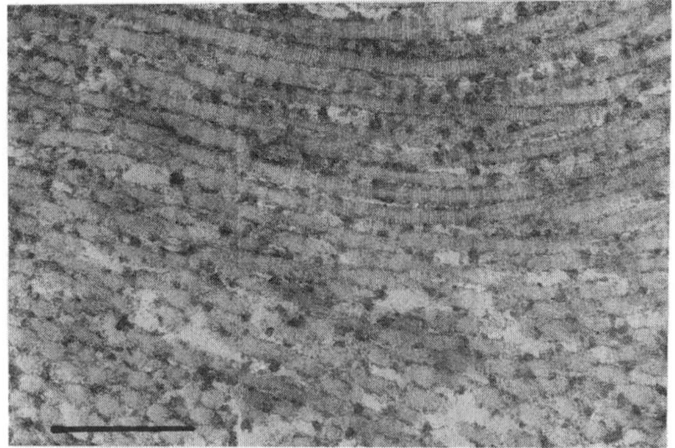

Fig. 2.   Electron micrograph before digestion

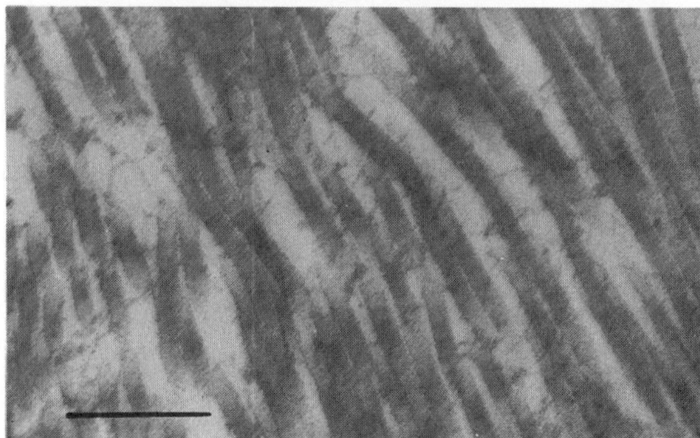

Fig. 3.   Electron micrograph after digestion with
         chondroitinase ABC

periodic lateral granules, 20-30 nm in diameter,were
observed on collagen fibrils (Fig. 2).   After digestion
with chondroitinase ABC, fine filaments and granular
substances have disappeared (Fig. 3).

Discussion

Both in human fibrotic lungs and in specimens from
fibrotic animal lungs that were experimentally produced,
an increment of the fraction of dermatan sulfate was
confirmed (9, 10).   Cantor and his associates showed that
the amount of ^{35}S taken up into GAG's of the hamster lung
after an intratracheal instillation of bleomycin was
increased (11).   Similar results were obtained in N-
nitrosomethyl-urethane induced pulmonary fibrosis (12).
Karlinsky found a marked increase of GAG's in the bleomycin lung of a hamster(13).   These data suggest the
occurrence of a change in the rate of synthesis of GAG's
prior to fibrogenesis of the lung.   As stated by
Karlinsky, of all sulfated GAG's, DS contains highest
percentage of iduronic acid, which enhances electrostatic
binding to collagen.   Most DS exists bound to collagen.
This hypothesis has been substantiated by our experiment
which showed that the lateral granules found in association with collagen fibrils remaind almost intact after
incubation with chondroitinase AC and disappeared after
incubation with chondroitinase ABC which degests HA, CHs
and DS.
The presence of detectable amounts of GAG's in BALF from
cases with sarcoidosis and pulmonary alveolar proteinosis
whose interstitial shadow of the lung persisted despite
treatments also suggested the participation of GAG's to
these findings.   The.presence of HA in bronchial secretions from asthmatic patients is an indicator of lung
injury as reported by Sahu and Lynn (14).   Thus it is
likely that more GAG's are present at the start of healing after lung injury.

In the present experiment an increase of FN in the acute
phase of bleomycin-induced experimental pulmonary fibrosis was confirmed.   Other investigators also found an
increase of FN in the acute phase of experimental pulmonary fibrosis together with an increase in number of
macrophages and fibroblasts (15, 16).   An increase of FN
in the phase of tissue repair and a decrease in the phase

of cirrhosis of the liver have also been reported (17).
FN is known also as a chemotactic factor for fibroblasts
(18). Thus the appearance of FN in the initial phase of
fibrogenesis seems to be very important. Both FN from
t'\ lung and FN in BALF were immunologically indistinguishable from human plasma FN. Hence the FN in BALF may
have been derived from plasma, although concomitant
presence of FN synthesized by connective tissue cells
could not be excluded.

References

1. Motomiya, M., Endo, M., Arai, H., Yokosawa, A., Sato,
   H., and Konno, K. Am Rev Respir Dis 111, 775-780,
   1975.
2. Bitter, J. and Muir, H.M. Anal Biochem 4, 330-334,
   1962.
3. Blumenkrantz, N. and Asboe-Hensen, G. Anal Biochem
   63, 331-340, 1975.
4. Rennard, S.I., Berg, R., Martin, G.R., Foidart, J.M.,
   and Robey, P.G. Anal Biochem 104, 205-214, 1980.
5. Yamaguchi, Y., Isemura, M., Yosizawa, Z., Kurosawa,
   K., Yoshinaga, K., Sato, A., and Suzuki, M. Am J
   Obstet Gynecol 152, 715-718, 1985.
6. Hunninghake, G.W., Kawanami, O., Ferrans V.J., Young,
   R.C. Jr., Roberts, W.C., and Crystal, R.G. Am Rev
   Respir Dis 123, 407-412, 1981.
7. Munakata, H., Isemura, M., Sato, N., Kikuchi, M.,
   and Yosizawa, Z. Int J Biochem 17, 301-308, 1985.
8. Takusagawa, K., Ariji, F., Shida, K., Sato, T., Asoo,
   N., and Konno, K. Histochem J 14, 257-271, 1982.
9. Motomiya, M., Arai, H., Sato, H., Yokosawa, Y.,
   Nagai, H., and Konno, K. Tohoku J Exp Med 115, 361-
   365, 1975.
10. Nagai, H., Arai, H., Ariji, F., Asoo, N., Ishikawa,
    T., Sato, H., Yokosawa, A., Motomiya, M., and Konno,
    K. Lung 154, 113-123, 1977.
11. Cantor, J.O., Bray, B.A., Ryan, S.F., Mandl, I., and
    Turino, G.M. Proc Soc Exp Biol Med 173, 362-366,
    1983.
12. Cantor, J.O., Bray, B.A., Ryan, S.F., Mandl, I., and
    Turino, G.M. Proc Soc Exp Biol Med 164, 1-8, 1980.
13. Karlinsky, B. Am Rev Respir Dis 125, 85-88, 1982.
14. Sahu, S., and Lynn, W.S. Biochem J 173, 565-568,
    1978.

15. Schoenberger, G.I., Rennard, S.I., Bitterman, P.B., Fukuda, Y., Ferrans V.J., and Crystal, R.G. <u>Am Rev Respir Dis</u> 129, 168-173, 1984.
16. Bray, B.A., Osman, M., Ashtyani, H., Mandl, I., and Turino, G.M. <u>Exp Mol Pathol</u> 44, 353-363, 1986.
17. Kojima, N., Isemura, M., Yosizawa, Z., Ono, T., Shinada, S., Soga, K., Aoyagi, Y., and Ichida, F. <u>Tohoku J Exp Med</u> 135, 403-412, 1981.
18. Hayashi, M., and Yamada, K.M. <u>J Biol Chem</u> 258, 3332-3342, 1983.

The Roles of Arachidonic Acid Cascade in the Pathogenesis of Idiopathic Interstitial Pneumonia (IIP)

Satoshi Kitamura and Jun Kobayashi

Department of Pulmonary Medicine, Jichi Medical School, Tochigi, Japan

In order to approach to the pathogenesis of idiopathic interstitial pneumonia (IIP), chemical mediators in BALF and in peripheral venous blood were analyzed. PGE2 and TXB2 were significantly elevated in peripheral venous blood. 6-keto-PGFla and 11-dehydro TXB2 tended to increase. In BALF, concentration of 6-keto-PGFla was significantly higher than that of control. Other chemical mediators also showed a tendency to increase. These results may suggest that arachidonic acid cascade metabolites play an important role in the pathogenesis of IIP.

We have some useful method for the diagnosis of idiopathic interstitial pneumonia (IIP), for example transbronchial lung biopsy (TBLB), open lung biopsy, bronchoalveolar lavage (BAL) and Gallium citrate scanning are available (1,2,3). But the pathogenesis of IIP has not been elucidated yet. TBLB or open lung biopsy do not offer any useful informations about pathogenesis of IIP. The analysis of BAL fluid (BALF) is not always necessary for the diagnosis of IIP, but is important to study the pathogenesis. Many kind of informations can be easily obtained from the peripheral area of the lung by BAL. Not only the cellular components, (alveolar macrophages, neutrophils, and lymphocytes) but also

the liquid components are useful for the analysis of
BALF. In this investigation we analyzed the liquid
components of BAL fluid in order to know the roles of
arachidonic acid cascades in the pathogenesis of IIP.

Subjects and methods

Six healthy control(HC), patients with 7 idiopathic interstitial pneumonia(IIP), 10 bronchial asthma
(BA), and 10 sarcoidosis(SA) were studied prospective-
ly. Age and numbers of smoker are showed in Table 1.
IIP patient was histologically confirmed by TBLB. Two
of these IIP patients were "inactive" and 4 patients
were "active" and needed therapy afterwards. Healthy
control was a group consisted of patients with hemosputum or other abnormal findings in chest X-ray but
have no apparent lesions in the lung.

Bronchoalveolar lavage (BAL) was performed via
right B3 bronchus using 50 ml of warmed saline three
times. Total cell count, recovery rate and cell differ-
entiations were measured by the total of BALF. Chemical
mediators were assayed using only the second fraction
of BALF by radioimmunoassay. Prostaglandin E2 (PGE2),
6-keto-Prostaglandin Fla (6-keto-PGFla), thromboxane B2
(TXB2),11-dehydro-thromboxane B2 (11-dehydro TXB2),
prostaglandin F2a (PGF2a), leukotriene C4 (LTC4), and
leukotriene B4 (LTB4) were assayed. Each value was
corrected by total protein of BALF and expressed per
1mg/ml total protein in BALF. In patients with IIP and
bronchial asthma, peripheral venous blood was also
assayed and was compared with those of healthy control.

Statistical analysis was performed by Student's
unpaired t-test and results were judged significantly
different when p value was less than 0.05.

Table 1. Profiles of cases in this study.

Groups	N	Ages	Smoker
Healthy Control (HC)	6	65±11	0
Idiopathic Interstitial Pneumonia			
(IIP)	7	58±11	5
Bronchial Asthma (BA)	10	46±13	4
Sarcoidosis (SA)	10	45±17	4

Results

A. Concentrations of Chemical Mediators in Periph
   eral Venous Blood of HC, IIP, and BA Groups.

Concentrations of PGE2 and 6-keto-PGF1a in peripheral venous blood are shown in Fig.1. The concentration
of PGE2 in HC, IIP, and BA are 65+29, 148+37, and 64+29
pg/ml respectively, and the values of IIP are statistically higher than those of HC (p<0.01). The concentrations of 6-keto-PGF1a in HC, IIP, and BA are 146+60,
448+370, 129+58 pg/ml respectively.
Concentrations of TXB2 and 11-dehydro-TXB2 are
shown in Fig.2. The concentration of TXB2 in HC, IIP,
and BA are 219+71, 339+51, and 240+97 pg/ml respective

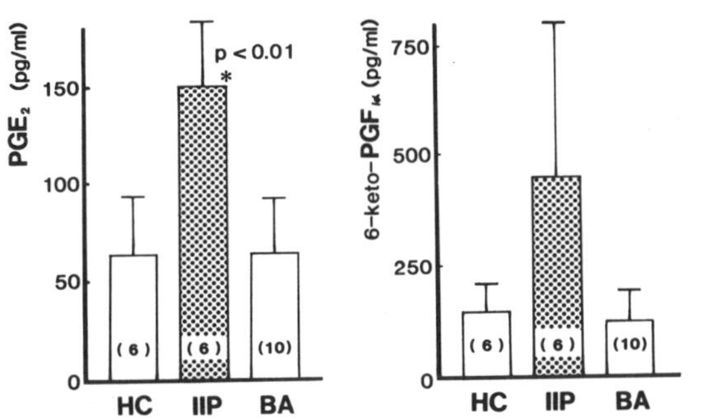

Fig.1 Concentration of PGE2 and 6-keto-PGF1a in
peripheral venous blood in HC, IIP and BA.

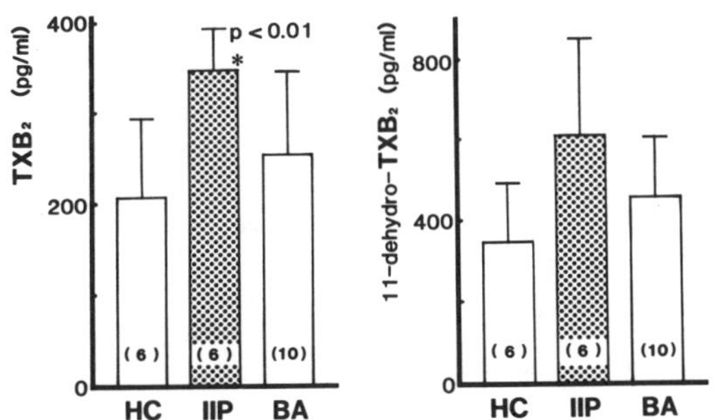

Fig.2 Concentration of TXB2 and 11-dehydro-TXB2
in peripheral venous blood in HC, IP and BA.

ly and the value in IIP are statistically higher than
those of HC (p<0.01). Concentrations of 11-dehydro-TXB2
in HC, IIP, and BA are 347+145, 604+254, and 457+159
pg/ml respectively. PGF2a was not detected.

B. Concentrations of Chemical Mediators in BALF in HC, IIP, BA, and SA groups.

Concentration of chemical mediator in BALF are
corrected by total protein of BALF and expressed per
1mg/ml of total protein. Concentrations of PGE2 and 6-
keto-PGF1a in BALF are shown in Fig.3. The concentrations of PGE2 in HC, IIP, BA and SA are 19.9+13.5,
43.3+23.0, 26.6+26.3 and 36.9+55.7 pg/ml respectively.
Concentration of 6-keto-PGF1a in HC, IIP, BA and SA

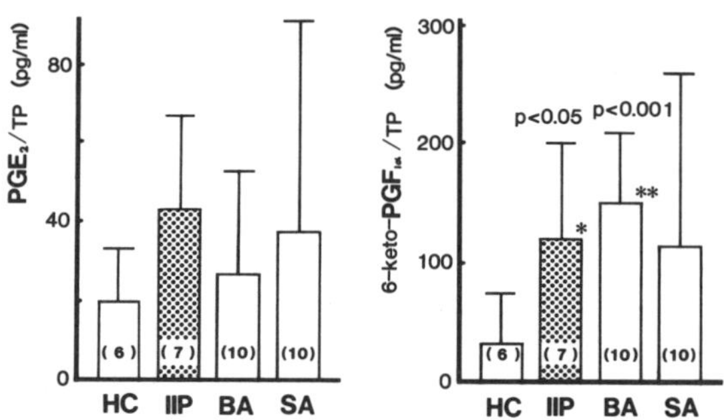

Fig.3 Concentration of PGE2 and 6-keto-PGF1a in BALF
corrected by total protein in HC, IIP, BA and SA.

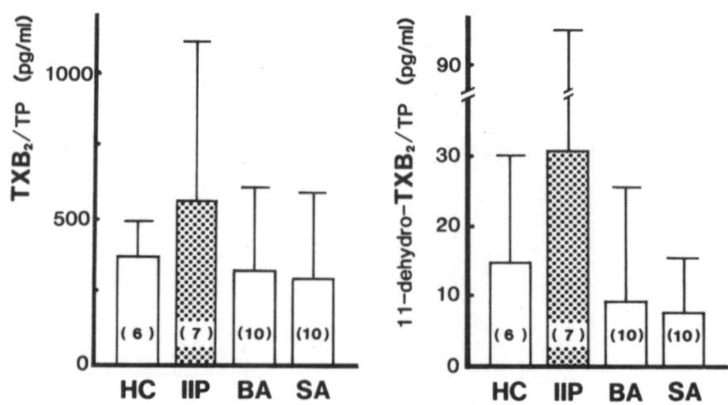

Fig.4 Concentration of TXB2 and 11-dehydro-TXB2 in BALF
corrected by total protein in HC, IIP, BA and SA.

are 26.7+46.9, 120+82, 149+62 and 114+147 pg/ml respectively. The values of IIP are statistically higher
than those of HC (p<0.05), and the values of BA are
significantly higher than those of HC (p<0.001).

Concentrations of TXB2 and 11-dehydro-TXB2 in BALF
are shown in Fig.4. The concentrations of TXB2 in HC,
IIP, BA and SA are 366+117, 560+545, 320+295 and 289+
294 pg/ml respectively. The concentrations of 11-de-
hydro-TXB2 are 14.2+16.0, 31.5+64.0, 8.9+17.5 and 7.0+
8.9 pg/ml respectively. Compared with HC, their values
tended to be higher, but significance was not found.

Concentration of LTC4 and LTB4 in BALF are shown
in Fig.5. The concentration of LTC4 in HC, IIP, BA and
SA are 0, 0.35+0.93, 0.15+0.48 and 0.09+0.3 pg/ml respectively. The concentration of LTB4 in HC, IIP, BA
and SA are143+53, 260+254, 232+169 and 164+95 pg/ml
respectively. Compared with HC, their values tended to
be higher, but significance was not found.

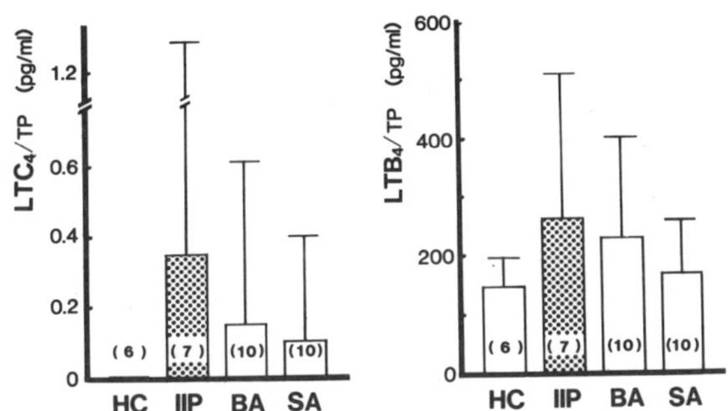

Fig.5 Concentration of LTC4 and LTB4 in BALF corrected by total protein in HC, IIP, BA and SA.

Discussion

IIP is a group of interstitial pneumonia with unknown etiology and poor prognosis. The concept of IIP
is regarded as one clinicopathological entity, because
its diagnosis is established when clinical features
and histological findings are compatible with so called
pneumonitis, and possibility of other diseases can be
excluded. Many similarities have been found in IIP patients when their entire clinical course, chest X-ray

and CT findings, pulmonary function tests, BALF and
laboratory findings are analyzed. But no common pathogenesis have been found and its pathophysiology has not
been clarified yet.

In this study, in order to approach to the pathogenesis of IIP, the roles of arachidonic acid cascade
were investigated. Assayed chemical mediators in peripheral venous blood and BALF were PGE2, 6-keto-PGF1a,
TXB2,11-dehydro-TXB2, LTC4 and LTB4. Concentrations of
these chemical mediator showed a tendency to be elevated in BALF and peripheral venous blood, compared
with HC and other deceases. Especially the concentrations of PGE2 and TXB2 in peripheral venous blood, and
6-keto-PGF1a in BALF are significantly higher than
those of control. According to the further analysis, as
is shown in Fig.6, concentrations of PGE2 and TXB2 in
peripheral venous blood have significant correlation
(r=0.88, p<0.001).

In IIP patients immunological systems seem to be
activated, because the immune complex has been found in
30% of patients. PGE2 is known to inhibit the function
of immunological systems by the activation or induction
of suppresser T-cells. In addition PGE2 is known to inhibit the antibody dependent cytotoxicity. It seems
likely therefore, that the increased PGE2 in peripheral
venous blood and BALF may act as a defense mechanism
against the inflammatory process.

The roles of TXB2, metabolite of thromboxane A2
have not been established yet in IIP. As is shown in
Fig.6, the interactions between PGE2 and TXB2 were

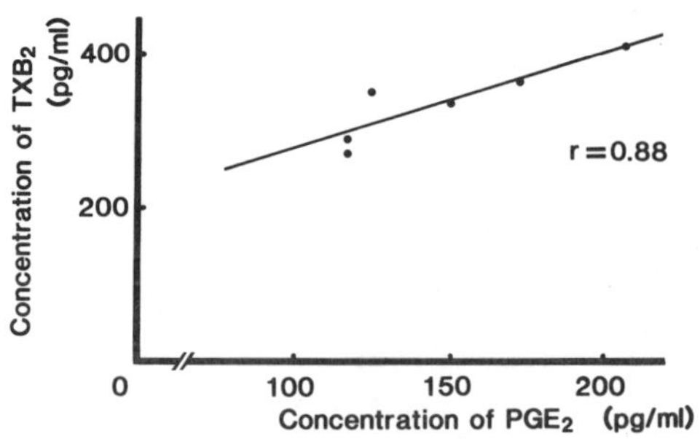

Fig.6   Correlation between PGE2 and TXB2
in peripheral venous blood.

suggested in this study, but the relationship of these two mediators has not been reported yet. 6-keto-PGF1a, stable metabolite of PGI2 was significantly elevated in BALF, but its roles have not been understood.

More subjects and further studies will be needed to establish the roles of these mediators in the pathophysiology and etiology of IIP.

References

1) Haslam PL: Bronchoalveolar lavage, Semin Respir Med, 6:55-70,1984.
2) Raynolds HY, Fulmer JD, et.al.: Analysis of cellular and protein content of bronchoalveolar lavage fluid from patients with idiopathic pulmonary fibrosis and chronic hypersensitivity pneumonitis. J Clin Invest,59:165-175,1977.
3) Anderson HA: Transbronchoscopic lung diagnosis for diffuse pulmonary disease. Chest, 73:734-736,1978.

V
TREATMENT

The Relationship of Bronchoalveolar Lavage Fluid Cellular Constituents with Histopathology and Therapeutic Responsiveness in Idiopathic Pulmonary Fibrosis

M.I. Schwarz, L.C. Watters, J.A. Waldron, R.E. Stanford, R.M. Cherniack, and T.E. King

University of Colorado Health Sciences Center and National Jewish Center for Immunology and Respiratory Medicine, Denver, Colorado, USA

There is a group of patients with IPF in whom BAL lymphocytosis is predictive of the underlying histopathology. In this group alveolar septal inflammation is prominent and honeycombing is mild or absent. In addition it is this group of patients who improve with corticosteroid treatment as measured by the clinical radiographic-scoring system. BAL neutrophilia on the other hand, does not predict the presence of alveolar inflammation or advanced fibrosis nor does it indicate therapeutic responsiveness.

INTRODUCTION

Bronchoalveolar lavage (BAL) is well established as a technique to sample the distal air spaces of the lung to investigate mechanisms of disease production and in some diseases to establish a diagnosis. What is less clear is whether BAL has utility in predicting the stage of disease activity (cellular vs. fibrotic disease) and the response to therapeutic intervention. The relationship between BAL cellular constituents an underlying histopathologic findings as well as response to therapy has not been well defined in idiopathic pulmonary fibrosis (IPF).

Tables and Figures were reproduced with permission of the American Review of Respiratory Disease

METHODS

I. Subjects

Twenty-six patients with untreated IPF were evaluated. The diagnosis
was based on a compatible clinical, radiographic and physiologic
picture and confirmed by open lung biopsy. Exclusions included
connective tissue disease, hypersensitivity pneumonitis, or a
significant occupational exposure.

Normal controls (18) underwent BAL and pulmonary function testing.

II. Determination of Clinical Impairment in IPF

Prior to open lung biopsy at 6 and 12 months a history, chest
radiographic, and physiologic evaluations were performed.

III. Quantitation (Initial and Follow-up) of Clinical Impairment

Impairment was assessed by means of a clinical-radiographic
physiologic scoring system (CRP) [1]. In this system 8 variables
were measured including: the type of activity to produce dyspnea (20),
the profusion of infiltrates, the presence of pulmonary hypertension,
and the extent of honeycombing on chest radiograph (10), FVC (12),
FEV1 (3), thoracic gas volume or FRC (10), DLCO/VA (5), resting
A-aPO2 (10), exercised induced oxygen desaturation indexed to the
faction of predicted maximum oxygen consumption (30). Numbers in
parenthesis refer to maximal points assigned. The following
indicates the significance of the individual scores:

SCORE	CLINICAL STATUS
0 – 14	Healthy individual
15 – 29	Mild impairment, fairly normal existence
30 – 59	Employed, moderate impairment
60 – 79	Severe impairment
> – 80	Can't work, confined to home

A 10 point decrease in the CRP score was considered improvement, a
10 point increase was considered clinical worsening, and a less then
10 point change was considered stablization.

IV. Bronchoalveolar Lavage and Fluid Analysis BALF

This was performed as previously described [2].

V. Histopathologic Assessment of Open Lung Biopsies

Lung tissue was obtained from both the upper and lower lobes.
Multiple sections from each area were stained with hematoxylin-eosin
and Masson trichrome and independently evaluated and the diagnosis
confirmed by two pathologists. The following 11 features were scored:

alveolar septal inflammation, intraalveolar round cells, alveolar
septal fibrosis, honeycombing, smooth muscle proliferation,
inflammatory airway narrowing, type II cell hyperplasia, obstructive
pneumonitis, lymphoid nodules, thickened pulmonary arterioles, and
obliterative air way narrowing. Each pathologic feature was scored
in the following manner: 0=absent; 1=mild; 2=moderate; 3=severe.
The mean scores of two pathologists were used for the correlations
with lavage cell counts.

VI. Treatment and Follow-up
Following initial evaluation, BAL, and open lung biopsy 22 of the
26 patients began oral prednisone using the following protocol:
1.5mgm/kgm not to exceed 100mgm daily tor 6 weeks; 1.0mgm/kgm for
6 weeks; 0.5mgm/kgm/day for 3 months; gradual taper to 0.25mgm/kgm/day.

RESULTS

I. Demographic and Physiologic Features of the Study Population

TABLE I

	Healthy Controls	IPF
N	18	26
Age	32 ± 2	57 ± 2
Sex	12 W, 6 M	9 W, 17 M
Tobacco Use	7	12
Duration of	–	20 ± 5
Symptoms (mos)		
Phys Testing		
FVC % Predicted	99 ± 3	67 ± 4
Vtg % Predicted	100 ± 3	86 ± 3
DLCO/VA % Predicted	94 ± 7	60 ± 4
A–aPO2, mmHg	ND	22 ± 2
Exercise O2	ND	29.8 ± 4
Desaturation		

ND = Not Done
Data expressed as the means of ± SE

II. Bronchoalveolar Lavage Results
TABLE II

	Healthy Volunteers (n = 18)	Patients With IPF (n = 26)
Recovery of instilled, %	75 ± 2	54 ± 4
Total cells/ml x 10^{-4}	15.4 ± 2.2	31.8 ± 5.1
Alveolar macrophages:		
%	92 ± 1	69 ± 5
cells/ml x 10^{-4}	14.3 ± 2.1	20.9 ± 3.7
Lymphocytes:		
%	7 ± 1	17 ± 5
cells/ml x 10^{-4}	1.0 ± 0.2	7.4 ± 3.6
Neutrophils:		
%	0.7 ± 0.3	9 ± 2
cells/ml x 10^{-4}	0.1 ± 0.04	2.0 ± 0.5
Eosinophils:		
%	0.1 ± 0.1	5 ± 1
cells/ml x 10^{-4}	0.02 ± 0.01	1.4 ± 0.3

III. Correlation Between BAL, Cell and Histopathology
TABLE III

	Alveolar Septal Inflammation	Honeycombing	Smooth Muscle Hypertrophy
Total			
cells/ml	$- +$	$- 0.48''$	$-$
Macrophages			
%	$- 0.71\ddagger$	$0.39''$	$0.39''$
cells/ml	$-$	$-$	$-$
Lymphocytes			
%	$0.82\P$	$- 0.56\S$	$- 0.46''$
cells/ml	$0.65\cdot\cdot$	$- 0.42''$	$- 0.38''$
Neutrophils			
%	$-$	$-$	$-$
cells/ml	$-$	$-$	$-$
Eosinophils			
%	$-$	0.29^{++}	$-$
cells/ml	$-$	$-$	$-$

The other 8 histopathologic abnormalities assessed were also evaluated, but none of the correlations with BALF cellular contents achieved statistical significance.
+ Signifies that these correlations were evaluated but not significant
‡ $p < 0.0002$ " $p < 0.05$ .. $p = 0.0003$
§ $p < 0.005$ ¶ $p < 0.0001$ ++ $p = 0.16$

There is significant correlation between alveolar septal inflammation
and BAL lymphocytes whether expressed as a percentage or cells per
millimeter BAL lymphocytes also correlated negatively with either
honeycombing or smooth muscle hypertrophy. In contrast BAL neutrophils
and eosinophils whether expressed as a percentage or cells per
millimeter showed no correlations with any histopathologic abnormality.

Figure 1 indicates that BAL neutrophil percentage could not distinguish
between absent to mild alveolar septal inflammation from moderate to
severe alveolar septal inflammation. Neither could BAL neutrophils
distinguish between the severity of honeycombing (Fig. 2).

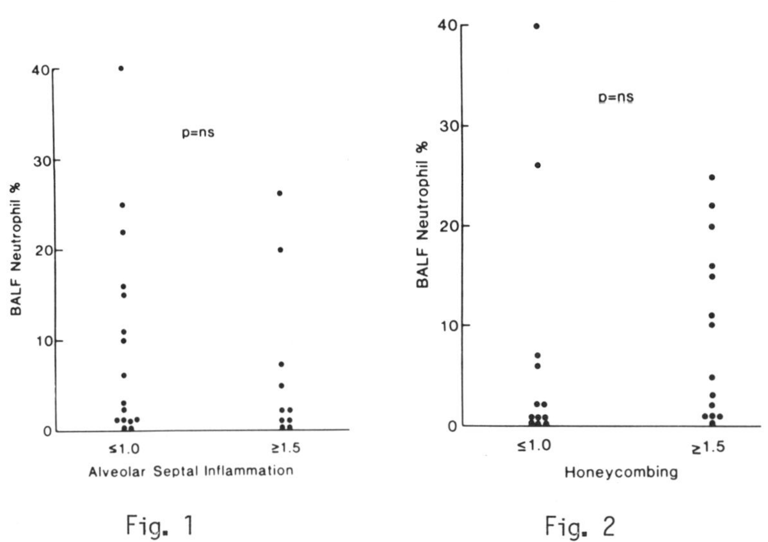

Fig. 1   Fig. 2

In contrast Fig. 3 illustrates that BAL lymphocyte content was
significantly increased in moderate to severe alveolar septal
inflammation and in absent to mild alveolar septal inflammation.
Similarily, if moderate to severe honeycombing was present lymphocyte
counts were significantly lower then if absent to mild honeycombing
was present.

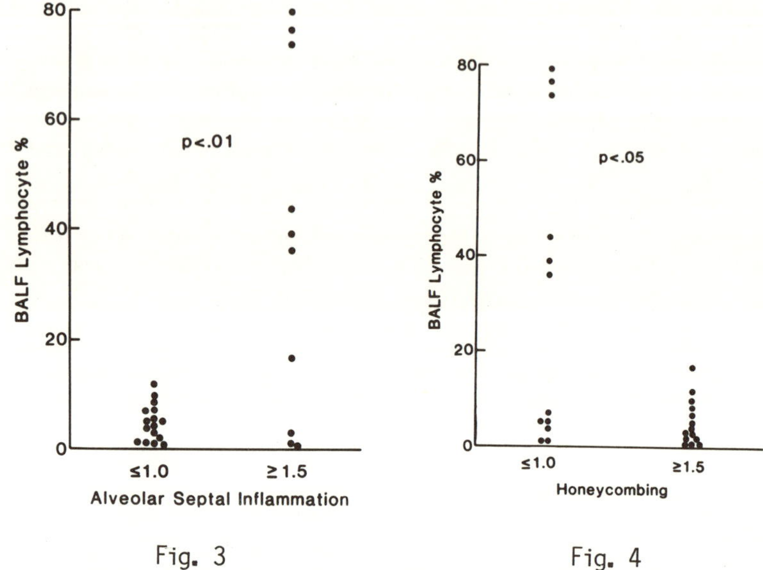

Fig. 3   Fig. 4

IV. Relationship Between Pretreatment CRP Score and Pretreatment Bronchoalveolar Lavage

TABLE IV

Pretreatment BALF Cellular Constituents	Pretreatment CRP Scores[†]			
	15–29	30–59	60–79	≥ 80
Patients, n	4	11	9	2
Total cells/ml × 10^{-4}	43 ± 17	31 ± 5	30 ± 11	19 ± 2
Macrophages				
%	66 ± 18	72 ± 9	69 ± 8	55 ± 4
cells/ml × 10^{-4}	36.54 ± 18.73	22.05 ± 5.28	15.37 ± 2.30	10.11 ± 1.74
Lymphocytes				
%	32 ± 19	14 ± 7	17 ± 8	6 ± 3
cells/ml × 10^{-4}	5.57 ± 2.37	5.76 ± 3.44	11.95 ± 9.70	1.17 ± 0.67
Neutrophils:				
%	1 ± 1	10 ± 4	7 ± 2	23 ± 3
cells/ml × 10^{-4}	0.36 ± 0.36	2.60 ± 1.11	1.25 ± 0.32	4.18 ± 0.84
Eosinophils				
%	2 ± 1	3 ± 1	7 ± 2	17 ± 9
cells/ml × 10^{-4}	0.94 ± 0.83	0.84 ± 0.25	1.87 ± 0.59	2.93 ± 1.40

The initial BAL neutrophil and lymphocyte counts did not predict the initial severity of clinical impairment as measured by the CRP score. Although higher neutrophil and lower lymphocyte counts were found in the subjects with the greatest degree of clinical impairment, this was not significant. On the other hand BAL eosinophil counts were increased in the subjects most severely impaired and this had statistical significance.

V. Relationship of Response to Treatment with Initial BAL Cell Contents

Of the patients with initial BAL lymphocytosis, 5 showed definite improvement when reevaluated at 6 months (Fig. 5) and this persisted for at least 1 year. As can be seen in Fig. 6 neutrophils could not predict therapeutic responsiveness. This was true for eosinophils.

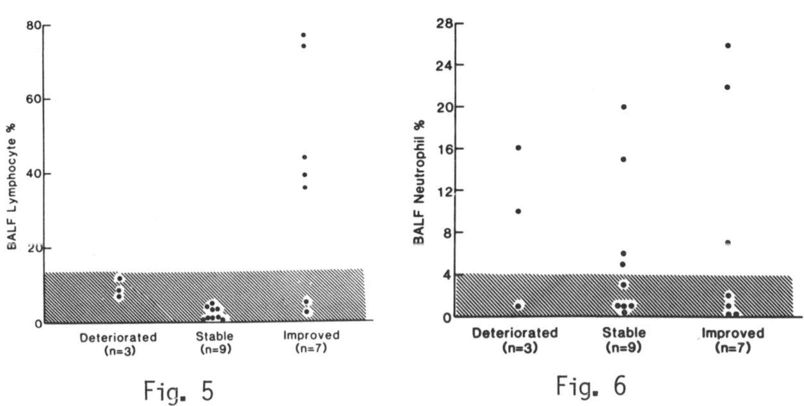

Fig. 5   Fig. 6

SUMMARY

There is a group of patients with IPF in whom BAL lymphocytes is predictive of the underlying histopathology. In this group alveolar septal inflammation is prominent and honeycombing is mild or absent. In addition it is this group of patients who improve with corticosteroid treatment as measured by the clinical radiographic-scoring system. BAL neutrophilia on the other hand, does not predict the presence of alveolar inflammation or advanced fibrosis nor does it indicate therapeutic responsiveness.

1. Watters LC, King TE, Schwarz MI, et al: A clinical radiographic and physiologic scoring system for the longitudinal assessment of patients with idiopathic pulmonary fibrosis. Am Rev Resp Dis 133:97–103, 1986.

2. Watters LC, King TE, Cherniack RM, et al: Bronchoalveolar lavage neutrophils increase after corticosteroid therapy in smokers with idiopathic pulmonary fibrosis. Am Rev Resp Dis 133:104–109, 1986.

Tokyo Criteria for Measuring Therapeutic Effect on Idiopathic Interstitial Pneumonia

Fumihiko Kitatani

National Kinki Chuo Hospital, Osaka, Japan

The project research members of Idiopathic Interstitial Pneumonia or IIp in Japan discussed how to determine objectove and subjective therapeutic effects on IIP.

This is because we often fiend that patients with chronic dyspnea note vague improvement fo their subjective symptoms when steroid are administered.

Furthermore, the improvement and the exacerbation accompany volume loss of affected lungs on chest X-ray, and it will also be useful in determining how and when the extent and the density of abnormal shadows change.

In 1977, we made "Tokyo Criteria" based on the findings experienced by a group of physicians in Tokyo.

Befor I futher describe this, I must mention the fact that the grade to determine the degree of chronic dyspnea has been evaluated by using modified Hugh-Jones' Classification.

As you can see on the Table 1 the degree of dyspnea is classified into five groups namely: Normal, slight, moderate, severe and very severe.

Table 1. Dyspnea Index of Modified Hugh-Jones' Classification

1st Degree – Normal :	Be able to work and walk as well as healthy at the same age can.
2nd Degree – Slight :	Be able to walk on the level 1 and as fast as the healthy at the same age can, but suffer from dyspnea by going uphill or stairs.

3rd Degree – Moderate : Even on the level land, unable to
                        walk as fast as the healthy can
                        but able to walk as far as 1 km
                        or more at one's speed.

4th Degree – Severe   : Unable to walk even up to 50 m
                        without taking rest.

5th Degree – Very severe : Suffer from dyspnea even during
                           conversation, dressing and also
                           one's minimal activity.

This classification has been modified by us so that
this may be conveniently and commonly used as valuable
index to determine the degree of dyspnea in Japan.

Well, than let me describe the following four conditions
as a part of our criteria.

1. Improvement by one grade or more in dyspnea grade according to modified Hugh-Jones' classification.
2. Increase of 10 Torr or more in PaO_2.
3. Increase of vital capacity by 15% or more.
4. Improvement in X-Ray findings.

The improvement is defind when the above all four conditions are met.

The stable is when two or three conditions are met.

The unchanged is defined when three conditions are
unchanged.

The exacerbation is define when more than two conditions
deteriorate.

As to the roentgenographic evaluation, the improvement
is diagnosed when the extent and the density of abnormal
shadows decrease regardless of any change of the shadow
patterns.

The exacerbation is diagnosed when the extent and density of the lesions increase or when nodular shadows
change to mixture of nodular and ring shadows or further
to predominant ring shadows with volume loss of the affected lungs.

In evaluating the clinical usefulness of our criteria,
we applied the criteria to the evaluation of the effectiveness of steroid treatment on histologically confirmed
107 cases with IIP.

There are 55 male and 52 female and the onset were at
age of 54.9±13.7 and ranging from 12 to 82 years old.

The results were: 12 cases or 11.2% of the whole subjects were improved and there were no death of IIP.

With these results, we conclude that this criteria, I
presented today, can be a useful index to determine the
therapeutic effect on IIP.

Treatment of Idiopathic Interstitial Pneumonia with Corticosteroids

Masahito Okayasu

Nihon University School of Medicine, Tokyo, Japan

In this paper I reported the result of
steroid therapy for IIP which was obtained
from the nationwide survey of special
research group for IIP granted by the
Ministry of Health and Welfare. It is
hard to say that steroid is effective for
IIP, however we can not simply deny its
effectiveness. At the present, steroid
therapy should be attempted to the cases
of IIP excluding the chronic stable cases
and those with honey comb lungs.

In the present paper, I am going to report the effect
of corticosteroid therapy on idiopathic interstitial
pneumonia (IIP). These results were obtained from the
nationwide survey of special research group for IIP
granted by the Ministry of Health and Welfare.
The first retrospective study was conducted for
3 years between 1974 and 1976.
In this survey, 133 cases of IIP who received the
steroid therapy for more than three weeks were chosen
from 183 cases who were diagnosed as IIP based upon the
pathological study of autopsy or biopsy specimens. The
protocols of steroid therapy were variable.
Table 1 shows the effectiveness of steroid therapy on
133 cases of IIP judged by physicians in charge. Marked
improvement was observed in 4.5% of cases, improvement
in 15.0%, and temporal improvement in 49.6%. In 12.0%

of cases, no remarkable changes were observed and
aggravation was found in 18.8% with steroid therapy.
Therefore, only 20% of cases revealed the improvement
with steroid therapy.

Table 1   Effectiveness of Steroid Therapy
N=133

	cases	%
markedly improved	6	(4.5)
improved	20	(15.0)
temporarily improved	66	(49.6)
unchanged	16	(12.0)
worse	25	(18.8)
total	133	(100.0)

Among 133 cases, 64 cases who had sufficient data
available were picked up and effectiveness of steroid
was re-analysed with these subjects. The results are
shown on Table 2.

Table 2   Effectiveness of Steroid Therapy
N=64

	initial	all courses(%)
markedly improved	2	2 (3.1%)
improved	6	6 (9.4%)
slightly improved	12	5 (7.8%)
unchanged	25	8 (12.5%)
worse	19	43 (67.2%)
total	64	64 (100%)

Therapeutic responses observed during initial 1 to 2
months after steroid therapy are shown in the column of
initial and the responses observed afterwards are
summarized as shown in the column of all courses. At the
initial stage of steroid therapy, improvement including
slightly improved were observed in 20 cases and worsening
with steroid was found in 19 cases. However, 43 cases,
that is 67.2% of all cases, revealed aggravations through
the all courses of steroid therapy.

The relationship between radiological classification of
IIP and the effectiveness of steroid is shown on Table 3.
Marked improvement was found only in cases of type I,
that is ground glass or cloudy patchy appearance with
active and early lesions.

Table 3   Relationship between Radiological Classification
and Steroid Efficacy

N=62

	I	I + II	II	II + III	III	III + I	III + I + II	total
markedly im.	2	0	0	0	0	0	0	2
improved	2	1	1	0	0	2	0	6
slightly im.	3	1	1	0	0	0	0	5
unchange t.	0	0	1	0	0	0	0	1
a.	1	0	3	0	2	0	0	6
worse t.	3	1	0	0	1	1	0	6
a.	7	9	8	3	8	0	1	36
	18	12	14	3	11	1	1	62

im.=improved   t.=temporarily im.   a.=all courses

Cases of type II that is mainly nodular and reticular
appearance on chest films mostly revealed no remarkable
changes with steroid therapy. Cases of type III that is
honey comb appearance tended to show no remarkable
changes and rather worsened with steroid. Abbreviation
of t described after unchange and worse indicates the
cases showed slight improvement during the initial course
after steroid administration.

Cases who revealed improvement and marked improvement
did not always receive the high doses of steroid and
average initial dose of predonisolone was 43mg ranging
from 30mg to 60mg/day. On the other hand, cases whose
progress worsened received 36mg of initial predonisolone
in average ranging from 10mg to 75mg. These doses were
not different from those of improved cases.

Table 4 shows the relationship between the duration
from the disease onset to the initiation of steroid
therapy and the classification of radiological findings
and efficacy of steroid therapy.

Table 4   Correlation of Duration from Onset,
X-P Classification and Steroid Efficacy

N=63

duration from onset	X-P classification	improved			unchanged	worse
		mark.	mod.	slight.		
2M. 12 cases	I	1	1			5
	II				1	1
	I · II					1
	I · III		1			1
2 6M. 5 cases	I			1		1
	I · II		1			
	II		1			1
6M. 1y. 13 cases	I		1	1	1	1
	I · II					4
	II				1	2
	I · III		1			
	III					1
1 2y. 10 cases	I	1		1		1
	I · II					2
	II			1		1
	III					3
2y. 23 cases	I					2
	I · II			1		3
	II				2	3
	I · II · III					1
	II · III					4
	III					7

Only 17 cases that is 27.0% of all cases received the
steroid therapy within 6 months of onset。 Marked or
moderate effect was observed in 8 cases and 6 out of 8
cases were started steroid therapy within 6 months.
Aggravation was observed in 35.2% of cases who started
steroid within 6 months and in 16.3% of case who
initiated steroid therapy after 6 months from the onset
and this difference was statistically significant.
Radiological findings revealed that type II and III that
is fibrotic change and honey combing were observed in
cases whose disease duration was only within 2 months.
It must be carefully considered that aggravation was
also observed in cases of type I.

R. Yoneda, who leaded the present study, pointed out
that patterns of response to steroid therapy could be
classified as A,B,C,D, and E, as shown in Fig 1.

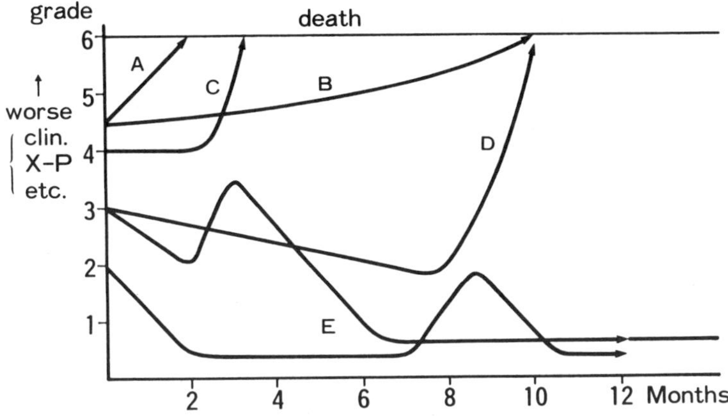

Fig. 1. Progress Patterns with Steroid
       Therapy   (R. Yoneda)

The grade of 1 to 5 in vertical axis was determined
mainly based upon the clinical finding and radiological
appearance, and grade 6 indicates the death of patient.
Pattern A indicates the patients who did not respond to
steroid at all and progressed rapidly and passed away.
   Pattern B indicates that these patients gradually
aggravated although clinical course was rather chronic.
   Pattern C indicates the cases whose progress did not
change in early stage of steroid therapy, then suddenly
aggravated.
   Pattern D indicates the cases who improved temporarily,
but, then, the progress suddenly got worse and died。
   Pattern E indicates the cases who responded to the
steroid therapy. In these cases, steroid was effective.
In some cases who showed pattern E response, temporal
aggravation was observed and these were considered to be
due to the procedure of reduction of steroid dosage.
   Second results were obtained from the nationwide
survey performed for 3 years between 1977 and 1979 by
the same research group for IIP. Total subjects were
107 cases including 55 male patients and 52 female
patients. Average age of onset of IIP was 54.9±13.7
years old. Among 107 cases, 9 cases were acute type and
98 cases were chronic type.

The duration from the onset of IIP to initial visit were within 6 months in 42 cases, 6 months to 2 years in 23 cases and more than 2 years in 42 cases. Initial doses of steroid varied among the subjects and average dose was 44.1±53.5mg/day. Duration of steroid administration ranged from less than 1 month to 7 years and 11 months. The criteria for the determination of effectiveness was already reported by Dr. Kitatani. Effectiveness of steroid therapy and prognosis are shown on Table 5. Improvement was observed in 12 cases, that is 11.2% of total cases. Progress was stable or unchanged in 13 cases, 12.1%, worsening was found in 67 cases, 62.6% and effectiveness was not judged in 15 cases, 14.0%. 75 cases died and 68 out of 75 cases deceased because of IIP.

Table 5   Effectiveness of Treatment and Prognosis

	clinical response	survival	dead		unknown
			underlying disease	other disease	
improved	12 11.2%	10	0	2	0
stable or unchanged	13 12.1%	7	3	2	1
worse	67 62.6%	8	55	3	1
no judgment	15 14.0%	3	10	0	2
	107	28	68	7	4

In 1984, questionnaire was sent to various institutes, and 195 cases of IIP were collected and following results were obtained on the basis of analysis of these patients.

Steroid therapy was judged as effective in 63.0% of IIP cases. In comparison, steroid was effective in 52.0% of sarcoidosis and 74.0% of collagen lung diseases as shown in Fig.2.

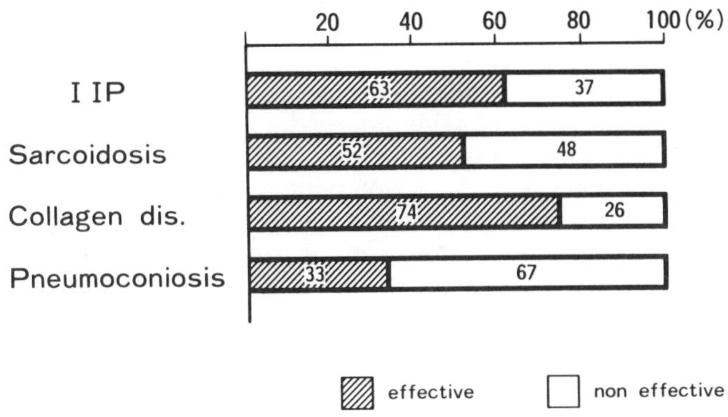

Fig. 2. Effectiveness of Steroid Therapy
(Ishida, Fukuchi *et al.*)

Fig.3 shows the efficacy of steroid therapy in relation
to the patient's age, however, no significant difference
in ages was observed between good responders and poor
responders.

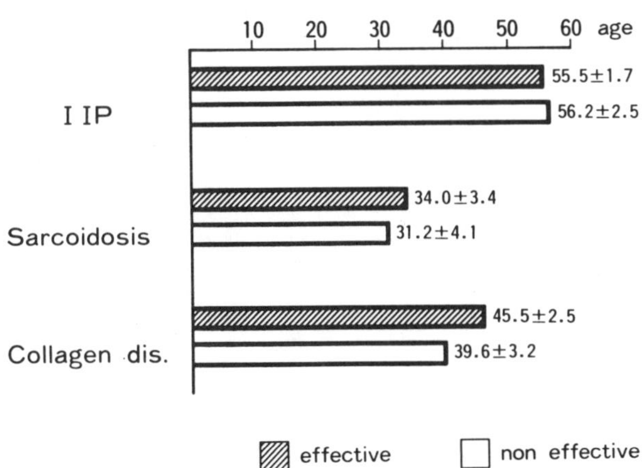

Fig. 3. Efficacy of Steroid in Relation
to Age   (Ishida, Fukuchi *et al.*)

The efficacy of steroid therapy was related to the duration from the disease onset to the therapy initiation.

In cases of IIP, effective cases tended to receive the steroid therapy in earlier course. Acute changes for the worse were observed in many cases, and the cause was aggravation of primary disease in 43.0% of cases, infection in 33.0% and reduction of predonisolone dosage in 20.0%.

In summary

I reported here the results of steroid therapy for IIP. These results were obtained from the nationwide survey of special research group for IIP granted by the Ministry of Health and Welfare. It is hard to say that steroid is effective for IIP. However, we cannot simply deny its effectiveness.

As I referred to the report from England by Turner Warwick et al[1], there are cases of cryptogenic fibrosing alveolitis who fairly respond to steroid and have longer survival than non-treated patients. Y.Kondo in Japan has also reported similar results, therefore, at the present, steroid therapy should be attempted to the cases of IIP excluding the chronic stable cases and those with honey comb lungs.

References

1.Turner-Warwick, M.Burrows. B, and Johnson, A.
   Thorax 35,593-599,1980

Clinical Study of Steroid Pulse Therapy for Idiopathic Interstitial Pneumonia

R. Yoneda and A. Kurashima

Tokyo National Chest Hospital, Tokyo, Japan

Idiopathic interstitial pneumonia (IIP) characterized by a divers clinical picture, want of disease spcificity even under clinical examination, and few telling parameters. Consequently, choice of treatment indications is extremely difficult. Often by the time a diagnosis of IIP is established, fibrosis is already advanced. Under such advaerse conditions, the consequences of steroid therapy seen still worse. A powerful impression got from study of histories is that almost invariably when treatment started with an initial prednisolone dosage of 20 to 30mg that in the absence of effect was then gradually increased, steroid response was nil, and death ensued.

In the light of this, we concluded that therapy was crucial, and that ample dosage with steroid was essential to adequate initial results. For this reson pulse therapy was thought to be possibly more effective and has been tried since 1978 with comparatively good results, although the limited number of cases makes evaluation difficult. Ideally, controlled trials are necessary, although difficult in practice.

In 1986 we were able to analyse a number of cases in which pulse therapy had been used. On the basis of clinical course, cases were arranged in three groups for purposes of orderly analysis. As shown in Table 1, there were acute chronic, and acutely exacerbated forms, the chronic beeing further divided into active and inactive.

All told there were 51 cases collected from 17 institutions. Sex, age and clinical course were as shown in

Table 1.

Clinical Course of IIP

I. Acute Form
II. Chronic Form
  a) Active
  b) Inactive
III. Acute Exacerbation Form

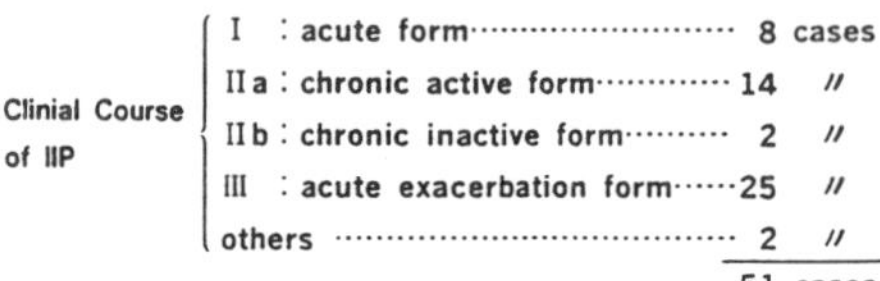

Table 2.

Questionaire Investigation of Steroid Pulse Therapy in IIP Patients

51 Cases from 17 Institutions
Male   : 39 cases, (average age 61.3 ys.)
Female : 12 cases, (″   ″   60.4 ys.)

Clinial Course of IIP
I   : acute form ················· 8 cases
IIa : chronic active form ············· 14 ″
IIb : chronic inactive form ········· 2 ″
III : acute exacerbation form ······ 25 ″
others ······································· 2 ″
51 cases

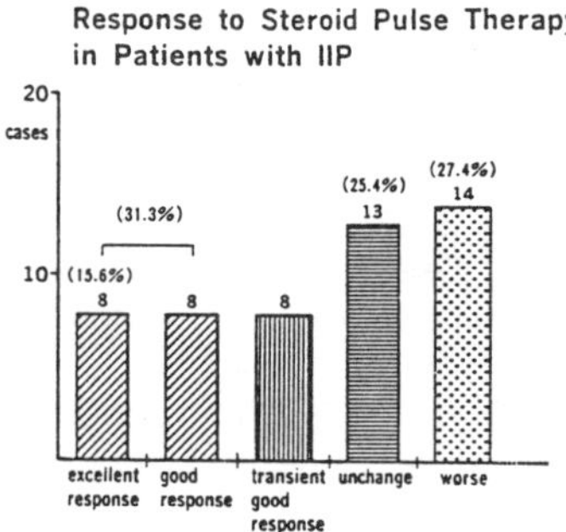

Response to Steroid Pulse Therapy in Patients with IIP

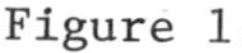

Figure 1.

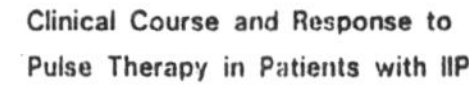

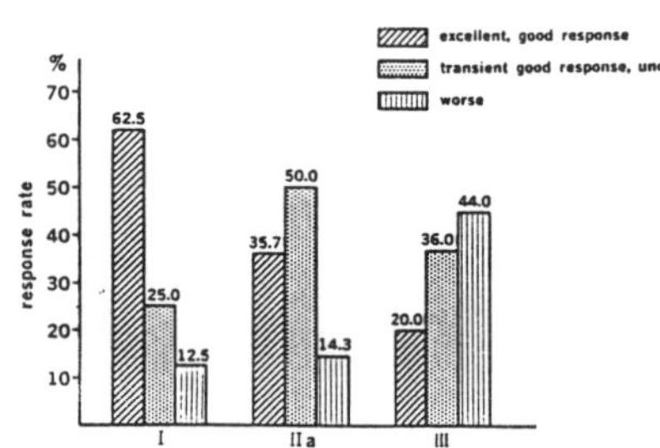

Clinical Course and Response to Pulse Therapy in Patients with IIP

Figure 2.

Table 2.   The number of cases of the chronic active form is notable; but most notable is the large number of the' acutely exacerbated. Most of these instances of aggravation occurred during tapering off of steroid dosage.

As shown in Fig. 1, respose was excellent to good in 16 cases, or 31.1%. In comparison to the results with common oral therapy described by the preceeding author, this response is fairly good. And it was noted that response rate for women was 41.7%, as against 28.2% for men, but this difference may not be significant.

Steroid therapy is not a radical treatment ofr IIP, but this is not to say that it is hopeless. Further analysis of the relationship of clinical course and steroid response is shown in Fig. 2. For group, that is the acute form response rate was high at 62.5%; for II-a, that is, the chronic active response rate dropped to 35.7%; and for group III, the acutely exacerbated, response was poor at only 20%. Moreover, on the negative side, 44% of this group became worse, a significant difference from the adverse rates for groups I and II-a. Thus, pulse therapy affords little help in cases of acute exacerbation.

Pulse therapy appears to be a relatively better method of treatment for IIP than the method of oral administration in use here to fore. Moreover, other than a facial flush observed in 11.8% of the cases, there were no remarkable or mahor side effects. Pulse therapy seems therefore to be a useful approach to treatmen of IIP. Guidelines seemingly appropriate are shown in Table 3. Pulse therapy for chronic active form were useful treatment as well as acute form. And indications marked with a dotted line show comparatively poor results.

Table 3.

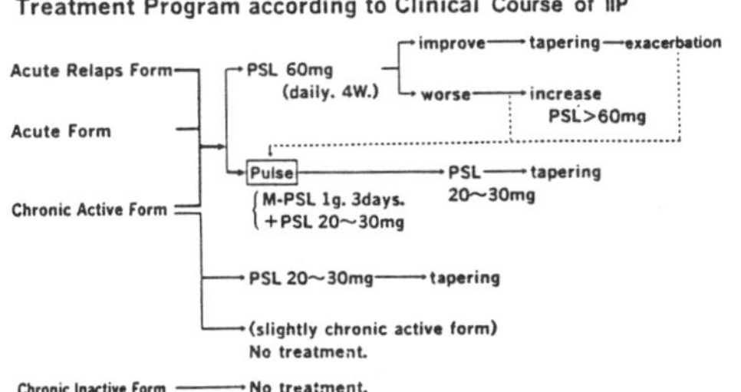

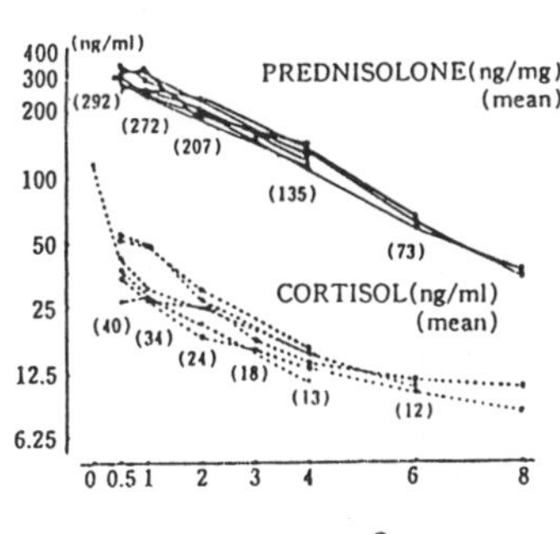

Prednisolone and Cortisol serum concentration-time curve after oral administration of Prednisolone (10mg) in healthy volunteers. (n= 7)

Figure 3.

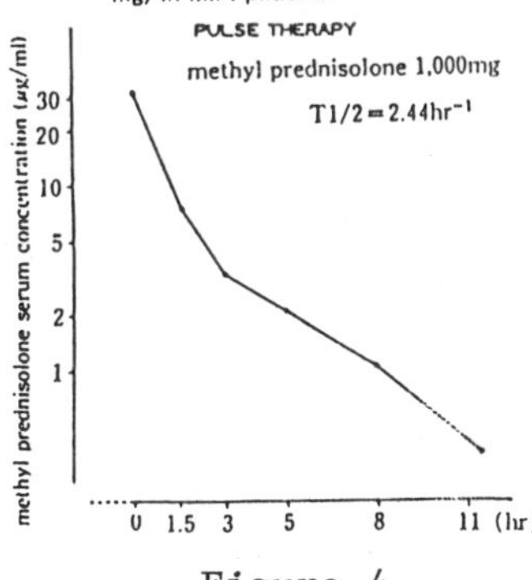

Methylprednisolne serum concentration-time curve after D.I.V. administration of methylprednisolone (1,000 mg) in I.I.P. patient.

Figure 4.

Furthermore, we tried to measure steroid concentration in the serum (Figs. 3,4). Figure 3 shows serum prednisolone and cortisol after ingestion 10mg prednisolone in healthy volunteers. And Fig. 4 shows serum concentration of methylprednisolone (100mg) in an IIP patient. Consequently, microgram level shown for pulse example indicates a concentration roughly 100 times the 10mg dose.

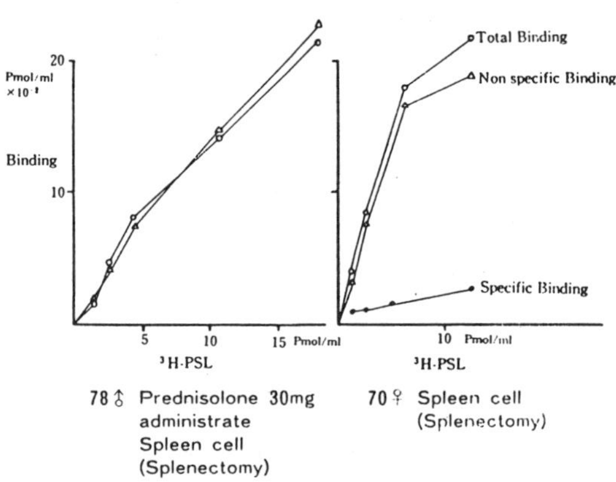

Figure 5.

In addition, steroid receptor assay was tried. The assay was measured by spleen cell from splenectomy and example with 30mg dose of prednisolone compared to control without steroid (Fig. 5). The difference between total binding and nonspecific binding quantities is small, indicating little specific binding.

The relationship between these results and pulse therapy are not easily explained.

The couse of IIP is unclear, and steroid actin is insufficiently understood. Accordingly, any absolute reliance on pulse therapy is unwarranted. It would seem well to consider treatment from a broader perspective with immunosuppressors such as cyclophosphamide or with inhibitors of fibrosis.

Meanwhile, early detection and treatment of and chronic form cases is important.

Prediction of Therapeutic Effects by Bronchoalveolar Lavage and Gallium Scintigraphy in Patients with Idiopathic Interstitial Pneumonia

Ikuro Kimura

Department of Medicine, Okayama University Medical School, Okayama, Japan

Prediction of therapeutic effect of corticosteroids was studied in patients with idiopathic interstitial pneumonia (IIP). In patients with IIP in active stage, bronchoalveolar lavage fluid (BALF) contained increased cellular components before treatments. Increased lymphocyte proportion in BALF indicated the good response in short period of therapy as in one month. However, the increased percentage of neutrophils in BALF indicated the poor response to the therapy especially in 6 months. Gallium scintigraphy was analyzed in relation with the response to therapy. The uneven uptake of radioactivity in the lung fields revealed the poor response although diffuse or relatively high uptake in the lower lung fields showed the good response to therapy. BAL and Gallium scintigraphy could be the useful means to predict the therapeutic effect of corticosteroids therapy.

Introduction
The fibrosing process in the alveolar wall in the patients with IIP has not been elucidated clearly. The treatment of IIP has not been achieved successfully

even with application of corticosteroids, though only a little population of patients with IIP could be relieved from the symptoms of dyspnea or disease progression under corticosteroids therapy. Furthermore, the prognosis of patients with idiopathic interstitial pneumonia is difficult to predict. One of the most reliable prognostic factors has been reported to be the effectiveness of the steroids therapy(1,2). So, the prediction of the therapeutic effect of corticosteroids in patients with IIP appears to be crucial for the prognosis. Therefore, the analysis of bronchoalveolar lavage fluids and gallium scintigraphy of patients with IIP before the treatments was performed in regard to the effects of corticosteroids therapy.

Subjects and Method

1. Fourteen patients with IIP were studied with bronchoalveolar lavage and thirteen patients with IIP were examined with gallium scintigraphy. Twelve normal volunteer and 38 patients with rheumatoid lung, hypersensitivity pneumonia and sarcoidosis were also studied as control.

2. Bronchoalveolar lavage(BAL): The bronchoscope (Olympus B-10) was positioned in a segment of the middle lobe(B4 or B5). A total of 200ml of sterile physiological saline was infused 50ml each, four times and aspirated by suction after each infusion. The lavage fluid was immediately centrifuged to separate cellular and protein components. The supernatant was carefully separated from the cell pellet for subsequent protein analysis as fibronectin and albumin. The cells were assayed for total number, viability and differential counts stained with May-Giemsa staining.

2. Quantification of Fibronectin: Fibronectin concentration in BAL fluid was measure quantitatively with enzyme linked immunoassay. Briefly, bovine serum albumin(BSA) precoated wells were filled with BAL fluid sample and peroxidase labeled antifibronectin rabbit serum. Mixture of sample and antiserum was transferred to the fibronectin coated wells and incubated for one hour. The wells were washed with Tween 20-PBS and ortho-phenylenediamine was added as substrate for peroxidase and measured with ELISA reader at 492nm(O.D.) The levels of fibronectin were obtained

from the standard curve sensitive to 10 ng/ml.
3. Neutrophil chemotactic activity: Chemotactic activity for neutrophils was measured with modified Boyden chamber method(3). The samples for neutrophil chemotactic activity were placed in the lower compartment separated from the upper compartment with nucleopore filter with 5 micrometer pore size. Neutrophils as target cells separated from normal volunteer with 6% dextran and Hypaque density centrifuge. Filters were placed on slide glass after one hour incubation at 37 C in CO2 incubator and stained with Giemsa staining. The number of neutrophils on the lower surface of filter was counted with high power fields. The summation of neutrophils count in 10 fields represented the chemotactic activity.
4. Ga scintigraphy: patients werc given 3mCi of gallium citrate intravenously. Seventy two hours later, gallium uptake of the lung fields was examined with whole body scanner. Gallium scintigrams were classified into 3 grades of uptake in lung fields from 0 as no uptake, I as moderate uptake and II showing uptake high as liver. For quantitative analysis of gallium scintigram, lung fields were separated into upper, middle and lower and each lung field was evaluated for the gallium uptake from 0 to 2 as gallium uptake score. Summation of gallium uptake score represent the total lung uptake of gallium.
5. Ga-BAL:BAL was performed right after the Ga scintigraphy. The radioactivities of BAL fluids and peripheral blood were measured with a single channel gamma counter. Volume of distribution and loss in recovery of BAL fluid were corrected by dividing the number of the counts in BAL fluid by the value of blood per milliliter to give the gallium index.
6. Evaluation of the effectiveness of corticosteroids therapy. The clinical and laboratory data as grades of dyspnea on exertion, partial arterial blood oxygen pressure, vital capacity and interstitial shadows in chest x-ray were examined periodically and the data before treatments start were compared with those in one month, 3 months and 6 months after treatments.
The effectiveness of the therapy was judged from the improvement or progression of these data as good or poor response, respectively.

Results
1) Cellular component of BAL fluids: Total cell counts
and differential cell counts of lymphocyte, neutrophil,
eosinophil and basophil were shown to increase in BAL
fluids of patients with IIP. The activity of fibrosing
process in patients with IIP were classified into two
types as active and inactive stage based on the
clinical and laboratory data of disease progression
within 3 months. BAL fluids of patients in active
stage contained increased total cell and each cell
populations more numerously than those of patients in
inactive stage.
2) Fibronectin levels in BAL fluids: Fibronectin levels
in BAL fluids was significantly high in patients with
IIP. Furthermore, the increase of fibronectin in
patients of active stage was statistically significant
in comparison with those of in active stage.
3) Fibronectin levels and cellular component of BAL
fluids: Fibronectin level and each cell density in BAL
fluid was examined. The significant correlations were
observed between fibronectin concentration and total
cell, alveolar macrophage and neutrophil density,
respectively, in BAL fluid.
4) Differential cell count in BAL fluids and the

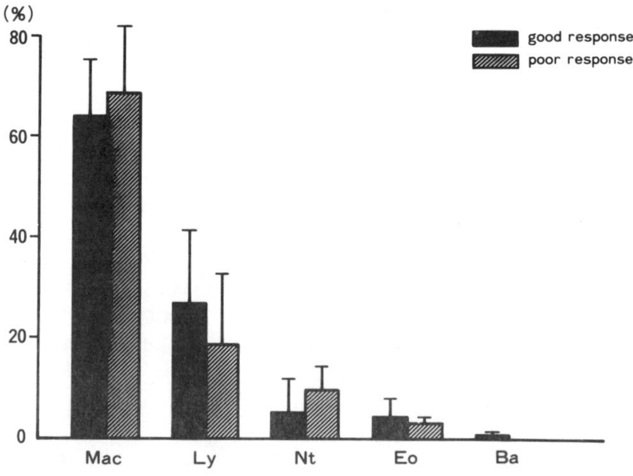

Fig. 1.   Differential cell counts in BAL fluids
before treatment in relation to the therapeutic
effect in one month

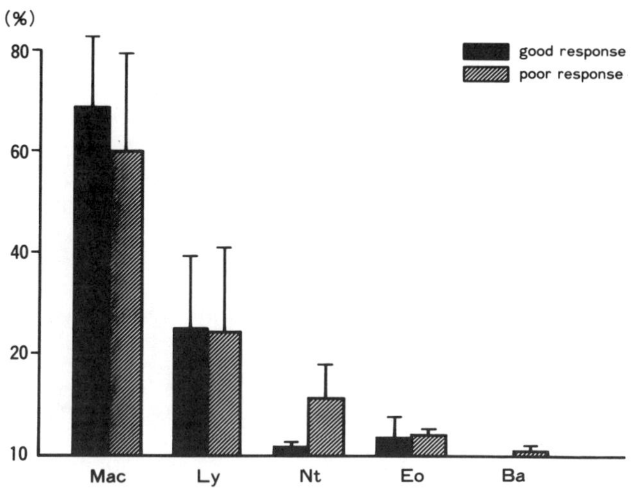

Fig. 2.   Differential cell counts in BAL fluid before treatment in relation to the therapeutic effect in 6 months.

response to the therapy: Cellular component of BAL fluids before treatments were analyzed in regard to the response to the therapy as good or poor response. Increased total cell count showed the good response. Increased lymphocyte in the differential cell count in BAL fluids showed also the good response in the short period as one month. But, no significant difference was observed in 6 months. On the contrary the increase of neutrophil in BAL fluids before treatments indicated the poor response in any period of the therapy(Fig.1,2). 5) Neutrophil percentage and response to the therapy: Patients were classified into two groups depending on the neutrophil percentage more or less 5 % in BAL fluids, tentatively. While 5 of 6 patients(83.3%) with

Table 1. Neutrophil Percentage in BAL Fluid and
        Responses to The Therapy in 6 Months

Neutrophil in BALF	Case No.	Response to therapy Good	poor
5%<	6	1(16.7%)	5(83.3%)
5%>	8	7(87.5%)	1(12.5%)

more than 5% of neutrophils showed the poor response, only one of 8 patients(12.5%) with less than 5% of neutrophils showed the poor response(Table 1).
6) Neutrophil chemotactic activity of fibronectin: Chemotactic activity of fibronectin for neutrophils were examined. Various concentrations of human fibronectin were applied for neutrophil chemotactic activity. Fibronectin showed the concentration dependent neutrophil chemotactic activity from 0.001 ul/ml to 10 ul/ml.
7) Gallium scintigraphy and BAL: BAL of patients with IIP was performed immediately after gallium scintigraphy. The radioactivity in BAL fluids correlated with the semiquantitative analysis of gallium scintigram.
8) Gallium radioactivity and cellular component in BAL fluids: The radioactivity levels of gallium in BAL fluids were compared with various cell density in BAL fluids. The significant correlations were obtained between the radioactivity and density of total cell and alveolar macrophage.
9) In vivo gallium uptake of cellular component of BAL fluids: Cells in BAL fluids obtained after gallium scintigraphy were separated with plastic culture plate into fractions of adhesive cells as macrophage rich and non-adhesive as lymphocyte rich. Most of radioactivity in BAL fluids was shown to be contained in macrophage rich fraction.
10) Distribution of gallium uptake in lung fields: The gallium scintigrams were evaluated in regard to the distribution of radioactive gallium in lung fields and classified into two groups, one with even uptake and another with uneven uptake. Four of 7 patients

Table 2.   Distribution of High Uptake of Ga
            Scintigram and Response to Therapy

Distribution of Ga	Case No.	Response to therapy	
		Good	Poor
upper<lower field even distribution	7	4(57%)	3(43%)
upper>lower field uneven distribution	6	1(17%)	5(83%)

with even gallium uptake showed the good response to
the corticosteroids therapy in 6 months. whereas only
one of 6 patients with uneven gallium uptake was
treated effectively(Table 2).
11) Gallium uptake before and after treatment in
relation to the therapeutic effect: The gallium
scintigrams were evaluated with score of gallium uptake
obtained by semiquantitative analysis. The patients
with high score both before and after treatment showed
the poor response. Furthermore, the decrease of scores
after the therapy might correlate with the therapeutic
effect(Fig3).

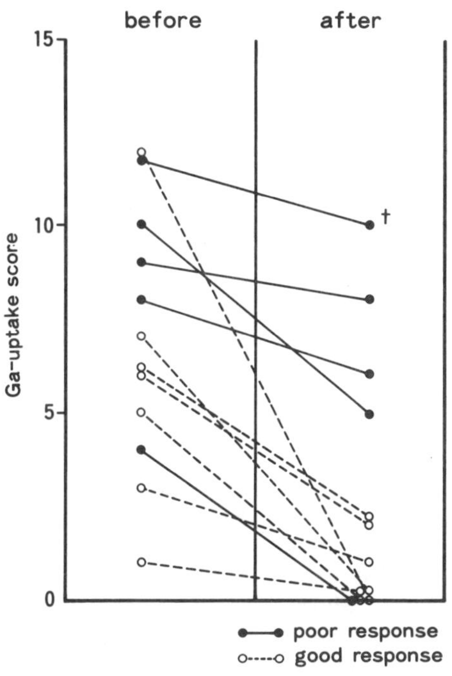

Fig. 3   Gallium uptake score before and after
treatment in relation to the therapeutic effect.

Discussion

Most of patients with IIP has been treated with
corticosteroids and partially with immunosuppressive
drugs. But, several studies on the clinical course of

patients with IIP treated with corticosteroids revealed
the poor prognosis(4,5). Although Crystal et al.
analyzed the precise mechanisms of fibrosing process in
patients with idiopathic pulmonary fibrosis, the real
etiology or fundamental factors regulating the fibrosis
were still obscure6.. Hence, there has been no
established treatment of these fibrosing lung diseases.
Analysis of survival data showed the longer survival in
younger patients and in patients with shorter duration
of symptoms, less radiographic abnormality, and less
impairment of pulmonary function(2). These data might
indicate the effectiveness of corticosteroids in the
early phase of the disease progression. The survival
rate of patients responded to corticosteroids therapy
was significantly higher than those uninfluenced by the
therapy(1,2). Before the treatments start it has been
difficult to predict the effectiveness. So, the
retrospective studies has been done on the cellular
component in BAL fluid before the therapy and the
response to the therapy within 6 months. Increase of
lymphocyte in BAL fluids indicated the good response
only in one month of the treatment. On the contrary,
increase of neutrophils in BAL fluids showed the poor
response through the period of 6 months. Neutrophils
has been shown to present in BAL fluid of patients with
interstitial lung diseases(6,7). Since neutrophils are
potent mediator of inflammatory processes with its
proteolytic enzymes and production of superoxide,
increase of neutrophils in BAL fluids would indicate
the accelerated process of fibrosis in lung tissue.
The mechanism of the accumulation of neutrophils in
lungs of IIP has not been clarified. Fibronectin which
increase in BAL fluids of patients with IIP especially
in active stage showed the neutrophil chemotactic
activity. Therefore, increased fibronectin levels
partly released from activated macrophages of patients
with IIP might play an important role in neutrophil
accumulation.
Gallium scintigraphy has been used for the evaluation
of various interstitial lung diseases(8,9). The higher
uptake of radioactivity in lung fields indicate the
active inflammatory processes in the alveolar wall. In
this study, gallium uptake in lung fields were analyzed
quantitatively by counting the radioactivity in BAL
fluids obtained after the gallium scintigraphy. The

radioactive counts of BAL fluids correlated with the grade of gallium uptake in lung fields by semiquantitative analysis. The radioactivity in BAL fluids was mainly contained in the cell fraction and this radioactivity correlated with macrophage density in BAL fluids. From these data it is likely that the gallium uptake in lung fields could be regulated by the activated alveolar macrophages. The relationship of gallium uptake in lung fields of patients with IIP and the therapeutic effect was studied. The high uptake of lung fields seems to indicate the poor response to the therapy. Furthermore, the larger the decrease of uptake after the therapy, the better response could be expected. In the examination of gallium distribution in lung fields, radioactivity showed not only even distribution or higher uptake in lower lung fields but also uneven distribution or higher uptake in upper lung fields. Although the reason for the uneven distribution of radioactivity in some patients has not been cleared, these patterns of distribution were shown to correlate with the therapeutic effects. The patients with even distribution showed better responses than those with uneven distribution.

Conclusion
 Prediction of therapeutic effects of corticosteroids therapy in patients with IIP could be achieved by the analysis of BAL fluids and gallium scintigraphy. At least, the increase of neutrophil in BAL fluids and the distribution of radioactivity in gallium scintigrams were shown to correlate with therapeutic effects indicating the usefulness for the prediction of prognosis.

Reference
1.   Stack,B.H.R., Choo-Kang,Y.F.J., and Heard,B.E. and Valle,M. Thorax 38, 349-355, 1983.
2. Tukiainen, P., Taskinen, E/, Holsti, P., Korhola,O., and Valle,M. Thorax 38, 349-355, 1983.
3.   Hunninghake,G.W., Gadek,J.E., Fales,H., and Crystal,R.G. J Clin Invest 66, 473-483, 1980.
4.   Livingstone,J.L., Lewis,J.G., Reid,L., and Jefferson,K.E. Quart J Med 33,71-103, 1964.
5. Turner-Warwick,M., Burrow,B., and Johnston,A. Thorax 22, 171-180, 1980.

6.   Hunninghake,G.W., Gadek,J.E., Lawley,T.J.,   and
Crystal,R.G. J Clin Invest 68, 259-269, 1981.
7. Weinberger,S.E., Kelman,J.A.,Elson,N.A., Young,R.C.,
Reynolds,J.D., Fulmer,J.D., and Crystal,R.G. Ann Intern
Med 89, 459-466, 1978.
8. Line,B.R., Hunninghake,G.W., Koegh,B.A., Jonas,A.,
Johnston,G.S., and Crystal,R.G. Am Rev Respir Dis 123,
440-446, 1981.
9. Braude,A.C., Cohen,R., Rahmani,R., Hornstain,A.,
Klein,M.,   Meindok,H.O.,   Chamberlain,D.W.,   and
Rebuck,A.S. Am Rev Respir Dis 130, 783-785, 1984.

VI
CLINICAL ASSESSMENT

Change of X-ray Patterns during the Course of Idiopathic Interstitial Pneumonia

Osamu Doi and Tokuro Nobechi

Department of Radiology, St. Luke's International Hospital, Tokyo, Japan

Chest X-ray films were reviewed in 23 cases
of IIP. There was the preponderance of
changing X-ray patterns from nodular or
ground glass shadows to reticulonodular
shadows and further to honeycombing.
Outer and lower lung zone distributions of
the lesions were predominant in many of the
cases although all lung zone distribution
were also seen in considerable number even
at the initial examinations.
Reduced volume of lower lobes were the other
important findings.
Remarkable ones were the presence of bullae
or cysts not only in upper lungs but in
lower lobes.

The Background of the Study and the New Survey

Fraser and Paré described roentgenographic patterns
of diffuse interstitial diseases in the text book. The
four basic patterns are ground glass (granular), reticular, nodular and mixed reticulonodular (1).
Mcloud also suggested a modification of the ILO/UC
system for pneumoconiosis and application of the system
to the diffuse infiltrative lung disease (2).
In 1974, the project team for the study of idiopathic interstitial pneumonia (IIP) was organized in Japan
and the nationwide survey was started.
Nobechi elaborated the table for descriptions of X-ray

findings of IIP for the survey and it has been widely used in our country for more than ten years (3).
Table 1. shows descriptions of chest X-ray findings. They are basically composed of nodular shadows including ground glass appearance, reticulonodular shadows and honeycombing. In addition, loss of lower lobe volume is picked up as the check item.
Table 2. shows the X-ray patterns seen at the initial examinations, at the time of biopsies and nearest the time of autopsies in the cases of the mass survey. There is preponderance of changing patterns from nodular or ground glass shadows to reticulonodular shadows, and further to honeycombing as time passed.
Table 3. reveals considerable number of cases with lower lobe volume loss seen even at the initial examinations and further increase in number toward the time of autopsies.

Since the beginning of 1988, re-survey of IIP has been performed in a relatively small group. Chest X-ray films and supplemental CT scans were reviewed in 23 cases proved or suggested either by open lung biopsy or autopsy. They were compared between the initial exam. and the other nearest the time of biopsy or reasonably near the date of autopsy. Minimum interval between the two exams. was two weeks and the maximum was almost eighteen years and the average, three years.

The Results and Discussion

1.   Exacerbation of X-ray findings from the initial one to the other were observed in 17 cases (74%).
2.   Similar to the previous survey, the X-ray patterns from the nodular or ground glass shadows to reticulonodular shadows, and to honeycombing in majority of chronic cases as seen in Table 4.
3.   Most of the cases showed the predominance of abnormal shadows in lower lung zones but 15 cases (65%) revealed the extention of the lesions to almost all lung zones even at the initial examinations.
4.   Nine cases (39%) showed predominant outer lung zone distribution of the lesions recognized even in PA views. But in some of them, the outer lung zone distribution became indistinct because of further extension of the lesions.

Table 1.   Descriptions of Chest X-ray Findings

Patterns

   I. nodular shadows
     a. fine nodular or ground glass
     b. coarse nodular
     c. patchy or coalescence of nodular shadows

  II. reticulonodular shadows

 III. reticular shadows or honeycombing
     a. fine reticular
     b. coarse reticular

 IV. reduction of volume
     a. elevation of hemidiaphragms
     b. downward deviation of minor fissure

Extent

    less than 1/3 of lungs......1
    1/3 ~ 2/3 of lungs......2
    more than 2/3 of lungs......3

Figure 1.   Illustrations of X-ray Findings

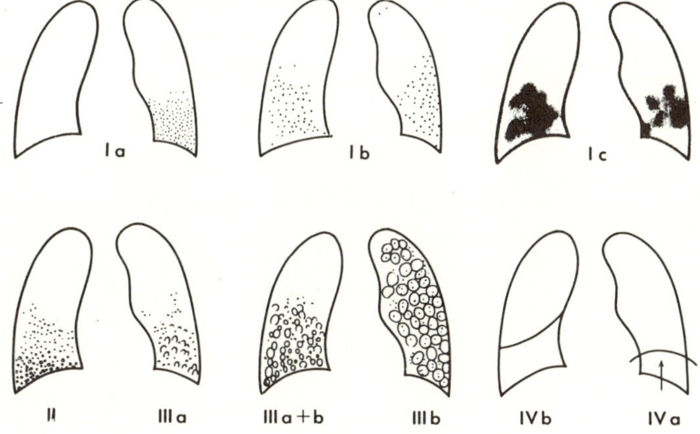

Table 2.   Change of patterns

	initial	biopsy	autopsy
I	38%	28%	13%
I + II	13	13	20
II	14	18	13
I+II+III	1	5	4
I+ III	6	5	19
II+ III	5	8	12
III	22	23	19
No.of cases	173	39	75

Table 3.   Reduction of lung volume

		(-)	(+)
initial	I + II	59 (52%)	55 (48%)
	III	32 (54%)	27 (40%)
biopsy	I + II	10 (45%)	12 (55%)
	III	8 (47%)	9 (53%)
autopsy	I + II	11 (32%)	23 (68%)
	III	13 (32%)	28 (68%)

Table 4.   Change of patterns (new survey)

	initial exam	last exam
0	1	
I	5	3
I + II	4	1
II	7	1
I + III	1	2
II + III	3	5
III	2	11
	23 cases	23 cases

5. Lower lobe volume loss was noted in 13 cases (57%) at
   the initial exam. and 18 cases (78%) at the other.
6. Mutiple bullae or cysts were seen not only in the
   upper lung zones (11 cases-48%) but occasionally in
   lower zones (5 cases-22%).
7. Supplemental CT scans made it easier to pick up or
   analyze the abnormal shadows, especially earlier
   honeycombing, subpleural zone distribution, lower
   lobe volume loss, or the presence of bullae or cysts.
In view of the results described above, items of outer
lung zone distribution and of bullae or cysts or even of
overinflation of lungs may be added to the original
table for descriptions of X-ray findings. CT is regarded as excellent tool to pick up the earlier lesions or
analyze the patterns and the distribution of the lesions
in avoidance of summation of the shadows in the conventional chest X-rays. It may also be of great help to
differentiate other disseminated lung diseases from IIP.

References

1.   Fraser. R.G. and Pare, J.A.P.: Diagnosis of
     Diseases of the Chest, W.B. Saunders, Philadelphia,
     pp 244-255, 1970.
2.   Mcloud, T.C. In: Pulmonary Diagnosis - Imaging and
     Other Techniques (Putman, C.E. ed.), Appleton-
     Century-Crofts, New York, pp 125-153, 1981.
3.   Nobechi, T. In: Naika Mook No.22 (Mikami, R. ed)
     Kenehara, Tokyo, 1983.

CT Images of Interstitial Pneumonia: Radiologic-Pathologic Correlations

Akira Suzuki, Hiroyuki Koba, and Seiya Katoh

Department of Internal Medicine (Section 3), Sapporo Medical College, Sapporo, Japan

In order to identify and classify the basic CT patterns of interstitial pneumonia, a radiologic-pathologic correlative study was performed using fifteen inflated and fixed lungs from autopsy and surgery. The abnormal patterns on the CT images of the specimens were classified into 7 categories. Important pathological changes which affected the CT images were alveolar collapse and airway dilatation. Based on the results of above study, we analyzed CT of 22 patients with IIP. Hazy density, micronodular densities, confluence of various sized ring like shadows and subpleural bullous changes were the most frequently recognized categories in the periphery of the lung.

The usefulness of CT in the evaluation of diffuse pulmonary diseases has been reported in recent years. With its cross-sectional plane imaging and superior contrast resolution, CT can correct the superimposition of structures and poor contrast resolution typical of plain radiography and thus complement it [1–4]. Also, in interstitial pneumonia, CT may be helpful in determining the pattern and distribution of lung involvement[5–7]. Honeycombing and reticular patterns have been reported as characteristic findings on CT in interstitial pneumonia.
However, the precise correlation between the CT findings and the structural changes associated with various stages of fibrosis has not been clearly demonstrated.

I. Pathologic—CT correlation in the specimens with interstitial pneumonia

This study was conducted to identify and classify the basic CT patterns of interstitial pneumonia which are correlated with alterations of lung structures by fibrosis using inflated and fixed lungs from autopsy and surgery.

Material and Method

Fourteen lungs from autopsied cases and one from surgery were inflated and fixed by Heitzman's method [8]. All of the specimens were pathologically diagnosed as interstitial pneumonia: chronic interstitial pneumonia-8, chronic interstitial pneumonia with collagen disease-2, drug induced pneumonitis-2, radiation pneumonitis-1 and acute pneumonitis-2. The slices of the specimens were scanned on a GE 9800 scanner using 1.5-mm collimation. Two mm thick slices of the specimens were radiographed using SOFT X-RAY APPARATUS. The CT and the soft X-ray radiographs of the specimens were compared with submacroscopic findings using the dissecting microscope as well as histologic findings.

Result

Morphological changes reflect CT images which are more than 0.5 to 1 mm in size. The changes were recognized at a submacroscopic level. In interstitial pneumonia, these submacroscopic changes are classified into two factors. One is a thickening of the alveolar wall as well as intra-alveolar exudate both of which do not cause prominent structural change of the lung structure. The other factor consists of structural changes in the lung due to fibrosis and collapse of alveoli, which is subclassified into volume loss and dilatation of airways. The dilatation of airways result in honeycomb at the end which is thought to be characteristic of interstitial pneumonia. The correlations between the histology and HRCT image are shown below in special reference to structural changes of the lung.

The photomicrograph of the specimen in Fig.1 shows a thickening• of the alveolar wall and intra-alveolar exudate without any prominent structural change of the lung. HRCT of the same specimen shows an increased density. Severity of cellular infiltration into the alveolar wall and/or intra-

alveolar exudate correlate with the density of opacity. These
histological changes are homogeneous and diffuse without major
structural change to make for an increased density in CT.

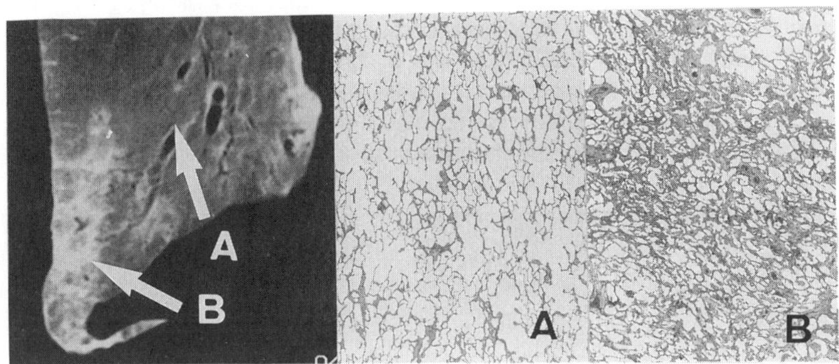

Fig. 1

However, collapse of almost all of the alveoli resulted from
alveolitis or fibrosis with less dilatation of the airways
which corresponds to a highly increased density with loss of
lung volume. The volume loss of the lung can be recognized from
deviation of the vascular or bronchial images. (Fig.2)

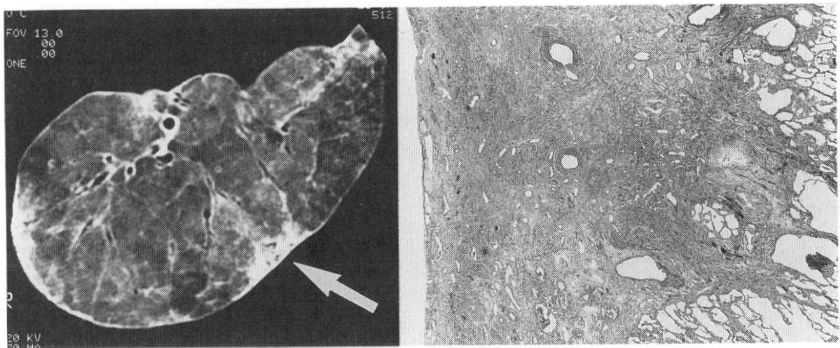

Fig. 2

The photomicrograph in Fig.3 shows irregular fibrosis and
dilation of the alveolar ducts and bronchiole 0.5 to 1 mm in
diameter. HRCT of the same specimen doesn't show a ring like
density but rather nodular densities. The dilated airways are
radiographically demonstrated as a ring shadow or tram line
whose sizes depend on the order of the bronchus and the
severity of dilatation. However because of the limitation of

spatial resolution power and summation effect even in thin slice section by HRCT, dilatation of small airways are demonstrated as fine nodular densities. The series of analysis using inflated and fixed lung suggested that size of dilated airways which can be recognized as ring like densities in thin slice section by HRCT is more than 1mm in diameter. So considering the various conditions in clinical practice, border size of airways whether it is recognized as ring like density or nodular densities is presumed to be between 1 to 1.5 mm in diameter.

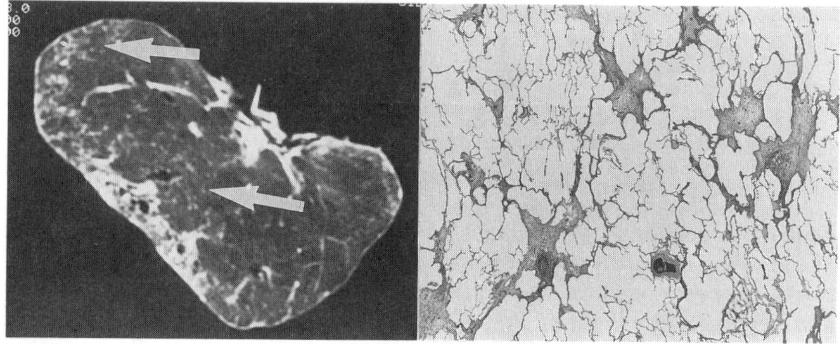

Fig. 3

The photomicrograph in Fig.4 shows atelectasis of the lung parenchyma due to a collapse and fibrosis of alveoli as well as dilatation of bronchi and bronchioles. HRCT of the same portion demonstrate air-bronchiologram in high density. The air-bronchiologram is thought to suggest the dilatation of bronchiole with atelectasis of adjacent alveoli because a simple consolidation usually never show such an air-bronchiologlams.

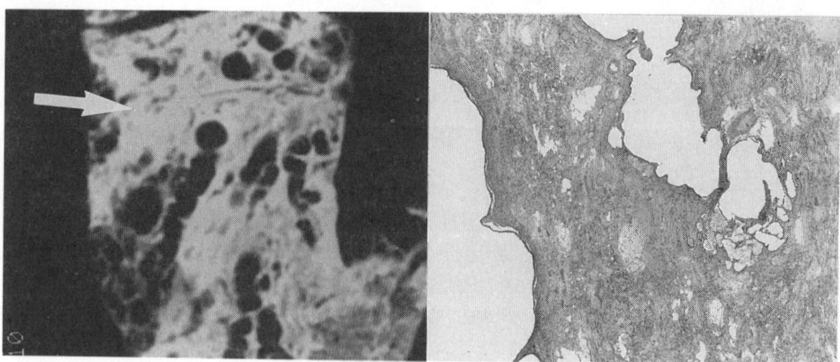

Fig. 4

The photomicrograph in Fig.5 shows dilatation of airways in various sizes which coincide with confluence of ring like densities in CT.

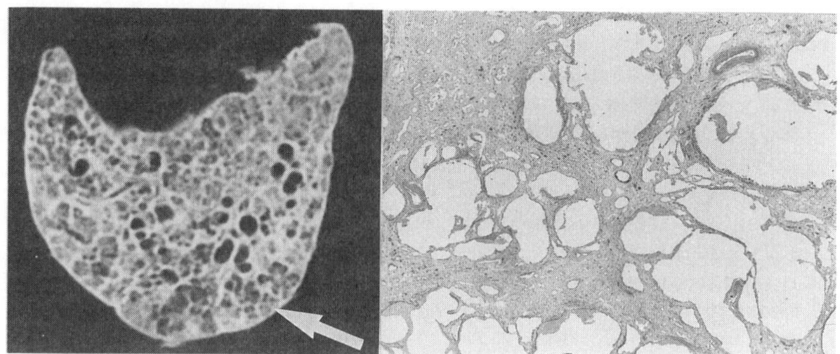

Fig. 5

The honeycombing which is thought to represent a terminal stage of fibrosis are recognized as coarse ring densities in HRCT.(Fig.6)

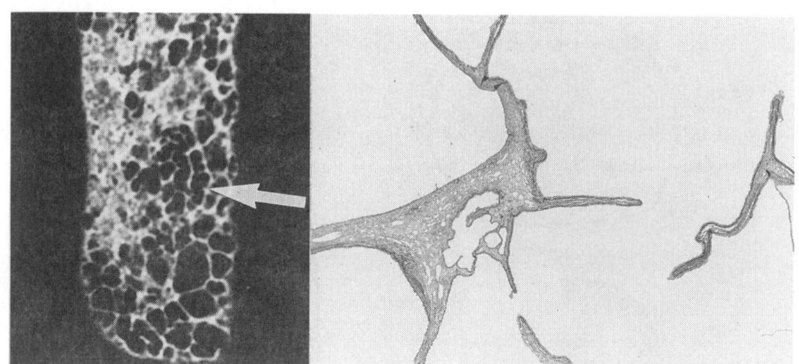

Fig. 6

II. Analysis on CT images of the patients with IIP

CT findings of IIP was analyzed using the categories based on the CT pathologic correlative study described above.

Patients and Methods

Twenty two patients with IIP who had been admitted to our hospital between 1981 and 1987 and followed up for more than one year are included in this study. All of them are definitely diagnosed under the clinical criteria by The Research Committee of interstitial lung diseases supported by the Japanese Ministry of Health and Welfare. CT was performed with GE CT/T9800 or Toshiba TCT 60A using 1.5 and 5-mm collimation.

The distribution of the lesion and parenchymal abnormal patterns on CT were analyzed.

In order to assess the distribution of the lesion, the lung was divided into several areas as demonstrated in Fig.7; upper, middle and lower lung field in axial direction, dorsal, ventral and mediastinal side as well as subpleural, middle and inner layer in transaxial plane.

The parenchymal abnormal patterns on CT was classified into 7 categories including subpleural bullous changes in addition to the results from the CT-pathologic analysis described above. The correlation between the CT findings and the submacroscopic structural changes of each category is summarized as below.

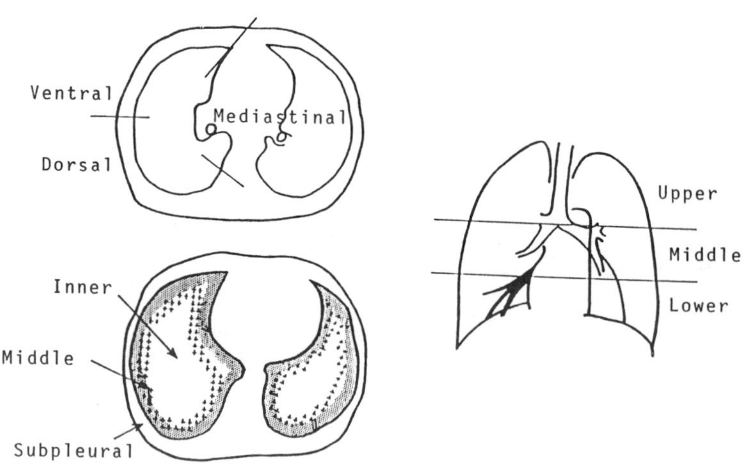

Fig. 7

A: patchy or homogeneous increased density (A1:hazy density, A2:high density); slight or no structural changes, thickening of alveolar septum and/or intra-alveolar exudate. B: high density with a decrease of lung volume; atelectasis due to alveolar collapse. C: micronodular or granular densities; dilatation of alveolar ducts and/or respiratory bronchioles, irregular fibrosis. D: air brochiologram with high density; atelectasis due to alveolar collapse and dilatation of bronchioles. E: confluence of various sized ring like shadows, 2- to 10-mm in diameter, so-called reticular pattern; various sized dilatation of bronchioles and/or bronchi. F: confluence of coarse ring like shadows, 5- to 15-mm in diameter; honeycombing. G: subpleural bullous changes; subpleural bullae. The categories from A to F are shown in Fig.8.

It should be noted that in this series of analysis, dilatation of airways of less than 2-mm in diameter was classified as category C (micronodular or granular densities), because dilatation of airways of 1 to 2-mm in diameter can be recognized by thin slice section of HRCT. Sometimes, however it looks like nodular or granular densities depending upon the slice thickness or the CT scanner.

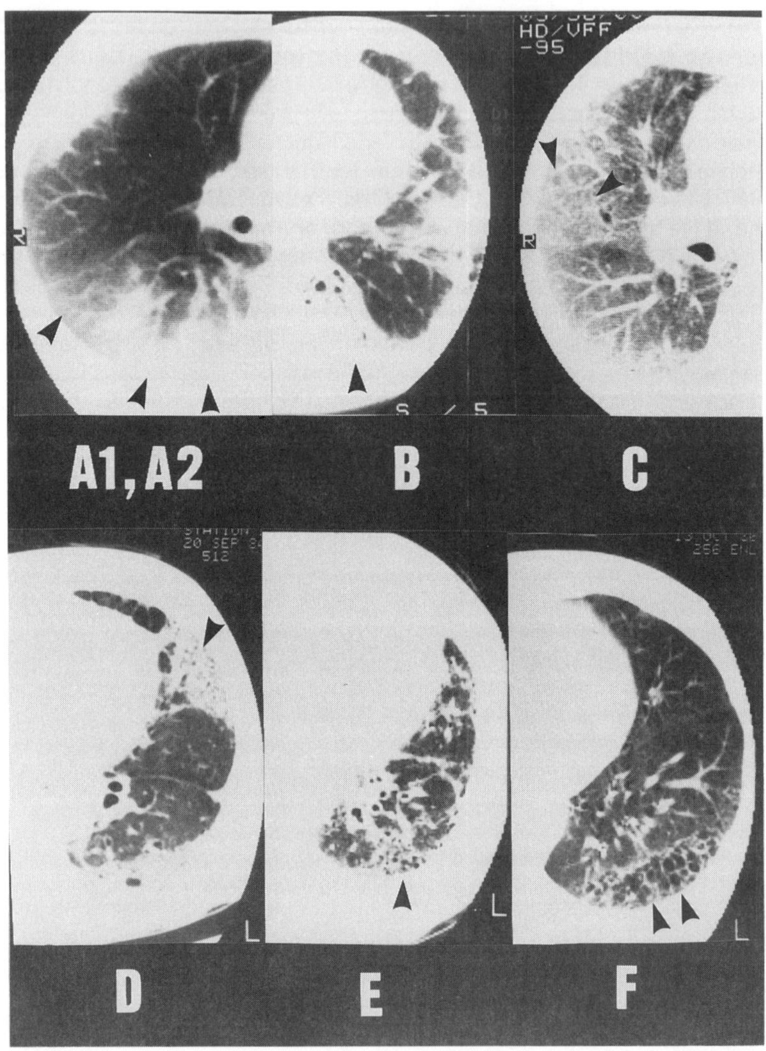

Fig. 8

Result

The results of analysis of all cases are shown in Tab. I.

Table I Summary of Analysis of All Cases

Case	Pt.	Age	Sex	Distribution	Categories
1	Y.I.	65	M	UML–DVM–SM	ECA1G
2	Y.K.	63	M	UML–DV–S	EA2CG
3	J.I.	72	M	UML–DVM–SM	A1CA2
4	Y.A.	53	M	UML–DS	EA1CG
5	K.H.	69	M	UML–DVM–SM	EA1C
6	M.Y.	62	M	UML–D–S	EAICG
7	T.S.	58	M	UML–DVM–SM	DC
8	H.T.	54	M	UML–DVM–SM	EDCA1G
9	S.O.	71	M	UML–DVM–SM	ECA1G
10	S.H.	65	M	UML–DV–SMI	CA1E
11	K.J.	60	M	UML–DVM–SMI	A1CE
12	T.M.	65	F	UML–DVM–SMI	A1CE
13	Z.N.	59	M	UML–D–S	SEG
14	K.H.	64	M	UML–DVM–S	EA1CG
15	I.K.	63	M	UML–DVM–SMI	A1ECG
16	S.K.	53	M	UML–DVM–SM	ECG
17	Y.K.	67	M	UML–D–S	CA1EBG
18	A.I.	60	M	UML–DVM–SM	CA1EG
19	M.S.	70	M	UML–DVM–S	A2D
20	I.K.	87	M	UML–DVM–S	EF
21	K.K.	56	M	UML–DVM–SM	SEFA1
22	J.S.	68	M	UML–DVM–SMI	FECG

U: upper, M: middle, L: lower
D: dorsal, V: ventral, M: mediastinal
S: subpleural, M: middle, I: inner

The analysis of distribution in a vertical direction proved
that the lesions were recognized in all upper, middle and lower
lung fields in all cases. The analysis of cross–sectional
planes showed that lesions exist predominantly at the dorsal
area followed by the ventral and mediastinal area in many of
the cases. Subpleural area was involved in all cases. (Tab. II)
This coincides with the marginal distribution which is
characteristic of this disease.

The frequency of remarkable categories in this study are
A1(slightly increased densities)–68%, C(nodular densities)–86%,
E(ring like densities of various sizes)–86%, and G(subpleural
bullous changes)–59%.(Tab. III) In many of the cases, these
categories co–exist in a patient.

Typical CT image of IIP is shown in Fig.9

<table>
<tr><td colspan="2" align="center">Table II
Incidence of Categories</td></tr>
<tr><td>Category</td><td>n/N (%)</td></tr>
<tr><td>A1</td><td>15/22 (68%)</td></tr>
<tr><td>A2</td><td>3/22 (14%)</td></tr>
<tr><td>B</td><td>1/22 (5%)</td></tr>
<tr><td>C</td><td>19/22 (86%)</td></tr>
<tr><td>D</td><td>3/22 (14%)</td></tr>
<tr><td>E</td><td>19/22 (86%)</td></tr>
<tr><td>F</td><td>4/22 (18%)</td></tr>
<tr><td>G</td><td>13/22 (59%)</td></tr>
</table>

Table III
Distribution of Lesion

Upper	22/22 (100%)
Middle	22/22 (100%)
Lower	22/22 (100%)
Dorsal	22/22 (100%)
Ventral	18/22 (82%)
Mediastinal	16/22 (73%)
Subpleural	22/22 (100%)
Middle	14/22 (64%)
Inner	5/22 (23%)

III. Discussion

CT has brought about marked progress in detecting morphological changes of the lung in the patient with IIP. Especially, CT clearly demonstrates the marginal distribution of the lesion on the horizontal plane which is characteristic of IIP. The severest lesion is seen in the subpleural area of the dorsal side in the lower lung field. These characteristic distributions of the lesion has been reported on conventional radiographs. However, use of CT help us to understand the three-dimensional distribution of the lesion in clinical practice. CT also demonstrated the paren-

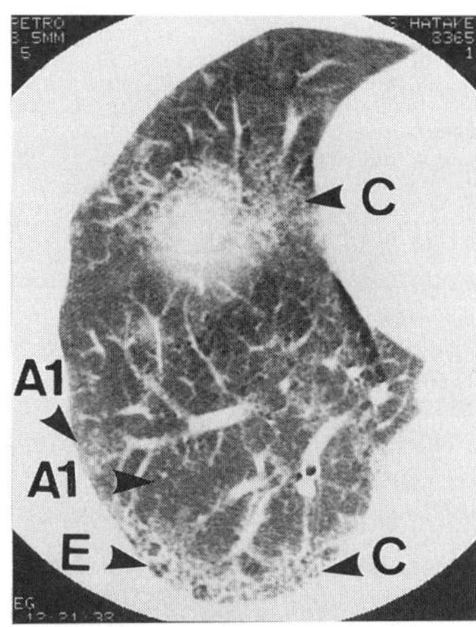

Fig.9

chymal abnormal patterns which correlated with structural changes of the lung in interstitial pneumonia. The thin slice plane by HRCT demonstrated structural changes of the specimens from 1 to 2 mm in size. The basic CT patterns in interstitial pneumonia could be classified into 7 categories. Our analysis on parenchymal patterns using the 7 categories proved that slightly increased density, nodular densities and ring like densities of various sizes are frequently recognized, which correspond to the series of

structural changes of the lung from alveolitis to honeycombing
due to fibrosis.   These findings revealed that various stages
of fibrotic process coexist and intermingle in the lung of a
patient with IIP.
 The role of CT will become increasingly important not only for
making the diagnosis in clinical practice but also as a method
to recognize the structural changes of the lung which is
essential to understand IIP.

Reference

1. Nakata H., Kimoto T., Nakayama T., Kido M., Miyazaki N. and
   Harada S.: Diffuse peripheral lung disease: evaluation by
   high-resolution computed tomography. Radiology 157,181-
   185,1985.
2. Todo G., Murata K., Itoh H. and Torizuka K.: Computed Tomography of Diffuse Pulmonary Diseases. Nippon Act. Radiol.46
   1281-1295, 1986
3. Zerhouni E.A., Naidich D.P., Stitik F.P., Khouri N.F. and
   Siegelman S.S.: Computed tomography of the pulmonary parenchyma. Part 2: Interstitial disease. J Thorac Imag 54-64,
   1985
4. Bergin C.J. and Muller N.L.: CT of Interstitial Lung Disease: A Diagnostic Approach. AJR 148:8-15,1987
5. Koba H., Mori T., Mori M., Sizyubou N., Watanabe H. and
   Suzuki A.: Radiologic Pathologic Correlation of Interstitial
   Pneumonia. Jpn. Clin. Radiol. 30, 971-978, 1985
6. Muller N.L., Miller R.R., Webb W.R., Evans K.G. and Ostrow
   D.N.: Fibrosing Alveolitis: CT-Pathologic Correlation.
   Radiology 162: 377-381, 1987
7. Suzuki A., Koba H., Katoh S. and Watanabe H.: Guideline of
   interpreting CT image of interstitial pneumonia. Annual
   Report in 1987 from The Research Committee of interstitial
   lung diseases supported by the Japanese Ministry of Health
   and Welfare, pp 94-96, 1988
8. Heitzman E.R.: The Lung. Radiologic-Pathologic Correlation.
   Mosby, St.Louise, pp 4-12, 1984

Is CT Useful in Differentiating between BOOP and Idiopathic UIP?

Koichi Nishimura and Harumi Itoh

*Chest Disease Research Institute, Kyoto University, and Department of
Radiology and Neclear Medicine, Kyoto University Hospital, Kyoto, Japan*

In order to clarify interstitial as
well as alveolar nature of BOOP and to
evaluate CT's ability to differentiate BOOP
fromd UIP, we performed a CT pathologic
correlative study in BOOP and idiopathic
UIP. The CT findings of BOOP were ①
marked increases in lung density with
central air bronchograms, ② a slight to
moderate increase in lung density, which is
observed in wide area of the lung field, and
③ clear demarcation between these two
areas and the normal lung. We concluded
that the interstitial nature of BOOP is less
clear on chest radiographs when compared
with the alveolar opacity of BOOP and that
CT findings are important to explain respiratory impairment in BOOP and will be
useful in differentiating BOOP from UIP.

1. Introduction

Bronchiolitis obliterans organizing pneumonia (BOOP)
is a new concept among diffuse infiltrative disorders
[1]. Pathologic features of BOOP are characterized by
bronchiolitis obliterans of respiratory and non-respira-
tory broncioles, organizing exudates in alveolar ducts
and alveoli and alveolar septal thickening with inflammatory cells [1,2,3]. There are two major radiologic
problems in the diagnosis of BOOP. One is that the key
radiographic finding of BOOP is alveolar opacity,

possibly caused by organized exudates in the terminal air spaces; however, this radiographic feature is contradictory to the established concept of an interstitial pattern of chest roentgenology. The other is that it is difficult to differentiate some cases of BOOP from usual interstitial pneumonia (UIP), because reticular shadows are noted on chest radiographs [2,3,4]. High resolution computed tomography (CT) has been reported to show better visualization of peripheral lung structures [5]. The purpose of this study was to clarify interstitial as well as alveolar nature of this disease through CT and pathology correlation and to evaluate CT's ability to differentiate BOOP from UIP.

2.   Subjects and Method

X-ray CT has been performed on most of the patients whose chest radiographs show diffuse infiltrative shadows for the last five years in our institute. From the results of open lung biopsy, done after getting CT images, nine of these patients were histologically disgnosed as having BOOP and 29 cases turned out to be of idiopathic UIP. Consequently, the CT images of the nine patients with BOOP could been compared with those of 29 cases of

Table. Clinical background and chest radiographic findings.

Findings	BOOP	UIP
Number	9	29
Male/Female	6/3	19/10
Age	57.2±6.9	58.0±9.7
Alveolar opacities	2 (22.2%)	0
Lobar	1 (11.1%)	0
Diffuse	1 (11.1%)	0
Interstitial opacities	2 (22.2%)	28 (96.6%)
Reticular	2 (22.2%)	22 (75.9%)
Reticulonodular	0	4 (13.8%)
Ground glass appearance	0	2 (6.9%)
Mixed alveolar and interstitial opacities	5 (55.6%)	1 (3.4%)

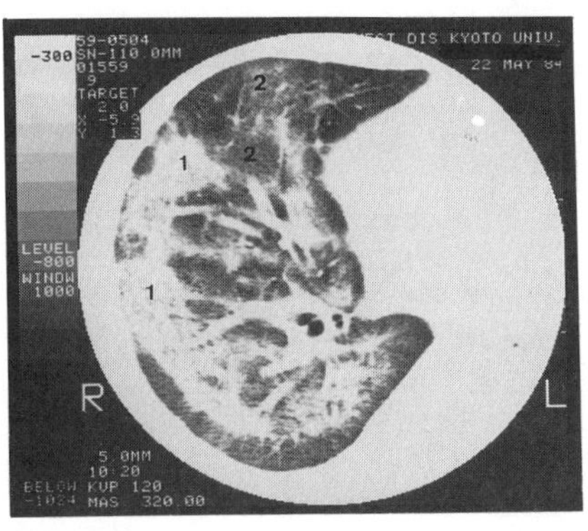

Fig. 1. A X-ray CT find-
          ing of BOOP
Two main CT findings are
observed in this CT image.
One is a marked increase
in lung density mainly in
the outer part of the lung
fields (marked as 1) with
central air bronchograms.
The other is slight to
moderate increases in lung
density in wider areas
(marked as 2).

idiopathic UIP, that is, idiopathic pulmonary fibrosis.
Their clinical background and routine radiographic
findings are shown in the table. The chest radiographic
findings of our cases of BOOP showed both alveolar and
intestitial opacities like previous reports[2,3,4].
However, we often found alveolar opacity in some areas
and interstitial opacity in the other areas of a chest
radiographic film, which we called mixed alveolar and
interstitial opacities[6]. We never observed alveolar
opacities on the chest radiographs of UIP. Reticular
opacities were seen on two cases of BOOP and three
quarters of the patients with UIP.

3. Results
1) CT-pathologic correlation of BOOP
    CT findings of BOOP (shown in Fig. 1 and 2) were as
follows: ① a marked increase in lung density mainly in
the outer part of the lung fields. Air bronchogram was

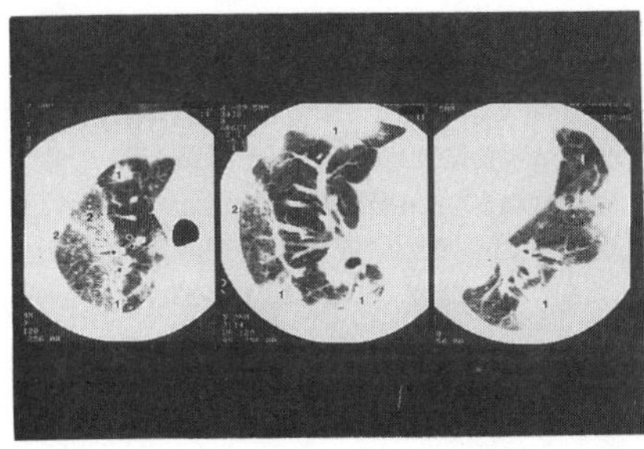

Fig. 2. A X-ray CT find-
          ing of BOOP
This CT image is also
formed by a combination of
much increased density
areas (indicated by 1) and
slight increased density
areas (indicated by 2).
Note their clear demarca-
tion from the normal lung
field.

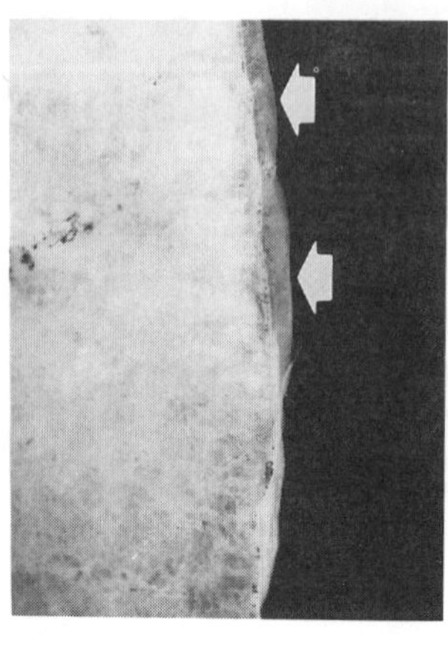

Fig. 3. Stereomicrophotogrraph of an inflated biopsy specimen taken from a case of BOOP

Note that all peripheral air spaces are narrowing and their walls are thicknened. In the upper half of this picture (↑), air apaces are filled with some materials. We supposed that the former finding was the cause of a slight increase in lung density and that the latter finding corresponded to a marked increase in lung density on CT images of BOOP.

always present. ② Slight to moderate increases in lung density, occurring in much wider areas of the lung field. ③ There two areas were cleary demarcated from the normal lung.

The corresponding pathologic features of a marked increase in lung density on CT images were organizing pneumonia with alveolar ducts and alveoli filled with organizing exudates. It was significant that, in the stereomicrophotograph of inflated biopsy specimens, some

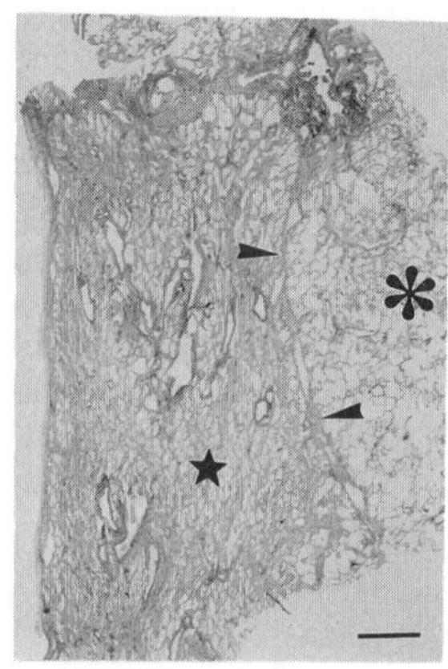

Fig. 4. Histological view of a biopsy specimen of BOOP under low magnification (elastica von Gieson stain)

Note that the boundary is detected between the two areas with different histologic findings due to interlobular septum (↑). Both organized penumonia in the left half (★) and septal and luminal alveolitis in the right half (✳) can be seen diffusely and alveolar walls can be hardly observed in each pulmonary secondary lobule. Bar is 1 mm.

peripheral air spaces were filled with branch-like yellowish-white materials (Fig. 3). These findings were the cause of air space consolidation on chest radiographs.

On the other hand, stereomicrophotographic views of open lung biopsy specimens obtained from the areas whose CT images showed a slight increase in lung density indicated that any peripheral air spaces were narrowing and their walls were thickened (Fig. 3). Histologically these were portions of the lung whose alveolar septa were thickened with inflammatory cells.

These histologic findings were seen diffusely and normal alveolar walls were hardly observed in the involved secondary pulmonary lobule (Fig. 4). Partially because of intervening interlobular seputa, the boundary was detected between two histological findings, in brief, organized pneumonia and mural and luminal alveolitis (Fig. 4). This histologic feature may correspond to the presence of the clear demarcation on CT findings. Because bronciolitis obliterans could not be identified on histological sections under low-magnification, we thought that bronchiolitis obliterans never played any role in the CT images.

2) CT-pathologic correlation of idiopathic UIP

Conversely, the major CT findings of UIP were as follows: (1) conglomeration of small cystic images with thick walls extending from the subpleural region toward the inner lung (20.7%, 6 out of 29 cases), (2) air bronchiolograms within areas of intense lung density (86.2%, 25 cases), (3) rugged pleural surface, or pleural or subpleural involvement (86.2%, 25 cases), (4) irregu-

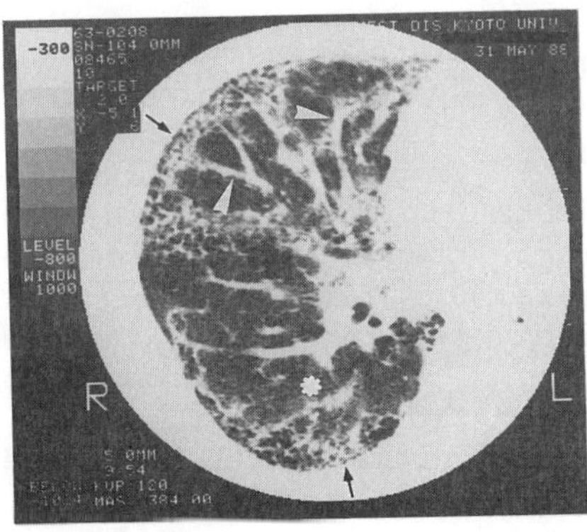

Fig. 5. A X-ray CT of UIP We can observe conglomerated cystic lesions (↑), enlarged vascular images (↓), rugged pleural surface and slightly increased lung densities (✳) on this CT image. These CT findings are certainly different from the CT images of BOOP shown in Fig. 1 and 2.

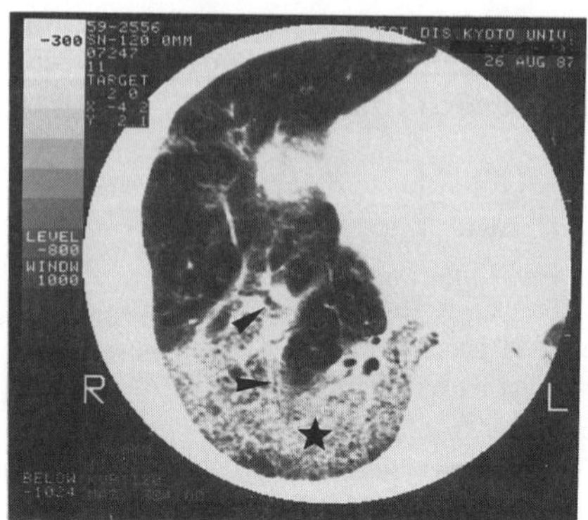

Fig. 6. A X-ray CT of UIP Air bronchiolograms within intense densities (★), bronchial wall thickening (⌇) and rugged pleural surface are detected in this CT image. The first finding corresponds to dilation of bronchioles, which is a process leading to honeycombing, that is, conglomerated cystic images.

lar enlargement of pulmonary vascular images (100%, 29 cases), ⑤ thickening of bronchial wall images (90.0%, 26 cases) and ⑥ slightly increased lung densities (96.6% 28 cases) (Fig. 5 and 6) [7].

From our CT-pathologic correlative study conglomerated cystic lesions on CT images turned out to be indicative of macroscopic honeycombing. It was thought that air bronchiolograms with intense densities corresponded to dilation of bronchioles in more than 1 mm diameter with fibrosis in their walls on the biopsy specimens. Because such a bronchiolar dilation is a process leading to honeycombing, we suppose that air bronchiolograms with intense densities are turning into conglomerated cystic images. Enlarged vascular images and bronchial wall thickening on CT were composed of fibrotic change of lung tissue surrounding pulmonary vessels and airways. Both subpleural fibrosis and

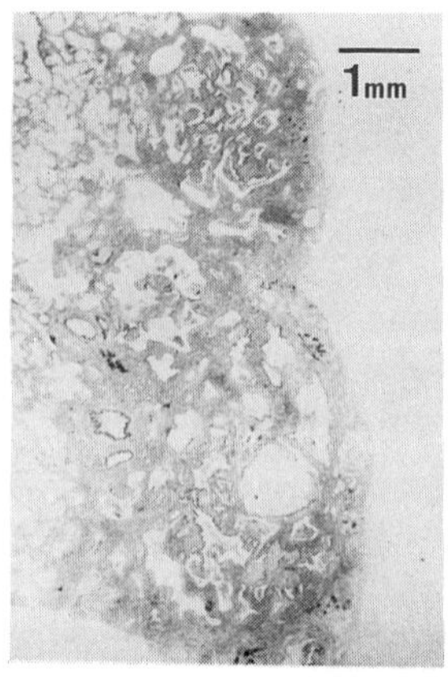

Fig. 7. Histologic view of a specimen obtained from the lung of UIP (hematoxylin eosin stain).
The dilation of bronchioles with fibrotic change is seen in this picture. This finding is thought to turn into honeycombing. This specimen was obtained from the area with air bronchiolograms with intense densities on the CT image.

honeycombing itself contributed to the rugged pleural surface.   Local fibrosis or inflammation of alveolar septa may have made lung density increase a little.

4. Discussion

Air space consolidation on chest radiograph of BOOP corresponds to a marked increase in lung density on CT images. These findings of BOOP are not the reflection of "interstitial" disease but caused by intra-alveolar organized materials. We think that the second CT finding, the slight to moderate increase in lung density, is more important to explain respiratory impairments in BOOP, suc as: sounding fine crackles, decreased vital capasity, decreased DLco and hypoxemia, because it is spread over wider areas of the lung field.

When slight to moderate increases in lung density on CT images can be detected by routine chest radiograph, they may be reflected by a slight decrease of X-ray transmission or ground glass like fine nodular shadows. As the low-grade film can not reveal such detailed findings, we had better call this radiographic finding of BOOP alveolar opacity instead of mixed alveolar and interstitial opacity. From the point of radiology, after studying CT-pathologic correlation, we can agree that BOOP should be categorized into the group of interstitial lung disorders.

It is not difficult to discriminate CT images of BOOP from those of UIP. The chief characteristics of those of UIP are conglomerated small cystic images, air bronchiolograms within intense densities, enlarged vascular images and bronchial wall thickening. On the other hand,

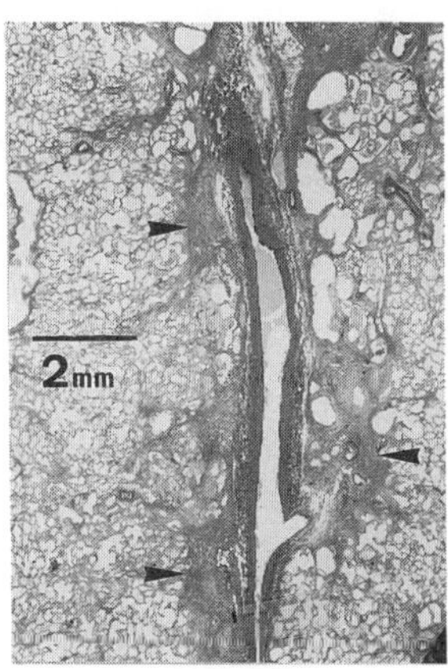

Fig. 8. Histological view of a biopsy specimen of UIP (elastica von Gieson stain).

Note fibrotic change of lung tissue surrounding pulmonary vessel ( ). This histologic finding causes enlarged pulmonary vascular images on the CT of UIP.

the main CT findings of BOOP are two types of increases in lung density. These differences are coincident with histological reports that honeycombing is usually detected in UIP but is seldom seen in BOOP. A slight increase in lung density is found on CT of both UIP and BOOP. This CT finding of BOOP is spread over wider areas and sharply stands out against the normal lung fields, because histologically in BOOP mural and luminal alveolitis is seen diffusely in the involved secondary pulmonary lobule. Some interlobular septa may contribute to the presence of such distinct borders on CT. These CT findings of UIP are often localized and their boundary against the normal area is unclear. The cause is that local fibrosis or inflammation of alveolar septa are patchily distributed and that normal alveoli remain in a secondary lobule [8]. These radiological findings of UIP are different from those of BOOP.

5. Conclusions

Our CT-pathologic correlative study has proved that the interstitial nature of BOOP is less clear on chest radiographs when compared with the alveolar opacity of BOOP and that X-ray CT reflects more actual pathological lesions than does routine chest radiography. These CT findings are important to explain respiratory impairments in BOOP. This new technique turned out to be useful in differentiating BOOP from UIP.

References
1) Epler,   G.R.,   Colby,   T.V.,   McLoud,   T.C., Carrington,C.B.,   Gaensler,   E.A.:   Bronchiolitis Obliterans Organizing Pneumonia. N Engl J Med 312: 152-158, 1985.
2) Katzenstein,   A.A.,   Myers,   J.L.,   Prophet,   W.D., Corley, III L.S., Shin, M.S.: Bronchiolitis ob- literans and usual interstitial pneumonia.   A comparative clinicopathologic study.   Am J Surg Pathol 10: 373-381, 1986.
3) Guerry-force,   M.L.,   Müller,   N.L.,   Wright,   J.L., Wiggs, B., Coppin, C., Pare, P.D., Hogg, J.C.: A comparison of bronchiolitis obliterans with organ- izing pneumonia, usual interstitial pneumonia, and small airways disease.   Am Rev Respir Dis 135: 705-712, 1987.
4) Chandler, P.W., Shin, M.S., Friedman, S.E., Myers, J.L., Katzenstein, A.L.: Radiographic manifestations

of bronchiolitis obliterans with organizing pneumonia vs. usual interstitial pneumonia. AJR 147: 899-906, 1986.

5) Itoh, H. et al. Recent progress of chest imaging. In: Biomedical imaging (Hayaishi, O. and Torizuka, K. eds.), Academic Press Inc. New York. pp. 249-271, 1986.

6) Heitzman, E.R. In: The lung: radiologic-pathologic correlations. 2nd ed, Mosby. St. Louise. 1984

7) Nishimura, K., Mio, T., Nagai, S., Kitaichi, M., Izumi, T., Oshima, S., Murata, K., Ithoh, H.: Radiological differential diagnosis between IPF and sarcoidosis by X-ray CT. Am Rev Respir Dis 135: A133 (abstract), 1987.

8) Carrington, C.G., Gaensler, E.A., Coutu, R.E., FitzGerald, M.X., Gupta, R.G.: Natural history and treated course of usual and desquamative interstitial pneumonia. New Engl J Med 298: 801-809, 1978.

Significance of Auscultatory Findings in Interstitial Pneumonia

Masashi Mori and Hiroshi Kino

Mitsui Memorial Hospital, Tokyo, Japan

Lung sounds were recorded from thirteen patients with interstitial pneumonia. In every patients late inspiratory crackles were heard but in two patients expiratory crackles were also heard. The initial deflection width(IDW) of the expiratory crackles were less than 1 ms and the directions of initial deflections were negative while those of inspiratory crackles were positive. The two patients died soon after the recordings were made. It is speculated that the expiratory crackles, are due to the sudden rupture of the mucous plugs obliterating the small airways and that the presence of expiratory crackles probably indicates the progression of the disease processes and may indicate a poor prognostic sign.

Since the age of Laennec auscultation of the lung has been one of the most important method of physical diagnosis. However, compared to the heart sound, the study of lung sounds remained rather neglected until recently when more sensitive microphones and better recording equipments became available. The purpose of this presentation is to discuss the clinical usefulness of lung sound analysis in pulmonary fibrosis and speculate the origin of expiratory crackles we observed in some of our

Materials and methods:
  Lung sounds recorded from thirteen patients with pulmonary fibrosis were studied. Seven patients were idiopathic, and the rest were pulmonary fibrosis secondary
to rheumatoid arthritis, systemic lupus erythematosus
and progressive systemic sclerosis.
The recordings were made by condenser microphones (ECM
150, SONY) mounted on an aluminum chest-piece (volume of
air-coupling space:0.785 ml) and attached to the chest
wall by double-stick adhesive tapes. The sites of recordings were both bases (mid-scapular line, 4-5 cm below
scapular angle), anterior chest wall (mid-clavicular
line, second intercostal space) and over the trachea.
The sounds were recorded on an FM tape-recorder(XR-510,
TEAC), and displayed on a multichannel recorder. For the
signal processing the sound signals were low-pass filtered (cut-off frequency:2 kHz), digitized (8 kHz, 10
bit), stored on a memory (256 kbyte /channel) and submitted to a microcomputer (PC9801, VM2).

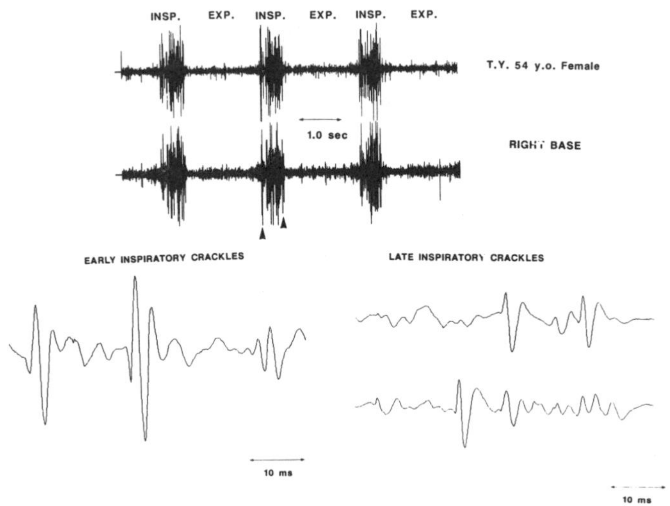

Fig. 1 Waveforms of early and late inspiratory crackles recorded from a 54 year-old woman with interstitial
pneumonia of unknown etiology. The directions of initial
deflections of inspiratory crackles were positive except
in some early inspiratory crackles, but were always negative in expiratory crackles.

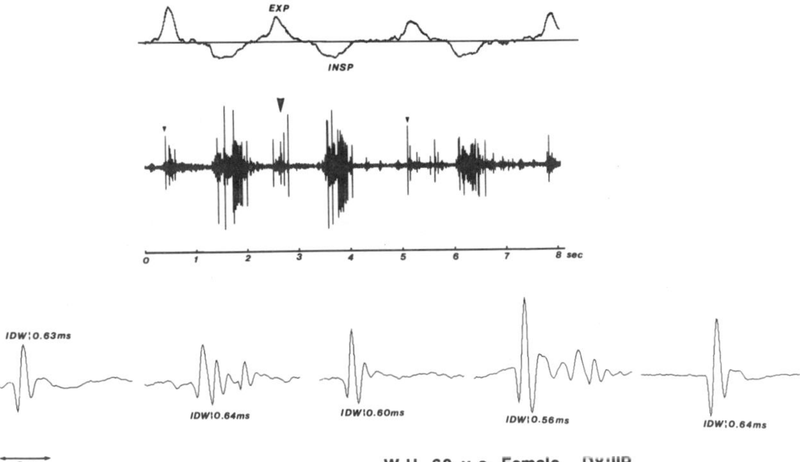

Fig. 2 Waveforms of expiratory crackles recorded from a
60 year-old woman with interstitial pneumonia of unknown
etiology. The IDWs (intitial deflection width) were less
than 1 ms and the directions of initial deflections were
negative. The patient died two months after this recording.

Results:
Inspiratory crackles were present in all patients
(fig.1), however, in two patients with idiopathic interstitial pneumonia expiratory crackles were also recorded
(fig.2). IDWs (initial deflection width) of these crackles, both inspiratory and expiratory, were less than
1 ms, so that by definition [1], they were classified as
fine crackles. The direction of initial deflection was
different in inspiratory and expiratory crackles, upward
in inspiratory and downward in expiratory. The direction
crackles, but in expiratory crackles it was always downward.
Discussion:
  Our observation of expiratory crackles in two patients
with idiopathic interstitial pneumonia is rather unusual
because in pulmonary fibrosis they are usually fine and
late inspiratory. Both patients died in about a year
after the recordings were made and at the autopsy severe
honeycombs and prominent goblet-cell metaplasia were
observed. It is speculated that the expiratory crackles

are due to the mucous from the goblet cells obliterating
the small airways. The presence of expiratory crackles
probably indicates the progression of the disease processes and may represent a poor prognostic sign.

   Recently Fredberg and Holford proposed stress-relaxation quadrupoles to explain the origin of fine crackles
[2]. They try to explain the polarity of the waveforms
by the opening and closing of the airways. However, the
production of snapping sound during expiration by the
closure of the airway is unlikely because the lung
becomes smaller so that the stress decreases during
expiration. Our theory is different. We speculate that a
small shock wave caused by the rupture of the mucous
meniscus is the origin of both the inspiratory and expiratory crackles we observed[3]. The direction of the
initial deflection is determined, as suggested by
Matsuzaki[4] and Abe[5], by the direction of the shock
wave, it is positive if it is toward the microphone and
negative if it is away from the microphone. Formation of
tion, due to the decrease in the diameter of the airway
during expiration.

References
1. International symposium on lung sounds. Synopsis of
proceedings. Chest 92, 342-345, 1987.
2. Fredberg, J.J., Holford, S.K.: Discrete lung sounds:
Crackles (rales) as stress-relaxation quadrupoles.
J. Acoust. Soc. Am. 73, 1036-1046, 1983.
3. Mori, M., Kinoshita, K., Morinari, H., et al: Wave-
form and spectral analysis of crackles.
Thorax 35, 843-850, 1980.
4. Matsuzaki, M., Ogasawara, H., Munakata, M., et al:
A phonopneumographical study of the direction of the
initial deflection of the waveforms of coarse crackles
and fine crackles.
Jap J Thoracic Dis. 20, 996-1002, 1982.
5. Abe, T., Kawashiro, T., Yokoyama, T.: Mechanism of
producing crackles studied by simultaneous recording
from oral cavity and chest wall.
8th International Conference on Lung Sounds, Baltimore,
Maryland, U.S.A., 1983.

Immunocytochemical Studies of Lung Biopsies

Patricia L. Haslam and Philip J. Townsend

Cell Biology Unit, Department of Cardiothoracic Surgery, National Heart and Lung Institute, London, UK

SUMMARY

Immunocytochemical studies of lung biopsies from patients with cryptogenic fibrosing alveolitis indicate that the majority of inflammatory cells in the interstitium are T-lymphocytes, and that cases with a predominance of the T-helper/inducer subset generally have a shorter duration of symptoms and a poorer prognosis than those with a predominance of the T-suppressor/cytotoxic subset. By contrast, B-lymphocytes are present in relatively small numbers except in the centres of lymphoid follicles which are found in some but not all cases. The presence of lymphocytes expressing IL2-receptors indicates that active lymphoproliferative responses are occurring in some areas and suggests that the lungs are the site of antigenic stimulation in this disease. Furthermore, the lung biopsy studies suggest that alveolar epithelial cells may be involved in antigen presenting function promoting the interstitial lymphoproliferative responses in CFA, since these cells show abnormally strong expression of HLA-DR antigens. The capacity of epithelial cells to enhance local cell mediated immune responses has been reported and this mechanism has been implicated in the pathogenesis of various organ specific autoimmune diseases. The lung biopsy evidence suggests that similar mechanisms may be operating in CFA where autoantibody production is also a feature.

INTRODUCTION

The etiology and pathogenetic mechanisms in cryptogenic
fibrosing alveolitis (CFA) are still not well
understood, although chronic inflammatory reactions in
the alveolar structures are clearly implicated in
inducing the tissue damage that leads to interstitial
pulmonary fibrosis. Bronchoalveolar lavage has
provided a safe and minimally invasive technique to
investigate components from the air spaces, and the
findings have focused attention on the role of
granulocytes and alveolar macrophages in the
pathogenesis of CFA because these are the main cell
types found in lavage samples from these patients (1).
However, it has long been known from conventional
histological studies of lung biopsies that lymphocytes
are the predominant inflammatory cell type infiltrating
the interstitial tissues near to the site of fibrosis,
while accumulations of alveolar macrophages are the
main feature in the air spaces (2). Many facts point
to the involvement of lymphocyte responses in CFA
including the frequent increases in serum
immunoglobulin levels, autoantibodies, circulating
immune complexes, and clinical associations with other
'autoimmune' connective tissue disorders(3).
Monoclonal antibodies and improved immunocytochemical
techniques are now available to characterise the
phenotypes of lymphocytes and other inflammatory cells
in situ, but studies in CFA have been limited by the
availability of open lung biopsy material and there is
still relatively little information (4, 5, 6). We have
now had the opportunity to apply these techniques to
study a comparatively large series of open lung
biopsies from 16 patients with CFA having lone lung
involvement and from 4 patients having fibrosing
alveolitis (FA) in association with other connective
tissue diseases (scleroderma in 3 and primary biliary
sclerosis in 1). Our aims were to investigate the main
types of lymphocytes and their subpopulations by
comparison with those in normal lung tissue (from 7
resected lungs); to explore whether the cells express
activation markers indicating that the lungs are the
site of antigenic stimulation; to consider possible
antigen-presenting cells; and to explore clinical
correlations.

MATERIALS AND METHODS

The mean age (± sd) of our 16 patients with lone CFA
was 52 ± 13 years and that of our 4 patients with FA
having associated connective tissue diseases was 49 ±
19 years. The 7 controls were of similar age. The
majority of the lone CFA patients and controls were
males and were either smokers or ex-smokers, while the
4 FA patients with associated disease were females and
3 were non-smokers. Most of the FA patients (15) were
untreated at the time of biopsy. The diagnosis in all
cases had been established on the basis of histology,
radiology, full lung function tests and case history
excluding any known causal agent.

Open lung biopsies were performed on all patients and
in addition to preparing blocks for conventional
histology, samples from each biopsy were coated in OCT
and frozen in isopentane cooled in liquid nitrogen and
stored at − 70° C.

For immunocytochemical staining, a series of $5\mu m$
sections were cut from each frozen tissue block using a
cryostat, air dried, then fixed for 5 minutes in
chloroform:acetone (1:1) prior to staining with a
battery of monoclonal antibodies using an indirect
immunoperoxidase staining technique employing 3,3-
diaminobenzidine tetrahydrochloride (DAB) giving a
brown reaction product to visualize the peroxidase-
tagged immunoglobulin attached to the monoclonal
antibodies (7). Pooled human serum was incorporated to
inhibit background staining.

The panel of monoclonal antibodies we have employed
were from the well characterised Becton Dickinson
series, including Leu 14 as a pan B-lymphocyte marker,
Leu 4 as a pan T-lymphocyte marker, Leu 3ab for T-
helper/inducer cells, Leu 2a for T-suppressor/cytoxic
cells, Leu M5 for macrophages and Leu M3 for monocytes.
In addition, we used a monoclonal to cytokeratin to
detect epithelial cells and monoclonals to detect cells
expressing surface markers associated with cell
activation or function, including IL2-receptors,
transferrin-receptors and HLA-D region antigens.

The results were recorded by using a semiquantatative
grading to score the frequency of positive cells
reacting with each monoclonal antibody in the different
histological locations. Interpretation of the
histology was aided by counterstaining the sections and
by including serial sections stained with Haematoxylin
and Eosin, Elastin van Gieson and Gomorri's Trichrome.
It was also possible, in the case of T-suppressor-
/cytotoxic cells, to determine the percentage
of positively stained cells in the interstitial tissues
by comparison with the total number of T-lymphocytes in
the consecutive stained section, by counting the
numbers of stained cells in randomly chosen high power
fields (x 25 objective) with the aid of an eye piece
graticule.

B-LYMPHOCYTES

Light microscopy observation of the stained sections
showed that very few B-lymphocytes were present in the
diffuse lymphocytic infiltrates in the interstitial
tissues of patients with CFA, or FA with associated
disease, and almost no B-lymphocytes were detected in
the controls. However, a few collections of
lymphocytes forming lymphoid follicles were seen in
sections from 2/3rds of the patients in both FA groups,
and B-lymphocytes were the predominant cells in the
centre of the follicles. There were also numerous
T-helper/inducer cells throughout the follicles but
T-suppressor/cytotoxic cells were less numerous and
mainly at the periphery. Cells expressing IL2-
receptors were also detected in some follicles
indicating that this was a site of active lymphocyte
proliferation.

Clinical correlations were explored and it was of
interest that 6 of the 7 patients in our study having
autoantibodies (all antinuclear antibodies and one also
having rheumatoid factor) were in the subgroup with
follicles. This subgroup also included all 5 patients
in the series who have died within 3 years following
their biopsy. No correlations were observed with other
clinical features including duration of symptoms at
biopsy, lung function measurements or grade of fibrosis
judged from the conventional histological stains.

T-LYMPHOCYTES

T-lymphocytes were the predominant cell type diffusely infiltrating the interstitial tissues of all patients and controls. Moderate numbers were seen in the controls and in the FA patients with associated disease but many patients with lone CFA had very numerous T-cells in the interstitium. T-lymphocytes were not seen in the air spaces. T-lymphocyte subsets were explored, and many T-suppressor/cytotoxic cells were detected in the interstitial tissues of all patients and controls. Their frequency grades were mainly moderate or numerous. However, using more accurate random field counting and expressing the results as a percentage of the total T-cells in the same fields, it was clear that the percentages of T-suppressor/cytotoxic cells were very variable in different cases in all groups. About half the patients with lone CFA had a predominance of T-suppressor/cytotoxic cells, and the duration of symptoms in most of these patients was greater than 2 years. By contrast, patients in whom less than 50% of the total T-cells were T-suppressor/cytotoxic cells had a shorter duration of symptoms ($\leq$ 2 years) and included 4 of the 5 patients in the series who have since died within 3 years. These correlations were significant (p < 0.02), and it is presumed that the patients with earlier disease and poorer prognosis have a predominance of T-helper/inducer cells in their biopsies. Considerable staining was observed using the monoclonal antibody to the T-helper/inducer subset, but accurate grading and counting were not possible because this antibody also reacted with many intra-alveolar macrophages. The variable reactivity of macrophages with T-helper/inducer monoclonals has been previously reported but does not appear to be well recognised, nor has sufficient attention been drawn to the problems this can cause in biopsy studies of cells <u>in situ</u>. A T-helper/inducer predominance might be an expected consequence of persistent antigenic stimulation in the lungs and our observations suggest that this might be the situation in CFA patients with more rapidly progressive disease.

ACTIVATED T-CELLS

Following induction of an immune response and T-lymphocyte activation, it has been shown from <u>in vitro</u> studies of blood lymphocytes that various surface markers indicative of activation are expressed at between 4 and 8 days following stimulation (8,9). These markers include IL 2-receptors, transferrin-receptors and HLA-D region antigens and while the first two are relatively short-lived and more indicative of the phase of lymphoproliferation, HLA-D region antigens persist for a longer time and can thus indicate past activation events. IL2-receptor expression is a more specific indicator of T-lymphocyte activation than expression of transferrin- receptors or HLA-D region antigens which are also expressed on other cell types, eg alveolar macrophages, either constitutively or following activation. No cells expressing IL2-receptors were observed in the controls but they were detected in small to moderate numbers in 69% of the patients with lone CFA and in one of the 4 patients with FA and associated disease. This observation, together with the observations on lymphoid follicles, is strong supporting evidence that lymphocyte activation is stimulated in the lungs of patients with CFA and argues against the view that lymphocytes may traffic to the lungs following their activation at some systemic site.

POTENTIAL ANTIGEN PRESENTING CELLS

<u>Alveolar macrophages</u>: T-helper lymphocytes recognise foreign antigens only when they are presented in association with MHC Class II products (HLA-D region antigens) on antigen-presenting cells (10). Although the majority of alveolar macrophages express HLA-D region antigens many workers have shown that they are very inefficient antigen-presenting cells compared with monocytes and macrophages from other sites in the body (11). Our immunocytochemical studies using a monoclonal antibody against macrophages, (Leu M5), confirm that macrophages occur in markedly increased numbers in the air spaces of many patients with CFA often appearing to form 'aggregates'. Macrophage 'aggregates' were a very prominent feature in 5 of our CFA patients but it is of interest that none of these

had autoantibodies and none have died in the subsequent
3 year follow-up period. This absence of especially
notable increases in macrophages in the patients having
increased T-helper/inducer lymphocytes and poorer
prognosis may imply that alveolar macrophages are not
playing a major role in antigen-presenting function in
CFA. We have also examined the intensity of expression
of HLA-D region antigens on alveolar macrophages in
bronchoalveolar lavage samples from patients with FA
using flow cytometry, and shown that there is no
evidence of any increased expression. By contrast, in
sarcoidosis, expression of HLA-D region antigens is
increased and the macrophages have been reported to
show enhanced antigen-presenting function (12, 13).
Thus, the identity of cells which aid the induction of
immune responses in the lungs of patients with CFA
still needs to be clarified.

Interstitial Monocytes: The monoclonal antibody
to macrophages reacted with most cells in the alveolar
spaces and also with smaller mononuclear cells in the
interstitium. However, cells reacting with a monoclonal
antibody to monocytes (Leu M3), were detected only in
the interstitium. Since blood monocytes have potent
antigen-presenting function compared with alveolar
macrophages, this raises the possibility that
infiltrating monocytes may be aiding the induction of
the lymphoproliferative responses in the interstitial
tissue sites in CFA patients. As far as we know, this
is the first evidence to implicate monocytes rather
than mature macrophages in the pathogenesis of CFA,
although monocytes have been implicated in sarcoidosis
(14).

Alveolar Epithelial Cells: Epithelial cells may also
be involved in antigen presentation in CFA since our
observations confirm the report of Kallenberg et al
(5) that epithelial cells lining the air spaces of
patients with CFA strongly express HLA-DR antigens.
Aberrant expression of HLA-DR on epithelial cells
has been implicated in stimulating delayed
hypersensitivity reactions in the skin as well as in
the pathogenesis of various organ-specific autoimmune
diseases, including autoimmune thyroiditis and primary
biliary sclerosis (15, 16). The evidence suggests that
gamma interferon released from activated T-lymphocytes

can induce the expression of HLA-DR on localised
epithelial cells enhancing the localised immune
response in the face of the normal systemic suppressor
mechanisms. The evidence also suggests that these
cells may be capable of inducing autoimmune responses,
and this could provide a possible explanation for
autoantibody production in CFA.

Because many different cell types in the lungs of
patients with CFA express HLA-DR antigens, it can be
very difficult to discriminate HLA-DR expression on
epithelial cells from that on other cell types. To
more accurately confirm that alveolar epithelial cells
in CFA express HLA-DR antigens we have, therefore,
extracted cells from lung biopsies of some patients and
shown using flow cytometry that cytokeratin positive
epithelial cells are also HLA-DR positive (17). In the
same study we have isolated such cells using the cell
sorter and shown by electron microscopy that they have
the ultrastructural features of Type II pneumocytes.

HYPOTHESIS

In conclusion, our findings are consistent with those
of Kallenberg et al (6) and Kradin et al (5) in that
T-lymphocytes are the predominant cells infiltrating
the interstitial tissues of patients with CFA, and that
B-lymphocytes are mainly confined to the centres of
lymphoid follicles. We have extended the findings of
previous workers by showing that the percentages of T-
suppressor/cytotoxic cells are very variable in
different patients, and that patients with lower counts
and an apparent predominance of T-helper/inducer cells
have a shorter duration of disease and poorer
prognosis. We have also confirmed that lymphocytes
expressing IL2-receptors are present indicating that
antigenic stimulation is occurring in the lungs of
patients with CFA, and that alveolar epithelial cells
expressing HLA-DR antigens may play a role in local
antigen presenting function and may promote autoimmune
responses in this disorder.

To explain these findings, we propose the hypothesis
that a persistant etiologic agent, possibly a virus,
within the interstitium of patients with CFA may
stimulate the host to mount a cell-mediated immune

response and that infiltrating monocytes probably
initially act as the antigen-presenting cells. Release
of mediators from activated T-lymphocytes and monocytes
would then recruit other inflammatory cell types to the
lungs resulting in chronic inflammation. We suggest
that this persistent inflammatory response leads to
locally high levels of the mediator gamma-interferon,
which causes alveolar epithelial cells to express HLA-D
region antigens giving them the capacity to enhance the
local immune responses. We further propose that the
local antigen-presenting cells, including epithelial
cells, by releasing the mediator IL1 may stimulate
fibroblasts to proliferate thus promoting the
interstitial fibrogenic response in CFA. Release of
fibroblast/pneumocyte factor from fibroblasts
stimulates epithelial cells to proliferate thus
providing a possible explanation for the Type II cell
hyperplasia in CFA patients.   The expression of HLA-D
region antigens on alveolar epithelial cells may also
explain the autoimmune responses in fibrosing
alveolitis.

REFERENCES

1. Crystal RG, Gadek JE, Ferrans VJ, Fulmer JD, Line
    BR, Hunninghake GW. Am J Med 70, 542-68, 1981.
2. Liebow AA & Carrington CB. In: Pulmonary Radiology
    (M Simon, EJ Pitcher, M LeMay, eds.) Grune &
    Stratton, New York, pp. 1102-1104, 1969.
3. Haslam PL & Turner-Warwick M. In: Scientific
    Foundations of Respiratory Medicine (JG Scadding, G
    Cumming, WM Thurlbeck, eds) William Heinemann
    Medical Books Ltd, London, pp. 451-472.
4. Campbell DA, Poulter LW, Janossy G, Du Bois RM.
    Thorax 40, 405-411, 1985.
5. Kradin RL, Divertie MB, Colvin RB, Ramirez J,
    Ryu J, Carpenter HA, Bhan AK. Clin Immunol
    Immunopathol 40, 224-235, 1986.
6. Kallenberg CGM, Schilizzi BM, Beaumont F, Poppema
    S, De Leij L, The TH. Clin exp Immunol 67,
    182-190, 1987.
7. Nakane PK. J Histochem Cytochem 16, 557-558, 1968.
8. Burns GF, Battye FL, Goldstein G. Cellular
    Immunol 71, 12-26, 1982.
9. Prince HE & John JK. Clin exp Immunol 67, 59-65,
    1987.

10. Benacerraf B. _Science_ 212, 1229–38, 1981.
11. Holt PG. _Clin exp Immunol_ 63, 261–270, 1986.
12. Campbell DA, Du Bois RM, Butcher RG, Poulter LW. _Clin exp Immunol_ 65, 165–171, 1986.
13. Venet A, Hance AJ, Saltini C, Robinson BWS, Crystal RG. _J Clin Invest_ 75, 293–301, 1985.
14. Hance AJ, Douches S, Winchester RJ, Ferrans UJ, Crystal RG. _J Immunol_ 134, 284–292, 1985.
15. Hanafusa T, Pujol-Borrell R, Chiovato L, Russell RCG, Doniach D, Bottazzo GF. _Lancet_ ii, 1111–15, 1983.
16. Bottazzo GF, Pujol-Borrell R, Hanafusa T. _Lancet_ ii, 1115–19, 1983.
17. Haslam PL, Townsend PJ and Parker DJ. _Cytometry_ supplement 1, 41, 1981.

Clinical Pictures Related to Different Types of Pulmonary Functional Impairment in Interstitial Lung Diseases: With Special Reference to Idiopathic Pneumonia

M. Kawakami, A. Chiyotani, K. Konno, and T. Takizawa

Department of Medicine 1, Respiratory Division, Tokyo Women's Medical College, Tokyo, Japan

Forty-two cases of interstitial lung diseases (ILD) with VC of less than 80% and $FEV_1/FVC\%$ of more than 70% were divided, according to lung volumes, into two groups, i.e., group A: TLC<80% and RV <120% and group B: TLC>80% and RV>120%. Most of the cases in group A had idiopathic interstitial pneumonia (IIP) and half of the cases in group B had also IIP. Functional analysis revealed that cases in group B had more possibly advanced small airway dysfunction and less advanced parenchymal disease. IIP diagnosed by the criteria proposed by the Research Group of Interstitial Lung Disease, Ministry of Health and Welfare Japan, seems various in pulmonary function.

Idiopathic interstitial pneumonia (IIP) is a disease of unknown etiology generally thought to be equivalent to idiopathic pulmonary fibrosis (IPF) and cryptogenic fibrosing alveolitis. The name, IIP, was proposed by the Research Group of Interstitial Lung Diseases, the Specified Disease of the Ministry of Health and Welfare, Japan (Research Group) [1]. According to the diagnostic criteria proposed by the Research Group, interstitial lung diseases (ILD) which accompany some related disorders such as rheumatoid arthritis are not included in IIP [2]. The criteria are composed of the following five items: 1) respiratory symptoms, 2) nature and distribution of infiltrative shadows and the degree of shrinkage of the lung on chest roentgenograms, 3) lung function including lung volumes, diffusing capacity and arterial oxygen pressure, 4) blood chemistry and immunology and 5) histological findings of the lung tissue obtained by biopsy or necropsy. For the definite IIP, three items including chest roentgenographic findings, or two items, chest roentgenographic and histological findings, are required to be fulfilled but the criteria do not always require lung biopsy.

Generally, various kinds of ILD including IIP are thought to have decreased lung volumes [3]. However, we have realized that it is not always the case in rheumatoid arthritis and even in IIP. In this study, we tried to divide our cases of ILD including IIP into two groups according to total lung capacity (TLC) and residual volume (RV) and to find the related clinical pictures.

Materials and Methods

Patients who had been diagnosed to have ILD based on respiratory symptoms, clinical course and clinical investigations carried out at Tokyo Women's Medical College Hospital, Tokyo, were used for the selection of the cases. All of them showed interstitial shadows such as fine granular, patchy, reticulonodular and/or honeycombing in the lung fields on chest roentgenograms. Transbronchial lung biopsy (TBLB) was performed in 29 cases. Diagnosis of IIP was made by the criteria of the Research Group [2]. The cases of rheumatoid arthritis (RA) fulfilled the criteria for classic or definite RA.

Forty-two cases with vital capacity (VC) of less than 80% (% predicted) and ratio of forced expiratory volume in one second (FEV_1) to forced VC ($FEV_1/FVC\%$) of more than 70% were selected. Then, they were classified into two groups based on the values of TLC and RV; group A: TLC of less than 80% and RV less than 120% and group B: TLC more than 80% and RV more than 120%. Clinical records concerning respiratory symptoms and smoking habits were reviewed.

Routine posterior-anterior chest roentgenograms taken
in close proximity to lung function tests were assessed.

Lung function tests were made when they were in
relatively stable condition. Functional residual
capacity (FRC) was obtained by helium equilibration
technique using a closed circuit. Respiratory
impedance (Z_{rs}) was measured by an oscillation method
at 3cps. Carbon monoxide diffusing capacity (D_{Lco})
was measured by single breath holding method. Closing
volume (CV) and closing capacity (CC) were measured by
single-breath N_2 washout method. Esophageal balloon
technique was used for pulmonary static (C_{st}) and
overall compliance ($C_{overall}$). Maximum expiratory
flow at 50% of VC ($\dot{V}_{max50}$) and 25% of VC ($\dot{V}_{max25}$)
were analysed using maximum expiratory flow volume
curve. Arterial oxygen and carbon dioxide pressure at
rest were also measured and alveolar-arterial oxygen
pressure difference ($AaDO_2$) was calculated by
alveolar equation. Standardization of the lung
function measurements was made regarding height and age
before statistical comparison; TLC, RV, and FRC were
standardized by the prediction formulae of Nishida et
al. [4], VC, of Sasamoto and Yokoyama [5], FEV_1, of
Yokoyama and Mitsufuji [6], CV/VC and CC/TLC, of Buist
and Ross [7], D_{Lco} of Nishida et al. [8], and
$AaDO_2$, of Yokoyama and Kawashiro [9].

Statistical analyses were made between the groups
concerning sex distribution, symptoms, smoking, and
roentgenographic findings. For the comparison of the
lung function measurements between the groups, cases
with matched VC (see Results) were selected.

Table I: Number of the case

Group A	23
Group B	19
Subgroup 1 (IIP cases in group A)	20
Subgroup 2 (IIP cases in group B)	9
Subgroup 3 (Non-IIP cases in group B)	9
Cases of matched VC in group A	18
Cases of matched VC in group B	12

Furthermore, the following three subgroups were also used for the analyses; IIP cases in group A (subgroup 1), IIP cases in group B (subgroup 2) and non-IIP cases in group B (subgroup 3). Chi-square test was applied to test the difference of the frequency of each sex, symptoms, smoking, roentgenographic findings between the groups, between subgroups 1 and 2, and between subgroups 2 and 3. Student's t test or Cochran-Cox's test was used for the comparison of lung function between the groups and between subgroups 2 and 3. The number of the case of each group, subgroup and the case with the matched VC are listed in table I.

Results

None of the cases had wheezing or was taking sympathomimetic agents or xanthines. None had valvular heart diseases. Twenty three cases were classified into group A and 19 cases, into group B. Means (standard errors of mean) of %TLC and %RV were 66.2 (1.5) and 80.4 (3.9) in group A and 108.6 (5.9) and 177.1 (16.1) in group B, respectively. The diseases and the number of the cases are listed in table II. Most of group A cases had IIP, whereas in group B, only half cases had IIP and the others had various kind of diseases such as collagen vascular disorders, hypersensitivity pneumonitis and sarcoidosis. Group A was more likely to include IIP than group B according to chi-square test (p<0.01). Also male patients

Table II: Disease and the number of cases

Group	A	B
Idiopathic interstitial pneumonia	20	9
Rheumatoid arthritis	1	3
Other collagen vascular disorders	1	1
Hypersensitivity pneumonitis	0	3
Sarcoidosis	0	2
Asbestosis	1	0
Drug induced pneumonitis	0	1
Total	23	19

Table III: Number of the cases and chi-square test

	Total cases		IIP		Non-IIP
	Group A	B	Subgroup 1	2	Subgroup 3
Male	15	6[*1]	12	5	1[*2]
Female	8	13	8	4	9
At onset					
Smoker	7	4	5	3	1
Nonsmoker	13	14	12	5	9
At lung function test					
Smoker	3	3	3	2	1
Nonsmoker	17	15	14	6	9
Cough	18	12	15	6	6
No cough	5	7	5	3	4
Exertional dyspnea	22	16	19	9	7
No dyspnea	1	3	1	0	3
Persistent sputum	4	2	4	1	1
No persistent sputum	17	15	14	6	9
Clubbed finger	9	3	9	2	1
No clubbed finger	14	16	11	7	9
Fine crackle	21	16	18	7	9
No fine crackle	2	3	2	2	1

Chi-square test was made between groups A and B, between subgroups 1 and 2, and between subgroups 2 and 3.
*1: Between groups A and B, p<0.05.
*2: Between subgroups 2 and 3, p<0.05.

tended to be included in group A whereas female patients, in group B (p<0.05), reflecting the fact

Table IV: Number of the cases with shadows
infiltrating predominantly in specific lung zones on
chest roentgenograms

Lung zone where shadows distribute dominantly	Total cases		IIP		Non-IIP
	Group		Subgroup		Subgroup
	A	B	1	2	3
Lower zone	17	14	15	7	7
Upper zone	2	2	2	2	0
Others	4	3	3	0	3
Peripheral zone	14	7	12	4	3
Not peripheral	9	12	8	5	7

Concerning chi-square test, see footnote of table III.
Concerning subgroups, see table I. No significant
trend was found in any conbination of the group and the
subgroup.

that most of the cases were female in subgroup 3 (table
III).

No consistent difference was seen in smoking
histories among the cases at the time of onset or at
the time of lung function tests (table III). No
consistent difference concerning frequency of symptoms
such as cough, dyspnea, chronic sputum lasting more
than two years, clubbed finger and fine crackles was
seen between groups A and B, between subgroups 1 and 2
and between subgroups 2 and 3 (table III).

Roentgenographic findings are summarised in table
IV. In many cases, the shadows were preferentially
distributed in the lower and lateral lung zones, but
chi-square tests did not reveal any trends between the
groups and between the subgroups.

VC was more severely reduced in group A than
group B (figure 1). Accordingly, for the comparison of
lung functions between both groups, the cases with
matched VC ranging from 40 to 65% were selected.

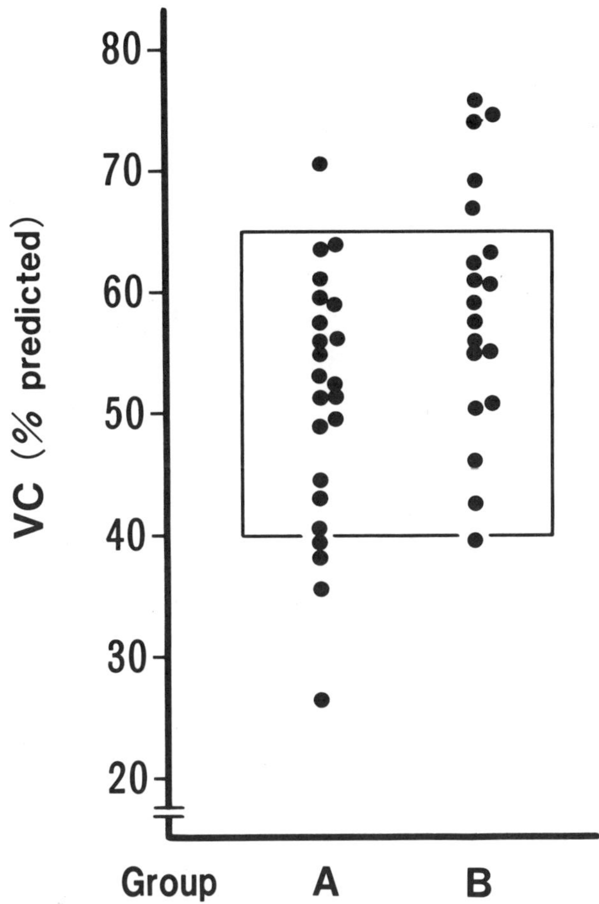

Figure 1. Distribution of vital capacity (% predicted).
Cases highlighted by the square were used for the
comparison of lung function measurements between both
groups.

Eighteen cases were selected from group A and 12 from
group B for this purpose (table I). Student's t test
revealed that in group B, $FEV_1/FVC\%$ and $\dot{V}_{max50}$ were
smaller whereas %FRC, %CC/TLC, $\%D_{Lco}$ and $C_{overall}$
were larger than group A (table V). Comparison between
subgroups 2 and 3 showed that %TLC, %CC/TLC and R_{us}

Table V: Mean (SEM) of lung function measurements

	Group A (18 cases)		Group B (12 cases)	
%VC	53.6	(1.6)	55.4	(1.9)
%FEV_1	69.9	(1.6)	71.8	(2.8)
FEV_1/FVC%**	88.9	(1.3)	82.0	(2.3)
%FRC**	71.8	(2.6)	132.2	(10.7)
%$\dot{V}_{max50}$*	86.6	(7.8)	60.3	(8.5)
%$\dot{V}_{max25}$	90.8	(14.1)	60.8	(15.2)
$\dot{V}_{max50}/\dot{V}_{max25}$	3.45	(0.36)	3.26	(0.28)
Z_{rs} (cmH_2O/L/sec)	4.76	(0.39)	4.79	(0.42)
delta N_2 (%)	2.99	(0.72)	4.33	(1.26)
%CV/VC	85.3	(15.8)	84.2	(18.0)
%CC/TLC*	116.0	(6.9)	137.2	(6.7)
%D_{Lco}*	43.9	(3.9)	60.7	(6.3)
D_{Lco}/V_A (ml/min/mmHg/L)	4.32	(0.39)	5.19	(0.58)
P_{Lmax} (cmH_2O)	42.7	(5.0)	33.2	(5.3)
C_{st} (L/cmH_2O)	0.064	(0.009)	0.091	(0.012)
$C_{overall}$ (L/cmH_2O)**	0.074	(0.006)	0.151	(0.023)
C_{dyn} (1 Hz/0 Hz)	47.4	(3.1)	59.2	(5.7)
R_{us} (FRC) (cmH_2O/L/sec)	2.33	(0.26)	2.29	(0.38)
P_aO_2 (Torr)	71.7	(2.6)	74.5	(2.5)
P_aCO_2 (Torr)	36.0	(1.2)	36.4	(1.1)
%$AaDo_2$	232.1	(23.4)	261.7	(42.5)

* $p < 0.05$, ** $p < 0.01$.

were significantly lower in the former than the latter
(table VI).

Discussion

It is generally accepted that patients with ILD
have decreased lung volumes [3]. It is surprizing that
45% of ILD cases had increased RV as well as normal or
rather increased TLC in this study. Concerning the
disease in group A, most cases had IIP whereas in group
B, only half had IIP and the others had various
diseases including collagen vascular disorders,
hypersensitivity pneumonitis and sarcoidosis. The

Table VI: Mean (SEM) of lung function measurements

	Subgroup 2 (IIP) (9 cases)		Subgroup 3 (Non-IIP) (9 cases)	
%VC	60.4	(4.1)	57.9	(3.1)
%FEV$_1$	75.9	(6.1)	73.4	(3.1)
FEV$_1$/FVC%	86.4	(2.0)	80.2	(2.9)
%TLC*	100.6	(4.9)	117.7	(6.3)
%FRC	126.5	(9.8)	141.6	(11.3)
%RV	165.9	(14.7)	190.8	(16.4)
%$\dot{V}_{max50}$	84.2	(13.0)	53.5	(10.4)
%$\dot{V}_{max25}$	82.3	(16.5)	57.2	(20.1)
$\dot{V}_{max50}/\dot{V}_{max25}$	3.18	(0.38)	3.09	(0.24)
Z_{rs} (cmH$_2$O/L/sec)	4.14	(0.31)	5.28	(0.45)
delta N$_2$ (%)	2.38	(0.64)	5.13	(1.72)
%CV/VC	63.1	(18.2)	101.2	(20.7)
%CC/TLC*	123.5	(5.7)	152.5	(7.8)
%D_{Lco}	59.5	(11.0)	60.7	(6.9)
D_{Lco}/V_A (ml/min/mmHg/L)	4.85	(0.95)	4.93	(0.65)
P_{Lmax} (cmH$_2$O)	34.2	(4.3)	31.7	(7.4)
C_{st} (L/cmH$_2$O)	0.102	(0.023)	0.112	(0.020)
$C_{overall}$ (L/cmH$_2$O)	0.127	(0.023)	0.179	(0.026)
C_{dyn} (1 Hz/0 Hz)	54.4	(8.3)	59.2	(6.5)
R_{us} (FRC) (cmH$_2$O/L/sec)*	1.45	(0.19)	2.93	(0.51)
P_aO_2 (Torr)	73.8	(4.9)	71.4	(2.7)
P_aCO_2 (Torr)	35.5	(1.4)	36.1	(2.5)
%AaDo$_2$	227.0	(39.8)	289.7	(49.9)

* p<0.05

results of lung function tests imply that group B had
more severely impaired small airway function and less
advanced interstitial alteration in lung parenchyma
than group A. Small airway disease is considered
frequently in relation to smoking habits. However,
this study suggests that the difference of the lung
function between the groups is not likely related to
smoking [10] (table III).
    There are pathological studies which show that

various kinds of ILD have abnormal small airways [11] such as IPF [12], rheumatoid lung diseases [13], pneumoconiosis [14], and hypersensitivity pneumonitis [15, 16, 17]. Intraluminal organizing and fibrotic changes occur not only within alveoli and alveolar ducts but also distal bronchioles frequently in various interstitial lung diseases [11] such as idiopathic pulmonary fibrosis, collagen vascular disorders [18] including rheumatoid lung diseases [13], hypersensitivity pneumonitis [16], pulmonary sarcoidosis, pneumoconiosis, and drug-induced pneumonitis [19, 20]. In the majority of cases with IPF, small airways are abnormal regardless of their smoking habits [12]. Fulmer and associates reported that 67% of the cases of IPF had narrowed small airways caused by peribronchiolar fibrosis, inflammation and bronchiolitis which were secondary to the interstitial process [12]. They found a significant correlation between these pathological findings and lung function measurements such as dynamic compliance and maximum flow-volume curve. Almost half of nonsmoking patients with sarcoidosis had small airway disease as well as elevated leukotriene B_4 production by peripheral blood mononuclear cells [21]. Bronchospasm is also suggested to occur in small airways of ILD. Lung function of our cases may indicate that a large number of cases had such pathological changes in peripheral airways as cited above.

About 70% of the cases studied had underwent TBLB but none underwent open lung biopsy. According to the diagnostic criteria of the Research Group, the open lung biopsy is not always mandatory; the reasons may be that (a) usual interstitial pneumonia (UIP), a microscopic requirement of IIP [22], is not always specific to IIP [13] and (b) TBLB, although it does not usually produce enough amount of specimen for the diagnosis of UIP, is much more popular than open biopsy. On the contrary, even if a patient is diagnosed to have IIP based on the criteria, it may still be necessary to rule out other diseases such as pneumoconiosis, diffuse panbronchiolitis [23], sarcoidosis and hypersensitivity pneumonitis before making definite diagnosis of IIP [2].

The diagnostic criteria for IIP have been realized by the Research Group to be sensitive in

finding out IIP cases whereas less specific
in diagnosing them [2]. This implies that our
subgroups 1 and/or 2 might include diseases other than
IIP. We had a question if the patients belonging to
subgroup 2 had the diseases of subgroup 3 in reality.
However, comparison between subgroups 2 and 3 showed
that both were likely to be different from each other,
i. e., in subgroup 3, female patients tended to be
included and subgroup 2 had significantly lower %TLC,
%CC/TLC, and R_{us} than subgroup 3.

Acknowledgement: The authors thank Drs. S.
Kameyama, K. Sakamoto, K. Aoshiba, K. Kobayashi,
and N. Sakai, Department of Medicine 1,
Respiratory Division, Tokyo Women's Medical
College, for cooperation in reviewing the
clinical records.

References

1.   Honma, Y. In: Report of the Research Group of
      Interstitial Lund Disease, Specified Disease of
      the Ministry of Health and Welfare, pp. 3, 1980,
      (in Japanese).
2.   Tamura, M. In: Report of the Research Group of
      Interstitial Lung Disease, Specified Disease of
      the Ministry of Health and Welfare, pp. 4-6, 1980,
      (in Japanese).
3.   Keogh, B.A. and Crystal, R.G. Chest 78, 856-865,
      1980.
4.   Nishida, O., Sewake, N., Kambe, M., Okamoto, T.,
      Takano, M., Aratani, Y., Shigeto, E., Sawake, H.,
      and Nishimoto, Y. Jap J Clin Path 24, 837-841,
      1976 (in Japanese).
5.   Sasamoto, H. and Yokoyama, T. In: Spirogram and
      clinical use, pp. 46, Igaku-shoin, Tokyo, 1959 (in
      Japanese).
6.   Yokoyama, T. and Mitsufuji, M. Chest 61, 655-661,
      1972.
7.   Buist, A.S. and Ross, B.B. Am Rev Respir Dis 107,
      744-752, 1973.
8.   Nishida, O., Kanbe, M., Sewake, N., Takano, M.,
      Kawane, H., Kodomari, Y., Arita, K., Nasuno, H.,
      and Nishimoto, Y. Jap J Clin Path 24, 941-947,
      1976 (in Japanese).

9.   Yokoyama, T. and Kawashiro, T. Kokyu to Junkan 30, 517–518, 1982 (in Japanese)

10.   Finucane, K.E. and Prichard, M.G. Aust NZ J Med 14,755–761, 1984.

11.   Basset, F., Ferrans, V.J., Soler, P., Takemura, T., Fukuda, Y., and Crystal, R.G. Am J Pathol 122, 443–61, 1986.

12.   Fulmer, J.D., Roberts, W.C., and vonGal, E.R. J Clin Invest 60, 595–610, 1977.

13.   Yousem, S.A., Colby, T.V., and Carrington, C.B. Am Rev Respir Dis 131, 770–777, 1985.

14.   Churg, A. and Wright, J.L. Human Pathol 14, 688–693, 1983.

15.   Reijula, K. and Sutinen, S. Pathol Res Pract 181, 418–29, 1986.

16.   Sutinen, S., Reijula, K., Huhti, E., and Karkola, P. Eur J Respir Dis 64, 271–82, 1983.

17.   Burke, G.W., Carrington, C.B., Stranss, R., Fink, J.N., and Gaensler, E.A. JAMA 238, 2705–8, 1977.

18.   Hakala, M., Paakko, P., Sutinen, S., Huhti, E., Koivisto, O., and Tarkka, M. Ann Rheum Dis 45, 656–62, 1986.

19.   Wolfe, F., Schurler, D.R., Lin, J.J., Polland, S.M., Smith, T.W., Montgomery, S.R., and James, D.L. J Rheumatol 10, 406–10, 1983.

20.   Holness, L, Tenenbaum, J., Cooter, N.B., and Grossman, R.F. Ann Rheum Dis 42, 593–6, 1983.

21.   Clancy, L., O'Laoide, R., Kelling, P.W.N., Power, J., O'Conner, P., and Kelly, P. Eur J Respir Dis 69 (suppl 147), 199–201, 1986.

22.   Yamanaka, A., Saiki, S., Yokoyama, T., and Yamaguchi, K. Saishin-Igaku 32, 1072–1078, 1977 (in Japanese).

23.   Honma, H., Yamanaka, A., Tanimoto, S., Tamura, M., Chijimatsu, Y., Kira, S., and Izumi, T. Chest 83, 63–69, 1983.

Comparisons of Clinical and Pathological Findings between Asymptomatic Individuals as Detected by Routine Health Examination and Symptomatic Patients in Idiopathic UIP

Takateru Izumi

Chest Disease Research Institute, Kyoto University, Kyoto, Japan

Thirty eight patients with idiopathic usual interstitial pneumonia (UIP) whose diagnosis was established by open lung biopsy were classified into three groups according to the modes of detection of the disease and the presence or absence of symptoms at the time of detection. And the manner of progression of UIP was examined by comparing the clinical and pathological findings. Our results indicate that UIP progresses as multiple fibrotic lesions increase in number and not as diffuse fibrosis advances over the entire lungs.

INTRODUCTION

Idiopathic pulmonary fibrosis (IPF) is a chronic interstitial lung disease with a poor prognosis. It begins with manifestations of exertional dyspnea and cough associated with diffuse infiltrative shadows in chest X-rays, and advances gradually with progression of lung fibrosis, resulting in death due to pulmonary insufficiency. Hisopathologically, the disease can be either UIP, which accounts for the majority of cases, or desquamative interstitial pneumonia (1).

To know the relationship between clinical and pathological findings in IPF is extremely important in clarification of the mechanism of progression of the disease and designing its treatment. However, serial evaluation of pathological findings of the disease is not possible in individual patients because open lung biopsy cannot be repeated many times. Therefore, to examine the progression of UIP, we compared clinical and pathological findings in three groups of patients classified according to the modes of detection and symptoms at the time of detection.

SUBJECTS AND METHODS

<u>Subjects</u>: This study includes 38 patients in whom a histological diagnosis of UIP (2) was established by open lung biopsy at Chest Disease Research Institute, Kyoto University. They were divided into the following 3 groups. Group I: 8 asymotomatic patients in whom the disease was detected through health examination (5 males and 3 females aged 54.0±13.2 years (mean±SD)). Group II: 9 symptomatic patients in whom the disease was detected through health examination (8 males and 1 females aged 59.6±5.5 years). Group III: 21 patients in whom the disease was detected by examination due to respiratory symptoms (15 males and 6 females aged 57.7±7.8 years). None of patients had received corticosteroids at the time of examination.

<u>Methods</u>: Clinical findings including the smoking history, clinical symptoms, physical findings, chest X-ray findings, pulmonary function tests, blood gas tests, laboratory tests, and bronchoalveolar lavage fluids (BALF) cell findings and histopathological findings were compared among the 3 groups. Histopathological findings were examined with regard to the severity of inflammation and fibrosis of the alveolar region. Degrees of alveolar septal inflammation, alveolar septal fibrosis, and honeycombing formation were evaluated according to four grade scales of 0 (absent), 1 (mild), 2 (moderate), and 3 (severe).

RESULTS

Table 1 summarize the characteristics of the subjects and results of various examinations.

There were no significant differences in sex, age distribution, and smoking habit among the three groups. There were no differences in the frequency of clubbing and rales among the 3 groups.

The involved area of abnormal   shadows in chest

X-rays was significantly larger in Group III than in Group I, extending over two-thirds or more of the both lung fields in more than half the patients in Group III but over one-third or less of the lung fields in more than half the patients in Group I.

Concerning the pulmonary function tests, FVC% was significantly reduced in Group III as compared with Group I. Restrictive impairment was noted in 60% of the patients in this group. DLco% was significantly lower in Group III than in Group I although it was reduced also in Group I in terms of the mean value.

As for the results of laboratory tests, CRP was positive in 40% of patients in Group III with a significant difference as compared with Group I, but no other differences were observed among the groups.

BALF cell findings were compared between UIP patients and age-matched healthy individuals aged 48-66 years (34 noncurrent smokers (NCS) and 20 smokers (S)). Currently non-smoking UIP patients showed increases in the number of recovered cells (0.77±0.47 vs.1.61±0.88; p<0.001), percentage of neutrophils (0.3±0.6 vs. 7.0±15.4; p<0.02), and percentages of eosinophils (0.2±0.4 vs. 8.5±19.6; p<0.02), but a decrease in the OKT4$^+$/OKT8$^+$ ratio (3.32±1.89 vs 1.69±1.12; p<0.005) as compared with healthy counterparts. Smoking patients showed a significantly higher percentage of eosinophils (0.1±0.2 vs 1.4±2.4; p<0.05) than healthy smokers. However, there was no significant difference in the number of recovered cells, percentage of lymphocytes, neutrophils, or eosinophils, or the OKT4$^+$/OKT8$^+$ ratio among Groups I, II, and III.

Histopathological findings in open lung biopsy specimens concerning alveolar septal inflammation, alveolar septal fibrosis, and honeycombing formation expressed as scores from 0 to 3 showed no differences among the 3 groups.

DISCUSSION

Serial evaluation of pathological findings in the same UIP patients is impossible. From the clinical experience that UIP is asymptomatic at first, despite abnormal chest X-ray findings but develops symptoms and progresses to respiratory insufficiency, Groups I, II, and III in this study are considered to correspond to Stages I, II, and III. of the disease.

TABLE 1. COMPARISONS OF CLINICAL AND PATHOLOGICAL FINDINGS AT THE TIME OF DETECTION IN IDIOPATHIC UIP

		Group I
Number (M/F)		8 (5/3)
Age, yr		54.8 ± 13.2*[1]
Smokers and ex-smokers		6 (75%)
Clinical		
Dry cough		0 (0%)
Dyspnea		0 (0%)
Physical		
Clubbing		2 (25%)
Rales		7 (88%)
Chest X-ray		
Area of abnormal shadows*[3]	1	5 (63%)
	2	2 (25%) } 1.5 ± 0.7
	3	1 (13%)
Pulmonary function and		
FVC % pred		99.3 ± 11.1
FEV_1/FVC %		77.9 ± 12.9
Obstructive impairment*[5]		2 (25%)
Restrictive impairment*[6]		0 (0%)
D_LCO % pred		63.5 ± 14.7
PaO_2 mmHg		87.3 ± 9.2
$PaCO_2$ mmHg		42.4 ± 3.4
Laboratory		
Blood sedimentation rate mm/hr		26.3 ± 17.4
CRP (+)		0 (0%)
Blood leukocytes/mm^3		7,440 ± 1,554
lymphocytes/mm^3		2,475 ± 861
Serum γ-globulin %		18.7 ± 4.9
LDH IU/ml		359.5 ± 67.1
CEA-Z ng/ml		3.5 ± 3.1
RA (+)		0 (0%)
Antinuclear antibody		1/7 (14%)
BALF cell		
Recovered cells	NCS*[7]	1.24 ± 0.18 (4)
x 10^5/ml	S*[8]	0.93 ± 0.66 (4)
Lymphocytes (%)	NCS	7.5 ± 4.0 (4)
	S	3.1 ± 0.8 (4)
Neutrophils (%)	NCS	3.5 ± 5.0 (4)
	S	1.5 ± 2.3 (4)
Eosinophils (%)	NCS	1.0 ± 1.1 (4)
	S	2.2 ± 3.5 (4)

IN THREE GROUPS BY THE MODES OF DETECTION AND SYMPTOMS

Group II	Group III
9 (8/1)	21 (15/6)
59.6 ± 5.5	57.7 ± 7.8
8 (89%)	16 (76%)
symptoms	
4 (44%) P<0.05*[2]	14 (67%) P<0.005
7 (78%) P<0.005	20 (95%) P<0.005
findings	
3 (33%)	11 (52%)
8 (89%)	19 (90%)
findings	
1 (11%) ⎫	1 (5%) ⎫
6 (67%) ⎬ 2.1 ± 0.6	8 (38%) ⎬ 2.5 ± 0.6 P<0.001
2 (22%) ⎭	12 (57%) ⎭
blood gas testings	
85.3 ± 14.8	73.8 ± 18.3 (20*[4] P<0.005
79.1 ± 8.3	80.3 ± 11.5
2 (22%)	1 (5%)
3 (33%)	12/20 (60%) P<0.005
60.8 ± 9.3	47.8 ± 15.5 (19) P<0.05
73.6 ± 9.2 (8) P<0.02	79.2 ± 10.3 (20)
42.3 ± 2.4 (8)	40.5 ± 4.9 (20)
tests	
36.3 ± 28.7	26.6 ± 23.5
2 (22%)	8/30 (40%) P<0.05
6,860 ± 1,615	6,830 ± 1,706
2,449 ± 829	2,195 ± 542
20.6 ± 4.5	21.4 ± 5.7
335.3 ± 127.9	412.1 ± 131.1
4.0 ± 2.6	3.2 ± 2.7
5/9 (56%)	2/19 (11%)
2/8 (25%)	4/17 (24%)
findings	
2.22 ± 1.58 (2)	1.72 ± 0.75 (13)
3.09 ± 1.68 (5)	2.27 ± 1.38 (4)
3.8 ± 0.2 (2)	8.9 ± 11.8 (13)
5.0 ± 5.4 (5)	7.9 ± 8.1 (4)
39.9 ± 30.1 (2)	3.0 ± 3.5 (13)
3.2 ± 3.7 (5)	3.2 ± 5.5 (4)
6.2 ± 6.2 (2)	5.0 ± 6.2 (13)
1.3 ± 1.9 (5)	0.9 ± 1.0 (4)

| OKT4$^+$/OKT8$^+$ | NCS | 1.86 ± 0.77 (4) |
| | S | 1.56 ± 1.16 (4) |

			Histopathological
Alveolar septal inflammation	0	2 (25%)	
	1	6 (75%)	0.8 ± 0.4
	2	0 (0%)	
	3	0 (0%)	
Alveolar septal fibrosis	0	0 (0%)	
	1	3 (37%)	1.6 ± 0.5
	2	5 (63%)	
	3	0 (0%)	
Honeycombing formation	0	0 (0%)	
	1	4 (50%)	2.0 ± 1.0
	2	0 (0%)	
	3	4 (50%)	

[1] Values are mean ± SD
[3] 1. under 1/3 in both lung fields
   2. 1/3 ~ 2/3 in both lung fields
   3. over 2/3 in both lung field
[5] FEV_1/FVC % < 70
[6] FVC % pred < 80
[7] NCS: Non current smokers
[8] S: Smokers

Interestingly, demonstrable alveolar septal inflammation was absent on histopathological evaluation except for a few patients in Group III. Also, there was no difference in alveolar septal inflammation, alveolar septal fibrosis, or honeycombing formation among three groups. These observation were in agreement with the absence of differences in BALF cell findings among the groups. From these findings, UIP appears to progress with the increase in the number of multifocal fibrotic lesions, resulting in decreases in DLco and FVC%, spread of abnormal X-ray shadows, and appearance of cough and dyspnea and not with advancement of diffuse alveolitis into diffuse fibrosis. Considering that the signs of

| 0.89 ± 0.30 (2) | 1.76 ± 1.23 (13) |
| 2.93 ± 4.19 (5) | 2.06 ± 1.39 (4) |

findings

2 (22%)		7 (33%)	
7 (78%)	0.8 ± 0.4	11 (52%)	0.9 ± 0.8
0 (0%)		2 (10%)	
0 (0%)		1 (5%)	
0 (0%)		0 (0%)	
3 (33%)	1.8 ± 0.6	7 (33%)	1.9 ± 0.7
5 (56%)		9 (43%)	
1 (11%)		4 (19%)	
0 (0%)		1 (5%)	
5 (56%)	1.7 ± 0.8	2 (10%)	2.4 ± 0.9
2 (22%)		5 (29%)	
2 (22%)		12 (57%)	

*[2] Significant difference compared group I
*[4] No tested

alveolitis were unremarkable, local fibrosis may not simply be a result of alveolitis but may be caused by abnormal proliferation of fibroblasts of unknown etiology.

REFERENCES

1. Crystal, R.G., Fulmer, G.D., Roberts, W.C., Moss, M.L., Line, B.R., and Reynold, H.Y. Ann. Intern. Med. 85: 769-788, 1976.
2. Carrington, C.B., Gaensler, E.A., Coutu, R.E., FitzGerald, M.S., and Gupta, R.G. N. Engl. J. Med. 298: 801-809, 1978.

Assessment of Severity of Interstitial Pneumonia of Unknown Etiology

J. Chretien, Th. Chinet, S. Labrune, C. Danel,
M.A. Collignon, and G. Huchon

Université René Descartes, Hospital Laennec, Paris, France

ABSTRACT

For all interstitial pneumoniae, there is a group of indices designed to evaluate the severity of the disease. According to the classification of interstitial disorders of unknown origin (nosologically defined and non-nosologically defined), specific indices of gravity may be considered. Their respective values are successively analyzed (indirect indices and indices allowing a more direct approach of anatomical lesions). The assessment of severity results in fact from a collection of various data.

Pulmonary interstitium comprises three components:(1) the <u>true interstitium</u> between the pulmonary capillary network and the alveolar surface which is a functional area participating in gas exchange, (2) the <u>tissue surrounding the airways and the pulmonary vasculature</u> which is a supporting tissue, (3) the <u>envelope wrapping the lung</u> and acting as a transmitter to the alveoli of the variations in thoracic volume and pressure (e.g. subpleural tissue).

Interstitial lung diseases represent the entire group of processes which diffusely affect the pulmonary interstitium. Pathologic involvement of interstitium may exhibit acute, subacute or chronic stages of inflammation. Nevertheless, whatever the triggering factors and the mechanisms, this involvement leads to an activation and multiplication of interstitial fibroblasts, followed by qualitative and quantitative collagen transformation due to a disorder in the collagen turn over (1). This evolution toward fibrosis represents the common denominator of all interstitial disorders of any origin and the main justification for their individualization. These processes alter the lung functions.

The cause and severity of the disease are variable and one of the most difficult dilemna for the clinician is to assess the prognosis and to decide whether anti-inflammatory treatment is required or not. Assessing the severity of the disease is a fundamental step in clinical practice. Two factors command the severity of the disease: <u>the degree of inflammatory process accounting for the activity and evolutivity</u> of the disease and the <u>degree of fibrosis</u>. However, the former may be reversible by therapeutical means, whereas the latter may be considered as definite and irreversible (2,3). Therefore, in managing patients with interstitial lung disease, it is necessary to assess the relative extents of inflammatory and fibrotic lesions, since they are considered respectively as reversible and irreversible (4).

Interstitial pneumonia of unknown etiology (IPUE) may be nosologically defined or not (5,6,7). The first group includes granulomatous diseases (e.g. sarcoidosis, histiocytosis X, Wegener's granulomatosis,...) and various non-granulomatous diseases (e.g. collagen vascular diseases, haemosiderosis, Goodpasture's syndrome,...). The group of non-nosologically defined interstitial pneumonia concerns essentially idiopathic pulmonary fibrosis.

In IPUE, the term "severity" currently used in clinical descriptions may be considered as including a set of information regarding 1) the degree of lung function impairment, and 2) the relative extents of inflammation and fibrosis. This set of information results from clinical data and biological investigations which can be classified into indirect and direct indices (8). <u>Indirect indices</u> are drawn from clinical data, general inflammatory syndrome, biochemical markers and lung function tests; <u>direct indices</u> reflect the changes in pulmonary structures and include non-invasive methods (radiological imaging, isotopic investigations, and bronchoalveolar lavage (BAL), as well as invasive techniques consisting in lung tissue sampling.

INDIRECT INDICES OF SEVERITY

* Indirect indices include first **the degree of the signs and symptoms of the disease:** cyanosis, degree of dyspnea, signs of cardiac right-sided failure (9). In multisystem diseases, the extent of the disease and the degree and rapidity of involvement of various organs (e.g. kidney, heart) may be an indirect index leading to therapeutic decision-making (10). The duration and course of the disease from its onset is also an important index to be considered.

* Information may also be drawn from the degree of **the general inflammatory process,** given for instance by sedimentation rate, serum immunoglobulins, free light chains and, in multisystem disorders, rheumatoid factor and anti-nuclear antibodies, which may also be present in one third of the patients with idiopathic pulmonary fibrosis.

* Inflammatory processes and granuloma formation and proliferation within the lung and within

other organs involved may be responsible for enzymatic activities expressed by **biochemical markers.** They are determined in blood, urine, BAL, or other fluids. Among the most commonly used, some are related to inflammatory cell activation: macrophage activation and transformation into epithelioid and giant cell, or lymphocyte activation. Others are related to collagen metabolism. They will be considered successively.

1) <u>Markers of cell activation</u>

- Markers of macrophage activation

Angiotension-converting enzyme (ACE) may be determined in blood (SACE), more directly in BAL with a good correlation between both, and in other fluids (tears, cerebrospinal fluid,...). This enzyme, a peptidyl-dipeptidase or kininase II, converts angiotensin I, an inactive decapeptide, into angiotensin II and inactivates bradykinin (11). In patients with sarcoidosis, ACE is detected in alveolar macrophages and at the surface of epithelioid cells, and consequently may reflect the development and extent of the granuloma (12,13). The majority of sarcoid patients have elevated SACE values albeit with variations in the proportion of increased SACE and mean values due to heterogeneity of the series. This heterogeneity concerns the type, site and intensity of clinical symptoms, the duration of the disease, the treatment (with or without steroids), and the extent of extrapulmonary involvement.

Serum lysozyme (=muramidase) is a low molecular weight bacteriolytic enzyme found in many cells but mainly in cells of the mononuclear phagocytic system, including epithelioid cells, and in polymorphonuclears. Serum lysozyme increases in diseases involving such cells especially when their number increases (14,15).

Carboxypeptidase (N) or kininase I has biochemical properties similar to those of ACE, inactivating bradykinin, anaphylatoxin, and fibrinopeptides (16).

Thermolysin-like neutral serum metalloendo-peptidase has recently been identified in human serum. The functions of this enzyme have not been clearly defined, but like ACE, it is a membrane-bound enzyme which is elevated particularly in sarcoidosis (17).

- Markers of lymphocytose activation.

Among markers related to lymphocyte activation, Beta-2 microglobulin in serum and BAL fluid has been extensively studied in sarcoidosis (18). It is a low molecular weight protein of about 20,000 daltons binding to HLA antigens on cell membranes, not specific of lymphocytes but increasing in serum of patients with lymphoproliferative disorders. Beta-2 microglobulin may be used as a marker in a disease such as sarcoidosis where granuloma formation results in an initial accumulation and activation of lymphocytes at different sites (10,19).

Adenosine deaminase is another marker of lymphocyte activity. Adenosine deaminase is necessary for differentiation of lymphoid cells and in particular T lymphocytes (11).

- Other markers of cell activation.

Transcobalamine II may be increased in the sera of sarcoid patients just as in lymphoproli-ferative or immune disorders, and may be considered closely related to the lymphocyte activity markers(11).

Neopterin is a pyrazinopyrimidin compound derived from guanosine triphosphate, a precursor of biopterin. Its determination in blood and urine has been proposed as an index of immune response in patients with various conditions involving the cellular immune system, and in particular the lymphocyte activation: activated T-cells release increased amounts of interferon which induces an increased production of neopterin in macrophages (20,21).

2) <u>Markers of collagen metabolism alteration</u>

They constitute indirect indices of abnormal collagen production and turn-over, and may be determined in serum, BAL fluid or urine.   Among the markers of collagen metabolism, four have been proposed for clinical use: collagenase, type III procollagen N-terminal peptide, hyaluronic acid, and fibronectin. They have been found to be elevated particularly in patients with sarcoidosis, but the determination of their practical value needs further investigation (11,22,23,24,25).

<u>In summary</u>, a large number of biochemical markers are available, but further studies are needed to determine their clinical application and prognostic significance in terms of sensitivity and specificity.

* **Lung function tests** determine the degree of respiratory impairment, and correlate satisfactorly with the extent of pathological involvement of lung structures. They show a restrictive pattern, with low lung volumes, increased elastic recoil pressure, reduced PaO_2 during exercice and low diffusing capacity (4,26).

Studies on structure-function relationships have shown that lung volumes correlate fairly to overall pathological process and to the degree of fibrosis (4). Results on the correlation between lung volumes and the degree of inflammation are confusing. Some authors consider that lung volumes bear no relation to the extent of inflammation, a point which is questioned in more recent studies (27).

Diffusing capacity correctly reflects overall disease process and fibrosis but not inflammation.

Arterial blood gases at rest bear no or little relation to overall disease process, inflammation and fibrosis, whereas arterial blood gases during exercice are good indices of overall pathological changes, inflammation and fibrosis. Static volume-pressure relationships follow overall pathological alterations and are rather specific for fibrotic process (4,26).

Finally, there is no evidence from these studies that determination of lung volumes, diffusing capacity and gas exchange at rest and during exercise can distinguish the relative contributions of inflammation and fibrosis to the functional impairment (4,27).

DIRECT INDICES OF SEVERITY

Direct indices allow a better evaluation of the anatomical lung features and therefore a better assessment of prognosis.

Among non-invasive methods, the first approach to anatomical interstitial lung abnormalities may be obtained by **lung imaging** on conventional X-ray examination and computed tomographic scan. The intensity and distribution of shadows (honeycomb pictures), the parietal abnormalities (retraction, pleural thickening), the enlargement of the trachea and major bronchi, the elevation of the diaphragm, and the dilatation of pulmonary arteries depend on the stages and degree of fibrosis (9). Computerized tomography helps to analyze the lesions anatomically.

Isotopic investigations comprise gallium scanning and more recently the determination of the respiratory clearance of

^{99m}technetium-labelled   diethylene   triamine pentaacetate (RC-DTPA).

1) <u>Gallium scanning</u> provides a more direct assessment of the inflammatory process, in particular granuloma formation and turnover, through accumulation of gallium (^{67}Ga) in activated macrophages (28,29). StanislasLeguern et al. have shown in animal model of granulomatous lung disease that mononuclear cells were responsible for ^{67}Ga uptake. This uptake was due to an increased number of mononuclear cells (30). This technique therefore helps to define the sites and extent of granuloma formation and the degree of inflammatory cell mobilization. It does not however indicate the degree of fibrosis nor the functional outcome.

2) Several studies have shown that <u>RC-DTPA</u> is increased in 25-60% patients with pulmonary sarcoidosis (31,32,33,34). Moreover, Dusser at al. have demonstrated that in patients with pulmonary sarcoidosis, when RC-DTPA is increased, there is pulmonary parenchymal involvement on chest roentgenogram, impaired lung function, and increased SACE, and that RC-DTPA correlates with SACE but not with luminal lymphocytic alveolitis (34). RC-DTPA is also increased in most patients with idiopathic pulmonary fibrosis (31,35). However, the clinical application and prognostic value of this new index remains to be established in the various types of interstitial pneumonia.

With **bronchoalveolar lavage** (BAL), it is possible to evaluate the degree of inflammation and the evolution toward fibrosis through 1) the cellular components, and 2) the fluid phase (36,37,38).

1) Studies of the <u>cellular component of BAL</u> include the evaluation of the intensity and the nature of the alveolitis, and the in vitro studies of cell-to-cell interactions. The

intensity and nature of the alveolitis have been related to prognosis in interstitial lung diseases. For instance, in idiopathic pulmonary fibrosis, it has been suggested that the proportion of neutrophils gives an indication of evolution toward fibrosis (38,39). In the pathogenesis of lung fibrosis, neutrophils may act by secretion of neutral proteases and oxygen radicals inducing fibrogenesis. However, elevated numbers of neutrophils may result from pulmonary infection. High <u>number</u> of lymphocytes and eosinophils suggests a more favourable response to therapy (39). Sequential studies of cell distribution in BAL provide interesting information regarding the evolution of the disease.

2) Studies of the <u>liquid component of BAL</u> include the dosage of biochemical markers of local cell activation in BAL fluid, and also the measurement of immunological compounds such as immune complexes, immunoglobulins and various cellular mediators, such as histamine or interleukins (40).

Invasive techniques are often necessary to evaluate the importance of inflammatory cells, particularly the number and distribution of immunocompetent cells and the respective parts of irreversible connective tissue alterations and reversible inflammatory process.

The <u>transbronchial biopsy</u> is the easiest and most repeatable procedure. It is mainly of use in sarcoidosis. <u>Lung biopsy under thoracoscopy</u> may give better lung specimens but needs general anesthesia. The best pathological documentation not only for diagnosis but also for therapeutic decision remains the <u>surgical biopsy</u>. Histological examination brings confirmation of interstitial pathology (particulary the extent and cell components of the inflammatory process, the degree of fibrosis) and assessment of bronchiolar and vascular alterations.

CONCLUSION

In summary, various types of indices may be used in clinical practice for IPUE investigation. These may be direct or indirect indices according to the anatomical approach of both inflammatory and fibrotic components. They must be discussed in terms of sensitivity and specificity, and considered as a whole for the assessment of prognosis and therapeutic decisions.

REFERENCES

1. Hance AJ, Crystal RG. Idiopathic pulmonary fibrosis. In:Flenley DC, Petty TL (eds) Recent Advances in Respiratory Medicine, vol 1 Churchill-Livingstone, pp 249-287 1984.

2. Hunninghake GW, Garett KC, Richerson HB, et al. Pathogenesis of the granulomatous lung disease. Am Rev Respir Dis. 130,476-96,1984.

3. Crystal RG, Bitterman PB, Rennard SI, Hance AJ, Keogh BA. Interstitial lung diseases of unknown cause. Disorders characterized by chronic cellular infiltration of the lower respiratory tract. N Eng J Med. 310,154-166,1984.

4. Keogh BA, Crystal RG; Clinical significance of pulmonary function tests. Pulmonary function testing in interstitial pulmonary disease. What does it tell us? Chest 6,856-65,1980.

5. Reynolds HV, Chrétien J. In Respiratory tract fluids: Analysis of content and contemporary use in understanding lung diseases. Disease-a-Month, Chicago 30-103,1984.

6. Hunninghake GW, Garret KC, Richerson HB et al. Pathogenesis of the granulomatous lung diseases. Am Rev Respir Dis, 130,476-496,1984.

7.   James DG. The granulomatous disorders. JR Coll Physicians Lond, 17,196-204,1983.

8.   Chrétien J. Interstitial lung disease. Clinical presentation. Postgraduate Medical Journal 1988 (In Press).

9.   Crystal RG, Fulmer JD, Roberts WC, et al. Idiopathic pulmonary fibrosis. Clinical, histologic, radiographic, physiologic, scintigraphic, cytologic, and biochemical aspects. Ann Intern Med, 85,769-88,1976.

10.   Chrétien J, Venet A, Israël-Biet D, Clavel F, Sandron D. Summary statement on disease activity assessment. In: Johnson Jones, C(ed) Xth International Conference on Sarcoidosis and Other Granulomatous Disorders, vol 1 A, NY Acad Sci, 81, 465-479, 1983.

11.   Selroos OBN. Biochemical markers in sarcoidosis. Clin Lab Sci, 24,185-216,1986.

12.   Lieberman J. Sarcoidosis. J Lieberman, ed. Grune and Stratton publ vol. 145-59,1985.

13.   Studdy PR, James DG. The specifity and sensitivity of serum angiotensin converting enzyme in sarcoidosis and other diseases. Experience in twelve centers in six different countries.   In: Chrétien J, Marsac J, Saltiel JC, eds.   Sarcoidosis and other granulomatous disorders, Paris Pergamon Press, 332-44,1983.

14.   Mordelet-Dambrine M, Stanislas-Leguern G, Huchon GJ, Baumann FC, Marsac JH, Chrétien J. Elevation of the bronchoalveolar concentrations of angiotensin-converting enzyme in sarcoidosis. Am Rev Respir Dis. 126,472-475,1982.

15.   Klockars M, Selroos O. Elevated muramidase levels in histiocytic medullary reticulosis. N Eng J Med. 294,901-902,1976.

16.   Rohatgi PK, Ryan JW. Serum angiotensin converting enzyme (SACE) and carboxypeptidase N

(CPN) activities in sarcoidosis and other chronic diseases. Am Rev Respir Dis. 125-115,1982.

17. Almenoff J, Skovrow ML, Teirstein AS. Thermolysin-like serum metalloendopeptidase. A new marker for active sarcoidosis that complement serum angiotensin converting enzyme. Ann NY Acad Sci. 465,738-743,1986.

18. Morishita M, Torii Y, Ichimura K, et al. Serum and bronchoalveolar lavage level of B2 microglobulin in patients with sarcoidosis. In: Chrétien J, Marsac J, Saltiel JC, eds. Sarcoidosis and other granulomatous disorders, Paris Pergamon Press, 366-388,1983.

19. Mornex JF, Revillard JP, Vincent C, Deteix P, Brune J. Elevated serum B2 microglobulin levels and C1q-binding immune complexes insarcoidosis. Biomedicine. 31,210-213,1979.

20. Eklund A, Blashke E. Elevated serum Neopterin levels in sarcoidosis. Biomedicine 164,325-332,1986.

21. Lacronique J, Auzeby A, Barbosa MLA et al. Urinary neopterin as a new marker of lymphocytic alveolitis in pulmonary sarcoidosis. Am Rev Respir Dis. 133,A24,1986.

22. GADEK JE, Kelman JA, Fells et al. Collagenase in the lower respiratory tract of patients with idiopathic pulmonary fibrosis. N Eng J Med. 301,737-741,1979.

23. Watanabe Y, Yamaki K, Yamakawa I, Takagi K, Satake T. Type III procollagen N-terminal peptides in experimental pulmonary fibrosis and human lung disease. Eur J Respir Dis 67,10-16,1985.

24. Hallgren R, Eklund A, Engstrom-Laurent A, Schmekel B. Hyaluronate in bronchoalveolar lavage fluid: a new marker in sarcoidosis

reflecting pulmonary disease. Br Med J 290,1778-1781,1985.

25.   Rennard Sl, Crystal RG.   Fibronectin in human bronchopulmonary lavage fluid. Elevation in patients with interstiail lung disease.   J Clin Invest. 69,113-122,1982.

26.   Fulmer JD, Roberts WC, Von GAI R, Crystal RG.   Morphologic-physiologic correlates of the severity of fibrosis and degree of cellular infiltration in idiopathic pulmonary fibrosis. J Clin Invest. 63,665-676,1979.

27.   Chinet Th, Jaubert F, Dusser D, Danel C, Chrétien J, Huchon GJ.   Effects of inflammation and fibrosis on pulmonary function in interstitial pneumonitis.   Bull Eur Physiopathol Respir. 23,349S,1987.

28.   Dige-Peterson H, Heckscher T, Herz M. 67-GA scintigraphy in non-malignant lung diseases.   Scand J Respir Dis. 53,314-319,1972.

29.   Huchon GJ, Berrisoul LG, Barritault LG, Venet A, Marsac J, Roucayrol JC, Chrétien J. Comparison of bronchoalveolar lavage and Gallium-67 Ing scanning to assess the activity of pulmonary sarcoidosis.   In: Chrétien J, Marsac J Saltiel JC, eds.   Sarcoidosis and other granulomatous disorders, Paris, Pergamon Press, 440-445,1983.

30.   Stanislas-Leguern G, Masse R, Jaubert F, Chrétien J, Huchon G.   Pulmonary gallium uptake in rats width granulomatosis induced by Complete Freund Adjuvant.   Exp Lung Res. 14,445-458,1988.

31.   Rinderknecht J, Shapiro L, Krauthammer M, Taplin G, Wasserman K, Uszler JM, Effros RM. Accelerated clearance of small solutes from the lungs in interstitial lung disease.   Am Rev Respir Dis. 121,105-117,1980.

32.   Jacobs MP, Baughman RP, Hughes J, Fernandez-Ulloa M. Radioaerosol lung clearance in patients with active pulmonary sarcoidosis. Am Rev Respir Dis. 131,687-689,1985.

33.   Dusser D, Mordelet-Dambrine M, Collignon MA, Barritault L, Chrétien J, Huchon GJ. Assessment of pulmonary epithelial permeability by clearance of an daerosolized solute and bronchoalveolar lavage in interstitial lung disease. Bull Eur Physiopathol Respir 20,223-227,1984.

34.   Dusser D, Collignon MA, Stanislas-Leguern G, Barritault L, Chrétien J, Huchon GJ. Respiratory clearance of ^{99m}Tc-DTPA and pulmonary involvement in sarcoidosis. Am Rev Respir Dis. 134,493-497,1986.

35.   Chinet Th, Dusser D, Collignon MA, Barritault LG, Chrétien J, Huchon GJ. Respiratory epithelium clearance of ^{99m}Tc-DTPA in idiopathic pulmonary fibrosis. Am Rev Respir Dis. 135,A414,1987.

36.   Crystal RG, Reynolds HY, Kalika AR. Bronchoalveolar lavage. The report of an international conference. Chest. 90,342-350,1986.

37.   Chrétien J, Venet A, Danel C, Israel-Biet D, Sandron D, Arnoux A. Bronchoalveolar lavage in sarcoidosis. Respiration. 48,222-230,1985.

38.   Daniele RP, Elias JA, Epstein PE, Rossman MD. Bronchoalveolar lavage: role in the pathogenesis, diagnosis and management of interstitial lung disease. Ann Intern Med 102,93-108,1980.

39.   Haslam PL, Turton CWG, Heard B et al. Vronchoalveolar lavage in pulmonary fibrosis. Comparison of cells obtained with lung biopsy and clinical features. Thorax. 35,9-18,1980.

40.   Casale TB, Trapp S, Wood D, Zehr B, Hunninghake GW. Elevated bronchoalveolar lavage fluid (BAL) histamin levels in interstitial lung diseases and association with disease activity. Am Rev Respir Dis. 135,A29,1987.

Closing Remarks

Michiyoshi Harasawa

I would now like to bring to a close this three-day international symposium on interstitial pneumonia of unknown etiology, and I would like to thank everybody involved for their cooperation.

This symposium has contributed much to understanding of the present situation concerning treatment of this disease, and has been very important in showing us the way that should be taken by future research. I would like to thank from my heart all of those involved in this symposium, and also to express my hope that future research will develop as the result of this meeting.

I would also like to express my thanks to the Japan Intractable Diseases Research Foundation for its cooperation in making possible this international symposium.

Author Index